Register
Access

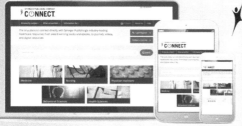

SPRINGER PUBLISHING COMPANY
CONNECT.

Your print purchase of *The Physician Assistant Student's Guide to the Clinical Year: Pediatrics* **includes online access to the contents of your book**—increasing accessibility, portability, and searchability!

Access today at:

http://connect.springerpub.com/content/book/978-0-8261-9535-7 or scan the QR code at the right with your smartphone and enter the access code below.

0MR9UL92

Scan here for quick access.

SPRINGER PUBLISHING COMPANY

View all our products at springerpub.com

TITLES IN *THE PHYSICIAN ASSISTANT STUDENT'S GUIDE TO THE CLINICAL YEAR* SERIES

Family Medicine

GERALD KAYINGO
DEBORAH OPACIC
MARY CARCELLA ALLIAS

Internal Medicine

DAVID KNECHTEL
DEBORAH OPACIC

Emergency Medicine

DIPALI YEH
ERIN MARTHEDAL

Surgery

BRENNAN BOWKER

OB-GYN

ELYSE WATKINS

Pediatrics

TANYA L. FERNANDEZ
AMY AKERMAN

Behavioral Health

JILL CAVALET

THE PHYSICIAN ASSISTANT STUDENT'S GUIDE

to the Clinical Year

PEDIATRICS

Tanya L. Fernandez, MS, PA-C, IBCLC, has been a physician assistant (PA) for 14 years, with a focus on underserved populations. She started her career in full-spectrum family practice and transitioned to pediatric and adolescent medicine as her patients began to grow their families. With an interest in promoting child and maternal health, she augmented her clinical skills by becoming an international board-certified lactation consultant (IBCLC) in 2014. She started teaching PA students in the clinical setting in 2006 and has been educating students ever since. Eleven years after graduating from the Child Health Associate/Physician Assistant (CHA/PA) Program at the University of Colorado, Tanya returned as faculty, where she now serves as the Clinical Course Director, is a liaison to the urban underserved health track, and is an assistant professor in the Department of Pediatrics. As the only PA program in the nation with an increased emphasis on pediatrics, the CHA/PA Program provides students with extended didactic and clinical experiences in specialty, hospital, and ambulatory pediatrics. In addition to curating the Stages of Life/ Patients and Populations longitudinal didactic curriculum, Tanya oversees the 3-year clinical education curriculum. Because of this role, she has a keen interest in students' self-directed learning while in the clinical curriculum.

Amy Akerman, MPAS, PA-C, has been a PA for 17 years, most of that time spent in primary care practice. She began her career working in Kodiak, Alaska, and then spent over 3 years in a general practitioner practice in Weston-super-Mare, England, as part of the National Health Service. She enjoyed helping to introduce the PA profession to the United Kingdom and still enjoys talking to patients and students about all the great things PAs can do. Amy joined the University of Colorado Child Health Associate/Physician Assistant (CHA/PA) Program in 2016 as the academic coordinator, global health track advisor and serves as an assistant director of the University of Colorado Interprofessional Education Council. Nationally, Amy serves on the Physician Assistant Education Association Government Relations Steering Committee. She enjoys talking with students about global health topics and professional and patient advocacy.

Maureen Knechtel, MPAS, PA-C (Series Editor), received a bachelor's degree in health science and a master's degree in physician assistant (PA) studies from Duquesne University in Pittsburgh, Pennsylvania. She is the author of the textbook *EKGs for the Nurse Practitioner and Physician Assistant*, first and second editions. Ms. Knechtel is a fellow member of the Physician Assistant Education Association, the American Academy of Physician Assistants, and the Tennessee Academy of Physician Assistants. She is the academic coordinator and an assistant professor with the Milligan College Physician Assistant Program in Johnson City, Tennessee, and practices as a cardiology PA with the Ballad Health Cardiovascular Associates Heart Institute. Ms. Knechtel has been a guest lecturer nationally and locally on topics including EKG interpretation, chronic angina, ischemic and hemorrhagic stroke, hypertension, and mixed hyperlipidemia.

THE PHYSICIAN ASSISTANT STUDENT'S GUIDE
to the Clinical Year

PEDIATRICS

Tanya L. Fernandez, MS, PA-C, IBCLC
Amy Akerman, MPAS, PA-C

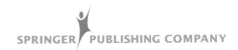
SPRINGER PUBLISHING COMPANY

Springer Publishing Company, LLC
11 West 42nd Street
New York, NY 10036
www.springerpub.com
http://connect.springerpub.com/home

Acquisitions Editor: Suzanne Toppy
Compositor: diacriTech

ISBN: 978-0-8261-9525-8
ebook ISBN: 978-0-8261-9535-7
DOI: 10.1891/9780826195357

21 22 23 / 5

The author and the publisher of this Work have made every effort to use sources believed to be reliable to provide information that is accurate and compatible with the standards generally accepted at the time of publication. Because medical science is continually advancing, our knowledge base continues to expand. Therefore, as new information becomes available, changes in procedures become necessary. We recommend that the reader always consult current research and specific institutional policies before performing any clinical procedure or delivering any medication. The author and publisher shall not be liable for any special, consequential, or exemplary damages resulting, in whole or in part, from the readers' use of, or reliance on, the information contained in this book. The publisher has no responsibility for the persistence or accuracy of URLs for external or third-party Internet websites referred to in this publication and does not guarantee that any content on such websites is, or will remain, accurate or appropriate.

Library of Congress Cataloging-in-Publication Data

CIP data is on file at the Library of Congress.
Library of Congress Control Number: 2019912895

Contact us to receive discount rates on bulk purchases.
We can also customize our books to meet your needs.
For more information please contact: sales@springerpub.com

Publisher's Note: New and used products purchased from third-party sellers are not guaranteed for quality, authenticity, or access to any included digital components.

Printed in the United States of America.

This book is dedicated to my husband, Jake, and my two beautiful children, Marissa and Alexander. Thank you for enduring many nights of warmed-up leftovers, missed story times, and unwatched movies because mom had "writing homework." I love you all more than words can express and am grateful for your support, your encouragement, and your willingness to let me try my hand at this writing thing. I also dedicate this book to my mother, who has believed in me since day 1 of life, has lived to tell the stories of my many harried pediatric milestones, especially the turbulent teenage years, and has been a constant support since as far back as I can remember. All of my adult life, she has endured my frantic phone calls when life seemed to be careening out of control, encouraged me to dip a toe in the water when I was hesitant about a new opportunity, and pushed me to be more than I ever thought I could be. Mom, you are my hero and a wonderful friend.

I would also like to dedicate this book to the outstanding University of Colorado Child Health Associate/Physician Assistant graduates who have paved the way for extraordinary careers in pediatrics, and to the soon-to-be graduates, who will carry on the program's legacy of top-of-the-line pediatric education. You all inspired me to write a book that would help other physician assistant students do what you do every day!

—Tanya L. Fernandez, MS, PA-C, IBCLC

I dedicate this book to my mom and dad, who instilled the love of reading and learning in me at a young age. My parents have always encouraged my educational and career endeavors and I would not be where I am without their advice. I also dedicate this book to my husband, Lee, and two children, Zoë and Harry. I appreciate your patience and understanding as I spent late nights and weekends working on this project. Thank you for your love and support.

—Amy Akerman, MPAS, PA-C

Contents

e-Chapter 8. Case Studies in Pediatrics
https://connect.springerpub.com/content/book/978-0-8261-9535
-7/chapter/ch08

e-Chapter 9. Review Questions in Pediatrics
https://connect.springerpub.com/content/book/978-0-8261-9535
-7/chapter/ch09

Peer Reviewers

Victoria Coppola, MHS, PA-C   Physician Assistant, Department of Emergency Medicine, Alfred I. DuPont Hospital for Children, Wilmington, Delaware

Annjanette Sommers, MS, PA-C   Associate Professor, School of Physician Assistant Studies, College of Health Professions, Pacific University, Forest Grove, Oregon

Foreword

Children are not just little adults. Their physiology is different. The diseases they get are different. Their response to treatment is different. Even the approach to history taking and physical examination for pediatric patients is different. Given that they are still growing and developing and that they are completely dependent on their caregivers, children present many other unique challenges. Understanding these differences is crucial to providing high-quality care to patients of all ages.

For me, the uniqueness of each patient is part of what makes pediatrics such an engaging and exciting specialty. Watching children grow and caring for the entire family add additional interest to my work in diagnosing illnesses and preventing disease. Every patient who comes in requires careful attention, and the differential diagnosis of fever in a 2-day-old newborn is very different than fever in a 2-month-old infant and again is different from the differential for fever in a 12-year-old recent refugee. Understanding these differences appropriately is medically necessary, but it also provides a greater sense of career fulfillment.

In this text, Fernandez and Akerman provide a concise yet complete approach to thinking through the care of pediatric patients. They appropriately highlight the differences between children and adults while also attending to the uniqueness of each patient. They combine their experience as clinicians with their expertise as educators to create a text that is both accessible and organized in a way that is easy to use for clinical rotations. The use of algorithms and a systematic approach to each complaint encourages critical thinking and attention to the details of each patient. Focusing on presenting complaints allows students to think like a clinician, starting with the patient's complaint and ending with the diagnosis, rather than the other way around.

Experience in caring for pediatric patients is essential for all physician assistant (PA) students. In the most recent statistical profile of certified PAs, 20% practice in family medicine, whereas a smaller number (3%) practice in pediatrics.[1] This means that nearly one in four graduating PAs will care for children. This number may increase greatly in the coming years as more pediatric practices and subspecialties begin to include PAs, and as the interest in employing PAs continues to rise.[2,3] In addition, because of the flexibility that the PA profession provides, a much greater number will care for children at some point in their careers. All PAs will be exposed to sick children even if it is just as a parent or friend.

Embracing the chance to learn about a clinician's role in caring for children is an exciting part of PA school. Just as children need support to grow and learn, this text provides a nice resource to help in your growth as an independent and competent clinician.

TAI M. LOCKSPEISER, MD, MPHE

REFERENCES

1. National Commission on Certification of Physician Assistants. 2017 statistical profile of certified physician assistants: an annual report of the National Commission on Certification of Physician Assistants. http://prodcmsstoragesa.blob.core.windows.net/uploads/files/2017Statistical ProfileofCertifiedPhysicianAssistants%206.27.pdf. Published May 2018.

2. Freed GL, Dunham KM, Loveland-Cherry C, et al. Nurse practitioners and physician assistants employed by general and subspecialty pediatricians. *Pediatrics*. 2011;128(4):665-672. doi:10.1542/peds.2011-0329

3. Freed GL, Dunham KM, Moote MJ, et al. Pediatric physician assistants: Distribution and scope of practice. *Pediatrics*. 2010;126(5):851-855. doi:10.1542/peds.2010-1586

Preface

For a physician assistant student, the clinical year marks a time of great excitement and anticipation. It is a time to hone the skills you have learned in your didactic training and work toward becoming a competent and confident healthcare provider. After many intense semesters in the classroom, you will have the privilege of participating in the practice of medicine. Each rotation will reinforce, refine, and enhance your knowledge and skills through exposure and repetition. When you look back on this time, you will likely relish the opportunities, experiences, and people involved along the way. You may find an affinity for a medical specialty you did not realize you enjoyed. You will meet lifelong professional mentors and friends. You may even be hired for your first job.

Although excitement is the overlying theme, some amount of uncertainty is bound to be present as you progress from rotation to rotation, moving through the various medical specialties. You have gained a vast knowledge base during your didactic training, but may be unsure of how to utilize it in a fast-paced clinical environment. As a clinical year physician assistant student, you are not expected to know everything, but you are expected to seek out resources that can complement what you will learn through hands-on experience. Through an organized and predictable approach, this book series serves as a guide and companion to help you feel prepared for what you will encounter during the clinical year.

Each book was written by physician assistant educators, clinicians, and preceptors who are experts in their respective fields. Their knowledge from years of experience is laid out in the pages before you. Each book will answer questions such as, "What does my preceptor want me to know?" "What should I be familiar with prior to this rotation?" "What can I expect to encounter during this rotation?" This is followed by a guided approach to the clinical decision-making process for commonly presenting complaints, detailed explanations of common disease entities, and specialty-specific patient education.

Chapters are organized in a way that will allow you to quickly access vital information that can help you recognize, diagnose, and treat commonly seen conditions. You can easily review suggested labs and diagnostic imaging for a suspected diagnosis, find a step-by-step guide to frequently performed procedures, and review urgent management of conditions specific to each rotation. Electronic resources are available for each book. These include case studies with explanations to evaluate your clinical reasoning process, and review questions to assist in self-evaluation and preparation for your end-of-rotation examinations as well as the Physician Assistant National Certifying Exam.

As a future physician assistant, you have already committed to being a life-long learner of medicine. It is my hope that this book series will outline expectations, enhance your medical knowledge base, and provide you with the confidence you need to be successful in your clinical year.

MAUREEN KNECHTEL, **MPAS, PA-C**
Series Editor
The Physician Assistant Student's Guide to the Clinical Year

Acknowledgments

We would like to acknowledge Melody Jones, PA-C, whose initial end-of-rotation (EOR) question ideas served as a springboard for some of the EOR exam questions included in the electronic material. This book would not be possible without the support and assistance of our editor, Maureen Knechtel. We would also like to acknowledge our mentors, Jacqueline Sivahop, MS, PA-C; Joyce Nieman, MHS, PA-C, MT(ASCP); and Tai Lockspeiser, MD, MPHE, for continually supporting this project and our desire to write this book despite curricular reinvention, a steep learning curve, and time that was not easy to carve out. We also thank our program director and friend, Jon Bowser, MS, PA-C. We could have never accomplished this without your blessing and support. Thank you!

TANYA L. FERNANDEZ
AMY AKERMAN

Introduction

The Approach to the Patient in Pediatrics

OVERVIEW OF THE PEDIATRIC ROTATION

WHAT TO EXPECT

As pediatric clinical experiences vary depending on the season and the setting, understanding the difference between outpatient and inpatient pediatric care is essential. The outpatient setting typically offers a smorgasbord of patient encounters, including well-child exams, acute and urgent visits, follow-ups, and chronic health condition management; the inpatient wards run the gamut from moderately ill children to those with life-threatening conditions and acute-on-chronic diseases that require medical and nursing care around the clock.

Inpatient Pediatrics

- Not all hospitals are equipped to treat children, so inpatient pediatric rotations tend to be limited to hospitals with robust pediatric training programs, such as those found on an academic campus, or those that specialize in children's care. However, if you are placed in a nonacademic pediatric inpatient setting for your pediatrics rotation, the hospitalists staffing the pediatric floor are typically pediatricians with an interest in acute and critical care.
- The inpatient census fluctuates throughout the year and is typically highest during the winter months when respiratory illnesses peak, but may spike during the summer with gastroenteritis and dehydration or in the autumn with asthma exacerbations.[1, 2] Seasonality could influence the number and types of patients that you carry. As there are usually more patients than there are hours in a shift, most students will care for between two and four patients at a time. A typical day may start as early as 6 a.m. for prerounding

and end as late as 7 p.m. after night handoffs. You may be expected to take call (stay the night in the hospital with the night shift), admitting and managing patients on the wards alongside a nocturnist, hospitalist, or a resident.

○ You may be asked to observe residents, work in tandem with another student or intern, or take responsibility for a cohort of patients under the supervision of your preceptor. You may have the ability to follow a patient from admission to discharge or you may acquire patients as team members move on and off service. You should expect that you will chart your patients daily, if not more than once a day. Because reading through each patient's chart is time-consuming and inefficient for residents and attendings, you should expect to give an oral "summary" of your patients during rounds. You will be expected to order and follow up on labs and imaging for your patients. Your job is to not only know your patients better than the residents do, but to present the patient using succinct, yet detailed, information that highlights the history of present illness (HPI) or the pertinent interim changes since the last report; physical exam findings; a prioritized/hierarchical assessment and a plan for admission, continued care, and/or discharge. Detailed information on what you should include in each type of note is covered later in this introduction.

Ambulatory Pediatrics

• Primary care pediatrics certainly sees its fair share of respiratory cases in the winter, diarrheal illnesses and injuries in the spring, a spike in well-child and sports physicals in the summer, and asthma exacerbations in the fall. These trends are generalizations and any given day in ambulatory pediatrics might range from well visits for children of various ages; follow-ups; and functional concerns like abdominal pain or headaches to rashes, minor injuries, and behavioral issues. Depending on the season and the scheduling patterns of the practice, you can expect that a pediatric preceptor will see between 25 and 35 patients a day, working standard office hours with occasional night clinics, after-hours call service, and weekends.

○ You should expect to see patients ranging in age from newborns to adolescents who come to the office for a variety of reasons. You should be comfortable with unpredictable schedules and unpredictable kids. Behind each exam door there may be a sleeping newborn, a crying kid, a surly teenager, or a worried parent. You will be expected to gather a history, perform a physical exam, create a differential diagnosis with a final assessment, and design a management plan for the patient. This may range from immunizations and anticipatory guidance to in-office nebulizer treatments and/or medication prescriptions. You will be expected to present and chart these visits in the typical subjective, objective, assessment, and plan (SOAP) note fashion and follow up with families with pending results or referrals.

WHAT YOUR PRECEPTOR WANTS YOU TO KNOW

As a large proportion of ambulatory pediatrics is focused around growth and development, understanding the developmental milestones and stages of development is an essential component of pediatric care. Although not the primary concern for a pediatric ward patient, having a good understanding of development is useful when serially evaluating children in the hospital setting. Growth and the direct and indirect measures used to monitor growth are primary concerns in both inpatient and outpatient pediatrics.

In the end, however, preceptors will likely care less about your intimate knowledge of obscure diagnoses of exclusion. Instead they want you to take ownership of your learning and your patients. Caring enough for your patients to learn about their conditions, follow up with their families, find culturally sensitive resources, and listen to the needs of the child and the parents are the keys to a successful pediatric rotation. Interest and enthusiasm will go furthest with preceptors when it is genuine and your questions are not related to facts that you can look up or memorize. Ask about the nuanced care that occurs in pediatrics, such as treatment plans that take socioeconomic, cultural, and parental beliefs into account or about the slight differences in presentation that alter the plan of care.

As with any area of medicine, preceptors want you to show your enthusiasm for the world in which they have chosen to spend their working lives. Show your enthusiasm by asking to see that walk-in patient or volunteering to stay after hours to finish reviewing labs and return phone calls with your preceptor. In an inpatient pediatric rotation, check in on your patients frequently, as their status can change quickly. Offer to go with them to a radiology appointment or bring a coffee to a mother who has been up all night worried about her child's breathing. That being said, there are some things that you just must know (or know where to find them in this book) to do well in the pediatric rotation, including:

- Understanding age-appropriate feeding, behavior, physical exam findings and common parental concerns will definitely help the student rotating in pediatrics.
- Recognizing common pediatric conditions and understanding their management.
- Identifying and differentiating between the well, mildly ill, and seriously ill patient.

What Previous PA Students Wish They Knew Before This Rotation

Students in a primary care pediatrics rotation often retell stories of that special patient or of making an unusual diagnosis, but the bread and butter of daily life in pediatrics may not be as legendary. It is found in those seemingly mundane, run-of-the-mill encounters that occur and on which students have reflected, wondering whether things might have gone better or been more efficient if they had only:

- Understood the classification of patients by age. Preceptors refer to patients by categories. Differentiating between ages of patients can help you understand how your preceptor thinks. Box I.1 refers to classifications of patients by age.

Box I.1 Classification of Pediatric Patients by Age

Newborn or neonate (birth to 30 days)	Middle childhood (5–10 years old)
Infant (1–12 months)	School-aged children (5+ years old)
Early childhood (12–60 months)	Adolescence (11–21 years old)
Toddlers (2–3 years old)	Tweens/preteens (11–13 years old)
Preschoolers (3–5 years old)	Teens (13–19 years old)
	Young adults (18–21 years old)

- Had a good working knowledge of immunization and catch-up schedules. As much of the day in ambulatory pediatrics is centered around preventative-care visits, knowing the basic vaccination schedule will save you countless hours looking up the same thing over and over again.
- Memorized developmental milestones. Perhaps it is not necessary to memorize all of them, but knowing at least one or two key milestones for each developmental stage serves to provide a solid foundation for each well-child visit. This will also help you provide appropriate anticipatory guidance to families.
- Read a high-quality parenting book before the rotation began. One of the most difficult parts of a pediatric rotation may very well be the anticipatory guidance and parental counseling that comes with well and acute visits. If you do not have children or your children are older, it can be difficult to

provide families with advice on managing common maladies or what to expect as an illness runs its course.

- Understood the hierarchy of the inpatient pediatric wards and asked about the expectations early in the rotation. The hospital setting, especially in an academic medical center, has a unique structure and expectations for PA students vary. Understanding where you fit and what your responsibilities are will help to keep you in good graces with everyone, from the attendings and chiefs to the residents and nurses.

- Practiced writing and presenting admission history and physical (H&P) exams and daily progress notes. Note writing in the inpatient setting may follow a traditional SOAP note outline, but the subjective section is not necessarily an OPQRST (onset, provocation, quality, radiation, severity/symptoms associated, timing associated with problem) HPI, but instead is actually the interim history and events that have occurred since the last note. The objective is still the physical exam, but it also includes an interpretation of the nursing notes, labs, consults, and imaging. Finally, the assessment and plan are typically derived by all the members of the team who provide input into the possible differentials and management of the patient. Depending on the setting of the hospital, this may be done by organ system or by problem(s).

- Set specific, measurable, and realistic goals for the rotation. Sharing those goals with your preceptor at the beginning of the rotation helps keep you accountable and will help your preceptors identify the areas you want to improve. Knowing where your weaknesses are helps preceptors or attendings direct their teaching and feedback. Asking for very specific feedback (e.g., "What should I do differently next time I do an abdominal exam on a ticklish 3-year-old?") from busy preceptors and attendings increases your chances of getting something more than, "You did a good job this week."

PERTINENT SPECIALTY-SPECIFIC PHYSICAL EXAMS

- The approach needed for a pediatric patient is quite different from that needed with an adult patient. Pediatric patients require patience, parental involvement, and at different ages may need the exam to be ordered differently.
  - For example, the child between the ages of 9 months and 3 years typically has some apprehension of strangers and will cry and try to climb on his or her parents when you try to examine him or her. Therefore, you may want to start with the least invasive physical exam component: observation.
    - The art of observation in pediatrics can not be underestimated. Observing a pediatric patient can provide a wealth of information without ever having to touch the child. You should observe parent–child interactions, a child's comfort level and overall appearance, breathing patterns and respiratory rate, and gait and movement of extremities. Many developmental milestones can be assessed by

observing a child with a book or something as simple as a tongue depressor.

○ Once you have made your observations, you will want to move to less invasive physical exam components, such as hip mobility and the abdominal exam, before moving to invasive maneuvers such as otoscopy.

> **CLINICAL PEARL:** Using distracting objects like toys or pictures and food can be helpful.

○ For a ticklish or painful abdomen you should warm your hands by running them under warm water before attempting the exam. One technique is to have a parent put his or her hand on the child's abdomen and you place yours on top of the parent's. Once the child warms up to the exam, then the parent can remove his or her hand and yours will then be on the abdomen and you will be able to palpate. Avoid the area of pain until the last part of the exam. A second technique is to have a patient put his or her hands on top of yours and to ask the patient to push down on your hand, which will allow you to do light and deep palpation. Move to the next area of the abdomen and repeat this technique. A final technique is to use your stethoscope to apply light and deep pressure to assess for pain.

○ Teaching parents how to help hold/stabilize the child during exams and immunizations: There are two important maneuvers that parents can do to help stabilize a child for an exam. The most versatile is the knee-to-knee position (Figure I.1). You and the parent will sit facing each other with your knees touching. The child will be on the parent's lap facing the parent and the parent will wrap their legs around the child's legs and hold their hands. The child is then laid back with the head in your lap. This position allows you to control the patient's head for an head, eyes, ears, nose, throat (HEENT) exam, but also may allow you to palpate the abdomen or auscultate the heart. The bear-hug technique has the parent sitting in a chair and the child on his or her lap facing away from the parent (Figure I.2). The parent uses one arm to come across the child's body, holding the arms at the child's sides. The other hand is used to hold the child's head against the parent's chest.

> **CLINICAL PEARL:** An extremely uncooperative child is not uncommon and requires creative thinking. This type of behavior is worth noting as it could signal a personality disorder or an underlying psychosocial concern. On the other hand, a completely submissive 3-year-old could signal that the child is critically ill.

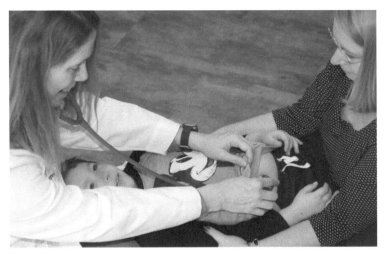

FIGURE I.1. Knee-to-knee exam.
With the child facing the parent, the provider and the parent sit opposite one another with their knees touching and then the child is laid down onto the provider's lap, while the parent uses his or her arms to control the child's legs and arms. This exam is ideally done for children between the ages of 2–5 years old.
Source: Photo courtesy of Tanya L. Fernandez, PA-C, and Amy Akerman, PA-C.

- Barlow and Ortolani maneuvers: The Barlow maneuver is used to detect whether an infant's hip can be dislocated posteriorly out of the hip acetabulum. To perform this, you will place your middle finger over the trochanter of the femur, bend the infant's knees, adduct the knees while pushing posteriorly. You are trying to feel whether the head of the femur is able to be dislocated, which sometimes can be described as a "click." The Ortolani maneuver is used to detect whether a hip is already dislocated and can be set back into the hip joint. To perform this, you will keep your fingers on the femoral trochanter, bend the infant's knees, abduct the knees while simultaneously applying anterior pressure on the femur. You are trying to feel whether the head of the femur moves back into the acetabulum, which sometimes can be described as a "clunk."
- Kernig's test and Brudzinski sign: Both exams are used to assess the amount of tension within the spinal cord and the meninges. They are often used when meningitis is suspected. The Kernig's test has the patient lying supine while you flex one of the knees and the hip to 90 degrees. Keeping the hip in this flexed position, you try to passively straighten the leg at the knee. A positive test occurs when the patient has pain with the attempt to straighten the knee and/or pain limits the range of motion at the knee. The Brudzinski sign is also performed with the patient lying in the supine position in full extension. You will grasp the occiput of the patient's head and

gently attempt to flex the neck. If flexion of the neck causes reciprocal flexion of the knees, this is considered a positive Brudzinski sign.

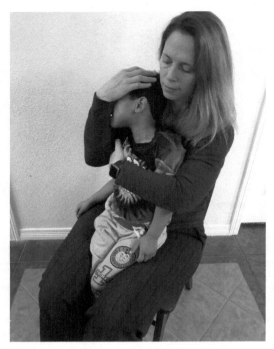

FIGURE I.2. K Bear-hug hold.
With the child sitting on a caregiver's lap, the caregiver uses one arm to hold both of the child's arms and the other hand to stabilize the child's head against the caregiver's chest.
Source: Photo courtesy of Amy Akerman, PA-C.

- Pneumatic otoscopy: Pneumatic otoscopy is an important technique to master because it can help you diagnose acute otitis media with effusion. Before you start, ensure that you have the correct ear speculum size for the patient's canal and that the bulb is attached to the otoscope. Gently pull the ear backward to view the tympanic membrane (TM). Insert the otoscope far enough to create a good seal. Gently squeeze the bulb on the otoscope to create positive pressure on the TM and observe TM mobility. Next, release the bulb to create negative pressure on the TM and observe TM mobility. Crisp movement of the TM with slight application of pressure is normal, whereas no movement or sluggish movement of the TM may indicate an effusion.
- Scoliosis evaluation (Adam's forward-bend test): This test is recommended by the American Academy of Pediatrics (AAP) to screen patients for scoliosis. To perform this exam, the patient stands with feet together, knees

straight, and arms hanging at the sides. The patient then bends forward at the waist until the spine becomes parallel to the horizontal plane. You will stand behind the patient, viewing the back and spine in the forward flexion position for asymmetry or any back or rib cage abnormalities, such as an elevation of the shoulders or rib cage.

- Cover–uncover test: This is an exam used to evaluate for signs of tropia (eye misalignment that is present all the time) and phoria (eye misalignment that is noted only when binocular vision is interrupted). Untreated, misalignment, or strabismus, will lead to amblyopia (loss of depth perception). This exam should be done a minimum of twice on each eye, with the first attempt focused on the uncovered eye and the second attempt focused on the covered eye after you pull your hand away. Ask the patient to look at your nose or try to have a small toy that the patient can fixate on; using your hand, cover the eye for 1 to 2 seconds. As this eye is covered, observe the uncovered eye for any shifts in fixation. Repeat on the opposite eye. Shifting of the uncovered eye toward the nose indicates exotropia, whereas shifting outward indicates esotropia; shifting upward indicates hypotropia and shifting downward indicates hypertropia. Repeat the cover and uncover maneuver, but this time focus on shifts in the covered eye when you remove your hand. If the patient's eye moves inward (nasally), this is esophoria; moving laterally indicates exophoria.[3]

- Visual accommodation testing: Accompanying the cover–uncover test is a test of accommodation (the ability to focus on near and distant objects). Pupillary changes, as the focus shifts from close to far objects, are a key finding in accommodation testing.

CLINICAL PEARL: For children who are verbal, you can place a sticker on your nose (or on a tongue depressor that you hold just in front of your nose) and ask the child to look at the sticker and tell you something about the sticker (e.g., Who is it? What color is the character?) and then look at a picture on the wall or have the parents stand behind you with a video on their smartphone. As the child's eyes move from the wall picture or video to the sticker on your nose, you should see that the pupil becomes myopic (smaller) and dilates with the transition back to the wall picture.

CLINICAL PEARL: Problems with accommodation and binocular vision may not be reported as abnormal in children, but rather as frontal headaches, blurry or double vision, words jumping or moving on the page, and poor attention and scholastic performance.[4]

USE OF INTERPROFESSIONAL CONSULTATIONS

Pediatrics is a collaborative specialty that often relies on interprofessional consultations to provide comprehensive, family-centered care to patients. Although referrals to pediatric subspecialists are most common, some of the interprofessional consultations that you may encounter in your pediatrics rotation include:

Audiologist

- Often patients with perceived or documented hearing issues, speech delays, and recurrent otitis media or persistent effusions are referred to audiology for formal hearing evaluation.

Dentist

- The AAP recommends that all pediatric patients establish a dental home by 1 year of age, so routine referrals to dentistry are common.[5] In addition, patients with malocclusions, injuries, caries, or dental infections are typically referred to a pediatric dentist for management.

Dietician

- A pediatric dietitian can help families understand the complexities of nutrition if a child has abnormal weight gain or loss, failure to thrive (FTT), enteral and parenteral nutrition needs, newborn/infant feeding disorders, elevated cholesterol, prediabetes, diabetes, tube-feeding requirements, or food allergies.

Care Coordinator

- Developmental surveillance and screening are the standard ways to identify a child with an isolated developmental delay, as well as one with several domain delays. "Early intervention" is a term that covers the services and supports that are available to children younger than 3 years old with developmental delays and disabilities and their families. The care coordinator will typically arrange for a comprehensive evaluation and manage the services deemed necessary for the child.

Lactation Consultant

- A lactation consultant has specialized skills in breastfeeding management and may become involved with a breastfeeding mother before delivery, immediately after delivery, and for ongoing support during the breastfeeding period. Mothers with a history of breast surgery, breast asymmetry, history of breastfeeding difficulties with previous children or a mother who experiences breast or nipple pain and/or engorgement should be referred to a lactation consultant. Infants with difficulty latching and inadequate milk intake, preterm or premature infants, infants with inadequate weight gain, or maxillofacial abnormalities may benefit from a referral to lactation support.

Mental Health Providers

- Within this category are psychiatrists, neurodevelopmental psychologists, child and adolescent psychologists, and social workers. Children or adolescents with emotional or behavioral problems, school avoidance, self-harm, substance abuse, a diagnosed psychiatric illness, a history of abuse/neglect, or a patient who screens positively for depression should be referred to mental health providers, such as a psychologist or social worker, for ongoing concurrent care. Neurodevelopmental psychologists and psychiatrists can be a referral resource for children with attention deficit hyperactivity disorder (ADHD), oppositional defiant disorder (ODD), and conduct disorder (CD), as well as children with developmental delays who have phased out of early intervention services. Psychiatrists may manage medications for some children and teens.[6]

Occupational Therapist

- An occupational therapist may be involved in a pediatric patient's care if the patient has torticollis; is not meeting fine motor, gross motor, or social milestones; has trouble with play and social skills; demonstrates sensory integration or regulation issues; or has feeding difficulties. Preschoolers may require OT if there are concerns about visual perception or age-appropriate activities of daily living.[7]

Optometrist

- When visual acuity concerns or strabismus are detected, the first-line referral is typically to an optometrist, who can assess the patient for glasses or other therapies. Sometimes concerns about infections, tear ducts, blepharitis, entropion, and conjunctivitis may also be referred to optometry. Pediatric optometrists, often co-located with pediatric ophthalmologists, can perform simple procedures, can serve as a primary care provider for the eyes, and are often more available for appointments than ophthalmologists, who are physicians who diagnose, treat, and perform surgery for complex eye conditions.

Physical Therapist

- Physical therapists typically are asked to evaluate musculoskeletal problems such as gait and mobility, limited range of motion, and injury rehabilitation. Physical therapists can provide various modalities of treatment for patients with neuromuscular and musculoskeletal issues.

Podiatrist

- Podiatrists are equipped to treat a variety of issues that affect the feet. From tinea and warts to ingrown toenails and hallux valgus, podiatry can evaluate, manage, and treat various conditions, including those that may require orthotics such as flat feet, metatarsus adductus, crossing toes, and intoeing.

Pediatric Subspecialists

- Pediatric subspecialists are often needed for medical or surgical problems beyond the scope of a primary care pediatric provider. These may include an adolescent gynecologist if a patient has severe dysmenorrhea or needs a family-planning method that the office does not provide, such as an intrauterine device (IUD). Allergists become a big partner in the care of children who need allergy testing, immunotherapy, and/or desensitization, and otolaryngologists are a common referral resource for children with recurrent ear or throat infections.

Speech Therapist

- A speech–language pathologist (SLP) is most obviously helpful for children with speech delays. Speech delays are divided into expressive or receptive language impediment. Expressive delays can include no speech production by 18 months, unintelligible speech after 2 ½ years of age, distorted or omitted sounds, abnormal inflections or rhythm, or when voice sounds are aberrant. Receptive language delays are usually diagnosed when a child is not following simple directions by 18 months.[8] In addition, an SLP may be recruited to evaluate breastfeeding issues, especially when they are related to swallowing, assess a child for aspiration risk, and to help with chronic tonsillitis/pharyngitis.

CONFIDENTIALITY PRACTICES AND ETHICS

Pediatrics has somewhat unique confidentiality practices as the majority of the patients are minors without the ability to consent to procedures, immunizations, or testing. The vast majority of visits involve parents in some capacity, from providing all of the history and assisting with the exam to bringing the patient and providing insurance documentation. As pediatric patients enter the tween and teen years, however, confidentiality becomes a bit blurry, as these patients become more independent and do acquire the ability to consent to some services and treatments. This is especially true around those services that teens may need or want to keep confidential. Adolescent confidentiality laws vary by state. It is vital that you understand whether adolescents have the right to confidentiality around family planning or contraception, substance abuse treatment and mental health treatments in your state. The Guttmacher Institute is a national leader in data involving adolescent reproductive care and has a state-by-state breakdown of the laws surrounding reproductive healthcare in the United States.[9]

Starting at about age 12, tweens and teens should be offered an opportunity to meet and discuss individual concerns and ask questions about high-risk behaviors without parents in the room. "Although confidentiality is particularly important in the area of reproductive health, providing adolescents opportunities for private discussion with clinicians on any topic serves to increase adolescents' feeling of responsibility and their ability to navigate the healthcare system and be their own advocates. Finally, research has confirmed that when confidentiality is not assured, adolescents are likely to forego needed health care."[10]

However, you should know that not all visits can remain confidential and telling teens about these special situations up front is essential. There are some clear reasons that a pediatric provider might need to break confidentiality, including abuse, self-harm, and risk of harm to others. Pediatric providers also face ethical decisions when it comes to state statutory rape laws. As state laws vary in the extent to which a provider is mandated to report, "reporting of such sexual behavior under these criminal statutory rape laws is premised on ethical and other considerations."[7] Often the laws are ambiguous and rely on the provider's discretion to determine whether the sexual relationship is psychologically damaging or "sexual abuse." However, in 43 of 50 states, providers who fail to report suspected abuse can face civil and criminal liability.[11]

Finally, the hardest ethical place for a pediatric provider to be is between the adolescent patient and the parent with whom there has been a long-standing relationship. In the end, open communication among the patient, the parents, and the provider can eliminate the feeling of being torn between two parties. Ultimately, the adolescents are your patients and deserve to be able to build their own relationships with you, knowing that sensitive topics will be kept in confidence until they are ready to share them with their parents.

SAMPLE DOCUMENTATION

- Admission note: This is essentially a full H&P exam, including:
  - Chief complaint
  - HPI
  - Past medical history (PMHx), including birth history, hospitalizations, significant complications of illnesses, and immunizations
  - Past surgical history
  - Family history
  - Social history
  - Medications
  - Allergies
  - Review of systems (ROS)
  - Physical exam
  - Labs
  - Assessment
  - Plan
- Hospital service/daily progress note: This serves as a record of the hospital course and is quite similar to the oral presentation during rounds, but

typically includes far more detail than is presented during rounds. The note should include the following:

- ○ Admit date
- ○ Admit diagnosis(es) listed in order of importance
- ○ Hospital course
- ○ Physical exam
- ○ Problem list prioritized by importance
- ○ Assessment
- ○ Plan, including medication changes, lab tests, procedures, consults
- Discharge note/summary: This should be provided to the primary care provider as a detailed record of the patient's hospitalization and post-hospitalization needs. It includes the following:
  - ○ Admission and discharge dates
  - ○ Admission and discharge diagnoses
  - ○ Service discharging the patient, including service name, attending, and resident
  - ○ Referring provider
  - ○ Consults
  - ○ Procedures
  - ○ Summary of pertinent admission H&P and labs
  - ○ Hospital course, which is a summary of treatment and progress during hospitalization
  - ○ Discharge condition
  - ○ Disposition, which may indicate that the patient was discharged home, discharged home with home health for respiratory support, and so on
  - ○ Medications
  - ○ Instructions
  - ○ Follow-up
- Well-child exam note: The format of these vary by site, but in general, a well-child check (WCC) note should include the following:
  - ○ Information about nutrition, elimination, sleep, family/social history, and development
  - ○ The physical exam with vitals and growth parameters, in addition to the exam findings
  - ○ The assessment should address growth, development, and physical health, while the plan typically includes anticipatory guidance, screening tests, and immunizations, if needed
  - ○ Follow-up should be clearly specified
- Office visit progress note: This is your classic SOAP note, which contains the following:
  - ○ The subjective portion contains/includes a chief complaint; the HPI begins with who accompanied the patient to the visit, followed by the current complaint history, pertinent PMHx, family history, and social history; immunization status; medications; and allergies.
  - ○ The objective portion should include vital signs, general appearance, and pertinent body systems from head to toe.

○ Depending on your setting, the assessment may be as simple as your diagnosis or you may need to document your medical decision-making with differential diagnoses considered.

○ The plan should include specifics for the diagnosis (including any patient education provided), return precautions that detail where to follow up (i.e., the office vs. the emergency department), and a follow-up timeline should be documented (whether you want the patient to follow-up on a specific diagnosis or if only to remind the patient of the need to follow-up for routine well care).

Sample Hospital Rounding Presentation Template

As hospital rounding, especially in an academic medical center, is quite different from presenting a well or sick child in the ambulatory pediatric setting, students have been known to struggle with the oral presentation of patients. Table I.1 is a basic template that can be modified for your setting.

TABLE I.1 Inpatient Rounding: Oral Presentation Components

Component	Information Needed	Example
Brief patient introduction	Patient name, age, reason for admission, and hospital day and/or day of illness	This is Joe Johnson. He is a 15-month-old male admitted with right lower lobe pneumonia, now day of illness #3.
Overnight events	Changes in clinical condition, changes in treatment plan, and any major events	Overnight he had increased work of breathing requiring an increase in oxygen to 5 L.
Objective data	Vital sign trends (not just the range) Intake and output Current respiratory support Medications (scheduled and as needed [PRN]) Physical exam Lab data Imaging	Afebrile for 24 hours after 3 days of temperatures from 101°F to 102.5°F with a T_{max} of 104.3°, slight tachypnea at 30 bpm, but improved from high 40s and low 50s earlier on admission Improving oral intake, especially after suctioning, with six breastfeeding sessions × 10 minutes over the last 24 hours, seven wet diapers, and 1 stool diaper Currently on high-flow oxygen via nasal cannula at 5 L with oxygen saturations holding in the mid-90s Medications currently include aamoxicillin 400 mg/5 mL, 5 mL PO q 12 hours and PRN acetaminophen for fever, discomfort

(continued)

TABLE I.1 Inpatient Rounding: Oral Presentation Components (*continued*)

Component	Information Needed	Example
		On exam, the patient is sleeping comfortably with no signs of increased work of breathing; CVP: RRR without murmurs, capillary refill at 2 seconds, lungs with persistent right inferioposterior crackles, but no abdominal breathing, tugging, costal retractions, or nasal flaring; HEENT: copious clear nasal secretions with mild erythema, but O/P is clear; TMs mildly retracted bilaterally without serous fluid or erythema; abdomen was soft, NTND and no masses, guarding or tenderness noted; MSK was deferred at this time, but will be evaluated when child wakes CBC showed a neutrophilia with a left shift on DOI #2 CXR taken 2 days ago showed a RLL consolidation and pneumonitis
Assessment or impression	Complete summary of the patient, including patient name, age, pertinent history, reason for admission, and current status	Joey is a 15-month-old male with an increased oxygen demand overnight, who is admitted for pneumonitis and RLL pneumonia. He is currently stable on 5 L oxygen via NC, but continues to require frequent mechanical suctioning.
Plan (problem based vs. system based)	List problems in descending order of importance	1 Pneumonitis: Continue oxygen at current setting, monitor WOB, and suctioning needs; will plan a trial of decreased oxygen to 4 L this afternoon; if tolerated well, keep at 4 L for daytime and increase to 5 L at night 2 Pneumonia: Continue amoxicillin, day 2 of 7

bpm, beats per minute; CBC, complete blood count; CVP, cardiovascular and pulmonary; CXR, chest x-ray; DOI, day of illness; HEENT, head, eyes, ears, nose, throat; MSK, musculoskeletal; NC, nasal cannula; NTND, nontender and nondistended; O/P, oropharynx; PO, by mouth; PRN, as needed; RLL, right lower lobe; RRR, regular rate and rhythm; TM, tympanic membrane; WOB, work of breathing.

REFERENCES

1. Nelson DS, Walsh K, Fleisher GR. Spectrum and frequency of pediatric illness presenting to a general community hospital emergency department. *Pediatrics.* 1992;90(1):5–10. https://pediatrics.aappublications.org/content/90/1/5
2. Weiss KB. Seasonal trends in US asthma hospitalizations and mortality. *JAMA.* 1990;263(17):2323–2328. doi:10.1001/jama.1990.03440170045034

3. Kirkpatrick C, Klauer T. How to perform a basic cover test in ocular misalignment or strabismus [video]. http://EyeRounds.org/video/Basic-Cover-Test.htm. Published April 24, 2015.

4. Jhajj J. Testing children for accommodative and convergence disorders: to obtain accurate test results for pediatric patients, consider these clinical strategies. Review of Optometry website. https://www.reviewofoptometry.com/article/testing-children-for-accommodative-and-convergence-disorders. Published October 15, 2017.

5. Bright Futures/American Academy of Pediatrics. Engaging patients and families: periodicity schedule. https://www.aap.org/en-us/professional-resources/practice-transformation/managing-patients/Pages/Periodicity-Schedule.aspx

6. American Academy of Child & Adolescent Psychiatry. Recommendations for pediatricians, family practitioners, psychiatrists, and non-physician mental health practitioners. https://www.aacap.org/aacap/Member_Resources/Practice_Information/When_to_Seek_Referral_or_Consultation_with_a_CAP.aspx

7. The Understood Team. Understood for learning and attention issues. Occupational therapy: what you need to know. https://www.understood.org/en/learning-attention-issues/treatments-approaches/therapies/occupational-therapy-what-you-need-to-know

8. D'Alessandro DM, Michaels SA. What are the indications for a referral to speech therapy? PediatricEducation.org website. https://pediatriceducation.org/2006/08/14/what-are-the-indications-for-a-referral-to-speech-therapy. Published August 14, 2006.

9. Guttmacher Institute. Overview of consent to reproductive health services by young people. https://www.guttmacher.org/state-policy/explore/overview-minors-consent-law

10. Levine SB. Adolescent consent and confidentiality. *Pediatr Rev.* 2009;30:457–459. doi:10.1542/pir.30-11-457

11. Madison AB, Feldman-Winter L, Finkel M, McAbee GN. Commentary: consensual adolescent sexual activity with adult partners—conflict between confidentiality and physician reporting requirements under child abuse laws. *Pediatrics.* 2001;107(2):e16. doi:10.1542/peds.107.2.e16

ELECTRONIC RESOURCES

AAP Sports Physical form:
https://www.aap.org/en-us/Documents/PPE-Physical-Exam-form.pdf

AAP WCC forms:
https://brightfutures.aap.org/materials-and-tools/tool-and-resource-kit/Pages/default.aspx

Minor consent laws by state:
https://www.guttmacher.org/state-policy/explore/overview-minors-consent-law

1

Common Presentations in Pediatrics

INTRODUCTION

The pediatrics rotation should serve as a primary opportunity for you to see how variable "normal" growth and development is, and to get experience with common neonatal, childhood, and adolescent conditions. Understanding normal growth and development by age is a fundamental concept for students, as the variability can influence the differential diagnosis, the pertinent positives and negatives, the exam, and the management plan. It is imperative to demonstrate the ability to gather and manage subjective and objective data, recognize common presentation patterns, identify and prioritize problems, and form an appropriate differential diagnosis through deductive clinical reasoning. If these steps are accomplished effectively, you should be able to distinguish between most and least likely diagnoses for any given age and presentation. This is a skill that requires interplay of foundational knowledge and the nuanced understanding of how development influences care.

The history and physical examination remain the cornerstones of evaluation, whether the child presents for routine well-child care or with a different chief complaint. Following a systematic approach to each patient allows you to efficiently identify pertinent positives and negatives, formulate a differential diagnosis, and initiate a management plan. The following steps facilitate your arrival at the correct diagnosis.

1. Identify whether the child is well, ill, or toxic.
   a. Much of pediatrics centers on well-child care. As these patients do not typically present with a chief complaint or disease state, pediatric providers are charged with assessing whether the child's growth, physical health, and development are appropriate for the chronologic age.

   b. Differentiating well from ill or toxic is a significant part of pediatric algorithms. Table 1.1 shows the key differentiations used to distinguish a child by appearance.

> **CLINICAL PEARL:** The appearance of infants and children can be assessed using the mnemonic *CRASH*, which stands for **c**ry, **r**eaction to environment (consolable or inconsolable), **a**lertness/arousability, **s**ocial response, and **h**ydration.

TABLE 1.1 CRASH Assessment of Infants and Children by Appearance

	Well Appearing	**Ill Appearing**	**Toxic or Critically Ill Appearing**
Cry Quality	Strong cry or no cry Cries only briefly	Whimpers or sobs Cries off and on	Weak cry/moan/high-pitched cry Persistent crying or absence of crying due to state of alertness
Reaction to environment and parents	Consoled by parent Cooperative (as age appropriate)	Is difficult to console, but is eventually consoled by parent May be cooperative due to weakness or completely uncooperative	Inconsolable even with the parent Submissive/weak
Alertness/ Arousability	Alert or arouses quickly	Alert but irritable Difficult to arouse, but does awaken	Lethargic Unable to arouse or has difficulty staying awake/alert
Social response	Smiles	Briefly smiles	No smile, dull affect, or anxious affect
Hydration	Moist mucous membranes	Mouth slightly dry, but capillary refill time <2 seconds	Mucosa dry Capillary refill >2 seconds Cyanosis, mottling, or palor

Source: CRASH Assessment is a modification of the Yale Observation Scale described by McCarthy PL, Sharpe MR, Spiesel, SZ, et al. Observation scales to identify serious illness in febrile children. *Pediatrics.* 1982;70(5):802–809.

   c. When a pediatric patient does present with a problem, taking a thorough history of the chief complaint (keeping in mind developmentally appropriate skills and abilities) helps to generate a problem list. It is vital to identify and focus on the primary complaint that brought the patient in for evaluation. A helpful mnemonic for remembering the components of a primary complaint is OPQRST (**o**nset, **p**rovocation, **q**uality, **r**adiation, **s**everity, **t**iming associated with problem).

2. Ascertain whether you need to collect an interim or comprehensive history.
   a. An established, healthy child may need only an interim history, including medical, surgical, social, and family history, with updates to the medication and allergy list, as appropriate.
   b. A new patient or a new problem warrants collecting the pertinent past medical history (including birth and development history), surgical history, social history, family history, medication and allergy list, and a review of systems.
3. Prioritize problems and identify whether and how they relate to the chief complaint, separating those problems that do not relate to the chief complaint.
4. Summarize pertinent positive and negative findings, both subjective and objective.
   a. Performing a thorough history should help guide the focused physical examination, although sometimes a full physical may be warranted.
   b. Putting together the findings from these two steps should help guide and solidify a differential diagnosis.
5. Formulate and prioritize an appropriate differential diagnosis.
   a. It is helpful to list the differential diagnoses in descending order from most to least likely diagnosis. If this step is performed correctly, it should guide the initial management plan. Be sure to keep in mind "danger differentials" or those that carry a higher mortality risk.
   b. For a well child with no complaints, a differential should still be generated, including both growth and developmental diagnoses that could influence the child's long-term growth trajectory or developmental potential.
   c. A mnemonic that can be useful for generating a differential diagnosis is VITAMINS ABCDEK, which can be found in Table 1.2.

TABLE 1.2 VITAMINS ABCDEK as a Mnemonic for Generating a Differential Diagnosis

V	Vascular (vessel bleeding, vessel blockages, and hematologic issues)
I	Infective or postinfective
T	Trauma
A	Autoimmune or allergic
M	Metabolic (affecting lipids, carbohydrates, protein, micronutrients)
I	Idiopathic or iatrogenic
N	Neoplasms
S	Social (child abuse and social deprivation)

(continued)

TABLE 1.2 VITAMINS ABCDEK as a Mnemonic for Generating a Differential Diagnosis (*continued*)

A	Alcohol related
B	Behavioral disorders or psychosomatic
C	Congenital problems
D	Drug-related or degenerative disorders
E	Endocrine or exocrine problems
K	Karyotype or genetic disorders

Source: Modified from Zabidi-Hussin, ZA. Practical way of creating differential diagnoses through an expanded *VITAMINSABCDEK* mnemonic. *Adv Med Educ Pract.* 2016;7:247–248. doi:10.2147/AMEP.S106507

    d. Clinical reasoning will help you narrow the differential diagnosis, keeping in mind the SPIT approach to medical decision-making. *SPIT* stands for **s**erious, **p**robable, **i**nteresting, and **t**reatable.[1] Your short-list differential should include at least one diagnosis that is serious, one to three that are probable, one that is interesting/unique, and one that requires immediate treatment (it may be the same one that you provided in one of the other categories).

6. Initiate a management plan that may include diagnostic evaluation, screening tests, immunizations, and treatment, if indicated.

    a. Order diagnostic tests and laboratory studies appropriate for the differential diagnosis or the age of the patient.

    b. Review the patient's immunization status and administer needed immunizations if the patient meets the criteria for administration.

    c. Initiate a care plan based on the most likely diagnosis. Remember that the initial management goal is always to stabilize the patient.

The most common general presentations you can expect to encounter in pediatrics include abdominal pain, cough and/or breathing difficulties, fever, growth and development concerns, refusal to use a limb, and skin changes.

ABDOMINAL PAIN

As one of the most commonly coded visits in pediatrics,[2] abdominal pain is an essential presentation to understand in both the inpatient and outpatient setting. Most abdominal pain in pediatrics is acute, with viral etiologies of gastroenteritis being the most common diagnosis. However, chronic abdominal pain sometimes leaves providers scratching their heads at the numerous return visits for the same issue. With the complex pathophysiology of solid and hollow organs, pain receptors and the peritoneum, the history and physical exam are extremely important tools used to uncover the clues to make a differential and a final diagnosis.

> **CLINICAL PEARL:** Not all "bellyaches" are truly of abdominal pathology. Diabetic ketoacidosis; psychosomatic symptoms; and pulmonary, renal, and pelvic pathology can also cause abdominal pain.

Differential Diagnosis

The differential for abdominal pain becomes increasingly complex with increasing age of the patient, so differentiating abdominal pain by age will enhance the likelihood of creating an appropriate differential. Table 1.3 provides a differential diagnosis for the most common causes of abdominal pain by age.

History

Similar to all other areas of pediatrics, your initial evaluation should determine the severity of the illness (i.e., well vs. ill), but for abdominal pain it should also include an assessment of the child's hydration status (e.g., food and fluid intake, as well as output) and activity level (writhing in pain vs. lying still).

- When taking the history of a patient with abdominal pain, your priority is to identify those patients with an acute abdomen who may need surgical intervention. Although only about 5% of abdominal pain in ambulatory pediatrics is acute, upward of 30% of pediatric abdominal pain in the ED is surgical. The patient history is the cornerstone of diagnosis and can help identify red-flag signs or symptoms that would warrant further evaluation versus lower acuity problems.
- Age and gender are important risk factors for various problems arising from abdominal pain, as some conditions rarely occur outside of the newborn period (necrotizing enterocolitis, pyloric stenosis, and colic) and others never present before adolescence (ectopic pregnancy).
- Onset, duration, timing: Acute-onset pain occurs within seconds and is typically associated with rupture, perforation, or infarct. Rapid-onset pain, such as that associated with cholecystitis, intestinal obstruction, appendicitis, and ulcers, presents with increasing pain that occurs over minutes. Pain that is more gradual in onset occurs over hours or days and can be associated with a variety of intra-abdominal etiologies, so onset is not as helpful as location, character, and associated symptoms.[3]
- Provocation/alleviating factors: Position, movement, food, and defecation may all be provoking or alleviating factors, so it is important to ask about these.
- Quality: The character of the pain is useful in determining whether pain is visceral or peritoneal. Pain that is constant or intermittent, as well as colicky (short bursts of pain with increasing intensity that abruptly stops for a period of time), dull or achy, burning, stabbing, or pressure-like can help differentiate between serious abdominal pathology and less concerning conditions.

TABLE **1.3** Differential Diagnosis of Abdominal Pain by Age

<3 months	3–24 months	2–5 years old	6–11 years old	12–18 years old
Colic Milk protein allergy Pyloric stenosis*				
	Intussusception* Volvulus*			
Incarcerated hernia* Necrotizing enterocolitis* Testicular torsion*	Trauma*			
	Urinary tract infection/pyelonephritis			
	Constipation Foreign body ingestions (battery/toxin)* Gastroenteritis			
	Hirschsprung's	Strep pharyngitis Henoch-Schonlein Purpura (HSP) Mesenteric lymphadenitis		
		Appendicitis* Diabetic ketoacidosis (DKA)* Pneumonia Viral illness		
			GERD Hemolytic uremic syndrome (HUS) Inflammatory bowel disease (IBD) Peptic ulcer Poor nutrition	
			Functional abdominal pain School avoidance	Cholecystitis Dysmenorrhea Ectopic pregnancy* Ovulation pain Ovarian torsion* Pancreatitis PID Ruptured ovarian cyst Testicular torsion*

Note: Emergent intervention is indicated

DKA, diabetic ketoacidosis; GERD, gastroesophageal reflux disease; HSP, Henoch–Schonlein purpura, HUS, hemolytic uremic syndrome; IBD, inflammatory bowel disease; PID, pelvic inflammatory disease.

Adapted from the following sources: Leung AKC, Sigalet DL. Acute abdominal pain in children. *Am Fam Phys.* 2003;67(11):2321–2326. https://www.aafp.org/afp/2003/0601/p2321.html; Abdominal pain—differential diagnosis. In DynaMed [database online]. EBSCO information services. http://search.ebscohost.com/login.aspx?direct =true&db=dme&AN=116819&site=dynamed-live&scope=site. Updated June 07, 2017; Kim JS. Acute abdominal pain in children. *Pediat Gastroenterol Hepatol Nutr.* 2013;16(4):219–2241. doi:10.5223/pghn.2013.16.4.219; Baker RD. Acute abdominal pain. *Pediat Rev.* 2018;39(3):130–139. doi:10.1542/pir.2017-0089

- ○ Colicky pain is pathognomonic of a small bowel obstruction, with proximal lesions having shorter intervals between pain and distal obstructions having longer pain-free periods. Intussusception is a classic example of distal abdominal colic, whereas cholecystitis is a proximal example.
- ○ Distention or edema of the hollow viscus creates a dull or achy pain, much like pain with constipation.
- ○ Pain that improves with movement is likely visceral in nature (stretching of pain receptors in hollow organs), but peritoneal pain is aggravated by movement.
- ○ Pain that is associated with nausea, vomiting, pallor, and sweating tends to be visceral, whereas conversely these symptoms are not normally noted in peritoneal pain.

> **CLINICAL PEARL:** A useful technique used to identify whether pain is peritoneal or visceral is to ask a child lying on the exam table to try to push his or her belly button toward the ceiling and then suck in the belly button, like he or she is trying to make it touch the table. If the pain is visceral, the child will typically do this without a problem, but peritoneal pain will lateralize (and can often be identified visually), so you can locate the pain without actual palpation of the abdomen.[4]

- Radiation: Location of pain may help determine the origin of the pathology. For example, pain localized to the epigastric area typically represents an esophageal, gastric, or duodenal issue, whereas periumbilical pain represents a small intestine problem and lower abdominal pain represents a large bowel etiology. Figure 1.1 illustrates various differential diagnoses by location, recognizing that these are generalizations.
  - ○ Somatic/peritoneal pain is usually well localized, whereas visceral pain is poorly localized and may be generalized to a segment of the abdomen.

> **CLINICAL PEARL:** Children under the age of 5 years old are unable to localize pain well.

- Symptoms: Associated symptoms or a constellation of symptoms can be pathognomonic for conditions. Requiring urgent intervention and surgical consult, there are red-flag symptoms that you should remember to ask about and document as pertinent positives or negatives. These will help determine the most likely cause of the abdominal pain. See Table 1.4 for common associated symptoms, paying particular attention to the starred, red flag symptoms.

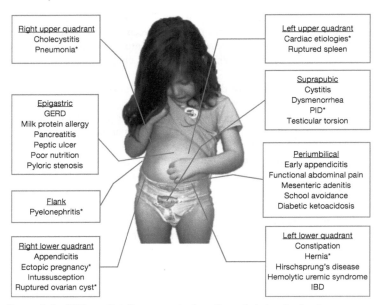

Figure 1.1 Differential diagnoses by location of abdominal pain.

*May present in contralateral quadrant or diffusely throughout the region.

GERD, gastrointestinal reflux disease; IBD, inflammatory bowel disease; PID, pelvic inflammatory disease.

Source: Created using information from Neuman MI, Ruddy RM. Emergency evaluation of the child with acute abdominal pain. In: Fleisher GR, et al, eds. *UpToDate* [database online]. https://www.uptodate.com/contents/emergency-evaluation-of-the-child-with-acute-abdominal-pain. Updated July 17, 2018.

TABLE 1.4 Symptoms Associated With Abdominal Pain and Diagnoses to Consider

	Associated Symptom	**Diagnoses to Consider**
Vomiting	Bilious vomiting*	Bowel obstruction (volvulus)
	Nonbilious and projectile vomiting	Pyloric stenosis
	Pain prior to the onset of vomiting*	Surgical abdomen
	Pain after the onset of vomiting	Medical abdomen

(continued)

TABLE 1.4 Symptoms Associated With Abdominal Pain and Diagnoses to Consider (*continued*)

	Associated Symptom	Diagnoses to Consider
Fever	Fever prior to the onset of pain	Infectious etiologies (gastroenteritis, strep pharyngitis, UTI, pneumonia)
	Fever after the onset of pain*	Appendicitis
	Fever and vomiting only	Mesenteric lymphadenitis
Genitourinary	Urinary symptoms (dysuria, urinary frequency, urinary urgency)	UTI or pyelonephritis
	Concurrent or anticipated menses	Dysmenorrhea Mittelschmerz
	Genital discharge	STI
	Vaginal spotting	PID Pregnancy
Blood in stool	Blood in the stool*	Ischemic conditions (i.e., intussusception (currant jelly stool)) Milk-protein allergy (flecks of blood)
	Bloody diarrhea*	Intussusception, volvulus, NEC, bacterial infection, HSP, IBD
	Abdominal distention*	Surgical, volvulus
	Hematochezia*	Obstruction
Other	Abdominal distention*	Surgical, volvulus
	Vomiting and diarrhea	Gastroenteritis
	Photophobia	Abdominal migraine
	Cough or shortness of breath	Pneumonia
	Sore throat	Respiratory etiologies such as Strep pharyngitis

*Red flag symptoms.

HSP, Henoch–Schonlein purpura; IBD, inflammatory bowel disease; NEC, necrotizing enterocolitis; PID, pelvic inflammatory disease; STI, sexually transmitted infections; UTI, urinary tract infection.

Adapted from: Hay WW Jr, Levin MJ, Deterding RR, Abzug MJ, eds. *Current Diagnosis & Treatment Pediatrics.* 24th ed. New York, NY: McGraw-Hill Education; 2018:652–668.

Other Medical History Specific to Complaint

- Chronic medical conditions, such as cystic fibrosis, may impact the differential for children with abdominal pain, whereas a history of intraabdominal surgery increases risk of adhesions and volvulus.
- Family history of chronic diseases may identify the child with an increased risk of a chronic abdominal issue (e.g., inflammatory bowel disease [IBD]), whereas a family history of appendicitis puts the child at increased likelihood of appendicitis as a viable differential (50% of children with appendicitis have a corresponding family history of appendicitis).[5]

- Social history is useful to identify factors that could contribute to abdominal pain. Bullying, depression, anxiety, and poor school performance can mask as abdominal pain. Poverty can point to food insecurity and poor nutritional choices.
- A dietary history is another key to your evaluation of a child with abdominal pain, as constipation is the most common cause of recurrent or chronic abdominal pain, and dietary habits can contribute to constipation. Cultural influences regularly appear in food choices, with spicy foods and caffeine commonly associated with gastritis and gastroesophageal reflux disease (GERD). Soda and sugar-sweetened beverages contribute to obesity, which is highly correlated with gallbladder disease.
- Sexual history for adolescent patients can help to pinpoint high-risk behaviors, which can be associated with sexually transmitted infections (STIs), pregnancy, ectopic pregnancy, and pelvic inflammatory disease (PID).

Physical Examination

After initial assessment and history have identified those patients with a high risk for a surgical abdomen from a less acute illness, a full exam, not just of the abdomen, is required.

- Inspection of the abdomen before palpation is obligatory in the pediatric patient, as this is often a challenging exam in pediatrics. Children with diffuse pain or guarding make their discomfort known to all and crying tenses the abdominal muscles, making a thorough exam more difficult. Before you auscultate, identify whether the abdomen is distended or scaphoid. A distended abdomen could represent a solid, fluid, or gas overload secondary to organomegaly, obstruction, or ascites. In addition, body habitus can be a good indicator of nutritional status. Abdominal breathing may indicate a pulmonary etiology, whereas positioning and guarding may help identify the location of pain. Note any visible lesions, masses or peristaltic waves; evidence of trauma or bruising; or previous surgical scars.
- Auscultating the abdomen may help you distinguish among hyperactive, hypoactive, and absent bowel sounds that may correlate to gastroenteritis, constipation, and obstruction, respectively. Reliability of bowel sounds in diagnosis, however, is limited.
- Palpation of the abdomen, using the techniques described in the introduction can help you localize pain to a quadrant and identify palpable masses, such as an olive-shaped mass in pyloric stenosis, or an enlarged sigmoid colon in constipation.
- Evaluating the oropharynx for tonsillar swelling, palatal petechiae, and tonsillar exudates can help you identify children who may have abdominal pain secondary to strep pharyngitis or potentially mononucleosis. Chest auscultation can help identify PNA or potentially myocarditis.

- The digital rectal exam, including checking rectal tone, can help you detect spinal cord injury, neuromuscular disease, constipation, fecal impaction, appendicitis, perianal abnormalities associated with IBD, and even a pelvic abscess.
- Pelvic exam may be necessary in pubertal females as a means of ruling out PID, collecting vaginal discharge samples for STI culture, and determining adnexal, ovarian, and uterine tenderness.
- Testicular exam is important to ensure that the abdominal pain is not referred secondary to a testicular torsion, a testicular appendiceal torsion, epididymitis, or hernia.
- Some of the special exam maneuvers that are important to the abdominal exam can help identify a diagnosis.
  - Rovsing's sign, pain in the right lower quadrant (RLQ) when pressure is applied in the left lower quadrant (LLQ), is a physical examination finding strongly associated with childhood appendicitis (positive likelihood ratio [LR+] = 3.52, 95% confidence interval [CI] = 2.65-4.68).[6]
  - Murphy's sign, pain in the right upper quadrant (RUQ) that is exacerbated by inspiration, is highly correlated with cholecystitis.
  - Rebound tenderness, pain that is intensified when pressure is released from the abdomen, is useful in determining peritoneal irritation.

Table 1.5 outlines some of the physical exam findings that may be correlated with diagnoses on the differential for abdominal pain.

TABLE **1.5** Physical Exam Findings Suggestive of Abdominal Diagnoses

	Physical Exam Finding	**Possible Diagnoses**
Inspection	Distended and shiny appearance	Peritonitis
	Surgical scars	Adhesions, volvulus
	Abdominal breathing	Pneumonia
	Peristaltic wave	Obstruction, pyloric stenosis
	Purpuric rash	HSP, HUS
	Jaundice	Hepatitis
	Scaphoid abdomen with abdominal breathing	Diaphragmatic hernia
Auscultation	Posterior crackles	Lower lobe pneumonia
	Gallop murmur heard at apex	Myocarditis
	High-pitched frequent bowel sounds	Small bowel obstruction
	Hyperactive bowel sounds	Gastroenteritis, diarrheal viral illness
	Hypoactive bowel sounds	Constipation
	Absence of bowel sounds	Ileus, perforation

(continued)

TABLE **1.5** Physical Exam Findings Suggestive of Abdominal Diagnoses (*continued*)

	Physical Exam Finding	Possible Diagnoses
Palpation	Epigastric tenderness	GERD, gastritis, peptic ulcer
	Palpable mass ("olive") in epigastric area	Hernia, pyloric stenosis
	(+) Murphy's sign	Cholecystitis
	CVA tenderness	Pyelonephritis, nephrolithiasis
	Flank fullness or mass	Wilms' tumor
	Localized abdominal pain (McBurney's point)	Appendicitis
	Suprapubic tenderness	UTI, pregnancy, dysmenorrhea
	Lateralized lower quadrant pain in a female	Ectopic pregnancy, ovarian torsion, ruptured ovarian cyst, ovulation pain
	Fullness and tenderness in LLQ	Constipation
	Bimanual	
	Cervical motion tenderness	PID
	Adnexal tenderness	Ectopic pregnancy
	Ovarian tenderness or enlargement	Ovarian cyst, ovarian torsion
	Uterine tenderness	Pregnancy, PID
Percussion	Dullness that shifts with changes in position (i.e., lateral decubitus)	Ascites
	Tenderness on percussion	Peritonitis
	Dullness in suprapubic area	Pregnancy, uterine mass, bladder distension
	Enlarged liver span	Hepatitis
	Dullness in lower lung field	Pneumonia

CVA, costovertebral angle; GERD, gastroesophageal reflux disease; HSP, Henoch–Schonlein purpura; HUS, hemolytic uremic syndrome; LLQ, left lower quadrant; PID, pelvic inflammatory disease; UTI, urinary tract infection.

Diagnostic Plan

The diagnostic plan that you create for patients with abdominal pain will vary depending on the differential diagnosis items; however, there are a few standard recommendations you should follow when evaluating abdominal pain.

- You should attempt to get a clean-catch UA from all patients, but if the child is too young or not yet toilet trained, a catheterized urine sample or suprapubic aspiration are gold standard for evaluating urine.
- Menarchal females should always have a pregnancy test, even if they deny sexual activity.
- If the history and physical warrant further investigation, the child is moderately to severely ill appearing, or when red-flag symptoms/signs are present with a high index of suspicion, the initial diagnostics should include a CBC with differential and erythrocyte sedimentation rate (ESR).

- A hemoccult stool test, stool cultures, liver function tests, electrolytes, renal function, and STI testing may also be indicated given the history and physical exam findings.
- If the patient presents with undifferentiated pain, a US can help you hone in on a differential diagnosis.
- You may consider an abdominal x-ray if you suspect a foreign body (FB), although you may not visualize organic material on the plain films. Suspected renal stones (if radiopaque), abdominal masses, perforation (free air), and constipation (heavy stool load) can also be evaluated with abdominal plain films.

Initial Management

- Evaluate the ill-appearing child quickly.
- If patient is ill appearing, has signs of a bowel obstruction and/or presents with peritoneal irritation, stabilize patient with oxygen, correct volume losses and metabolic abnormalities, and provide pain control (preferably before surgical evaluation). Empiric intravenous (IV) antibiotics are usually started if there is a suspicion of a serious infection.[7]
- Online, point-of-care stratification tools, such as the Pediatric Appendicitis Score or Alvarado score, can help you determine the disposition of a patient with a suspected appendicitis (to the ED if in outpatient setting or getting a surgical consult if in the ED or inpatient setting). The tools may also help differentiate an appendicitis from mesenteric lymphadenitis.
- Reassurance and supportive care may be the management decision for well or mildly ill-appearing children; however, serial follow-ups/exams on a patient can identify those children who present early in the course of an illness and change rapidly.

Key Points

- Stratifying patients by age can help narrow the differential diagnosis for abdominal pain and ensure that the most appropriate preliminary diagnostics are performed.
- The most common causes of abdominal pain in children are typically self-limiting viral illnesses, such as gastroenteritis, but it is important that you do not mistake a common illness for a critical illness. Appendicitis is the most common surgical condition in children and missed diagnoses are most often initially diagnosed as gastroenteritis. More common in children younger than 5 years old, a missed diagnosis can lead to perforation, abscess, and sepsis.
- History and physical exam can greatly narrow your differential diagnosis, but often diagnostics are needed to confirm your suspicions.

COUGH AND BREATHING DIFFICULTIES

Patients present with complaints of cough or trouble breathing for a variety of reasons. A cough is a reflex mechanism that protects the lungs and is a forceful expiration that removes foreign or infected material from the airway. A cough may also be voluntary or may be produced by a reflex irritation of the nose, sinus, pharynx, larynx, trachea, bronchi, or bronchioles. Loss of the cough reflex can lead to aspiration or PNA.[8] Most young infants are not developmentally able to shift nasal secretions from their airway and will swallow them instead of expectorate them.

Differential Diagnosis

Although the differential for cough or breathing difficulties is extensive and may contain obscure or rare diagnoses, those listed in the text that follows are the most commonly encountered or life-threatening causes of cough that may have corresponding shortness of breath:

- Asthma
- Allergies
- Bronchiolitis (may be caused by several viral infections, but RSV is the most common)
- Bronchitis
- Croup
- Epiglottitis
- FB
- GERD
- PNA (Influenza, bacterial, viral)
- Postinfectious drainage
- Sinusitis
- Tuberculosis
- URI
- Whooping cough

History

Cough, with or without shortness of breath, is a concerning symptom for parents and providers alike, as it is often a symptom that is not well tolerated by parents, can be perceived as "contagious," and parents often use popular home remedies as go-to treatments. These home remedies and OTC cough medications can be dangerous for children. For these reasons, a careful history must be elicited from the parents and from the child, if possible.

- Onset, duration, timing: The onset and duration of symptoms and a gradual buildup for fewer than 5 days is typically associated with a viral illness, whereas abrupt onset may be related to an exacerbation of a chronic condition or a bacterial infection.

- Provocation/alleviating factors: Identifying triggers at the onset of the cough allows you to create a medical decision pathway. You should always investigate possible environmental or exercise triggers for the cough, as this may point toward a more allergic or inflammatory cause, whereas sick contacts are not uncommon for viral infections. Next, review with the patient or parent whether there are any exacerbating features such as seasonal changes, time of day, supine position, or activity. Relieving factors may include rest, certain medications, increasing fluid intake, change in environment, and body position.
- Quality: One of the key historical components of cough is the character of the cough. Often a good description of the cough itself can differentiate cough etiologies.
  - ○ Common descriptive terms for cough include "wheezing," "barking," "whooping," "productive" or "nonproductive," and "dry" or "hacking." For example, a barky cough may indicate croup; however, children with asthma may also present with a barky cough.
  - ○ If the cough is productive, ask the family about sputum characteristics.
- Radiation: In this presentation, region is less related to an anatomical site, but rather to locations or positions that potentially trigger the cough.
- Symptoms: Associated symptoms can further narrow a diagnosis. Let us use the barky cough example. If this cough is associated with mild fevers and a hoarse voice, you would feel confident differentiating it from the asthmatic's barky cough, which is associated with mild sputum production and chest tightness without fevers and improves with albuterol.
  - ○ Associated symptoms may also include chest pain, shortness of breath, wheezing, snoring, apnea, nasal drainage, fever, headache, fatigue, night sweats, and rash. Table 1.6 lists some of the commonly associated symptoms and diagnoses to consider when evaluating a patient with an acute cough.

TABLE 1.6 Common Causes of Acute Cough and Associated Symptoms

Associated Symptoms	Common Causes
Acute cough and fever	Pneumonia, bronchitis, bronchiolitis
Acute onset of choking and coughing; stridor	Aspiration of foreign body
Acute cough and nasal drainage	Sinusitis, postnasal drainage
Acute cough and wheezing; no fever	Reactive airway disease/asthma

  - ○ Red-flag signs/symptoms for cough include neonatal age, sudden onset, dyspnea, recurrent chronic wet cough, hemoptysis, fever, night sweats, weight loss, FTT, feeding problems, recurrent PNA, abnormal chest exam, and continuous, unremitting or worsening cough.[9]

Other Medical History Specific to Complaint

- Family history: A strong family history of atopy can increase the chances for an asthma diagnosis. Also consider family history of cystic fibrosis, cardiomyopathies, interstitial lung disease, esophageal disorders, and any neurological or psychiatric disorders.
- Social history: There are many environmental factors that can contribute to a cough, so you should ask about smoking in the home, pets, age of the home, and mold. Socioeconomic status (SES) may also provide clues. A lower SES is inversely correlated with higher asthma rates and increasingly complex exacerbations.

Physical Examination

Although the cardiopulmonary exam is of utmost importance when evaluating a cough, it is important that you also evaluate body systems above and below the chest, as these can provide clues to help narrow your differential diagnosis. As with other pediatric conditions, an initial survey of the patient's status is critical to determining whether rapid interventions are necessary.

- Vital signs, including respiratory rate, heart rate, and temperature, as well as breathing pattern and pulse oximetry/SpO_2, should all be used to create your overall initial impression.
- Inspect the patient's chest with shirt removed. Inspect for size, shape, symmetry of chest, use of accessory muscles, retractions, nasal flaring, and/or pursing lips. Also, assess the patient's skin, nails, and mouth for cyanosis and fingers for clubbing.

> **CLINICAL PEARL:** To avoid producing anxiety, the parent may hold the child on his or her lap during the physical examination.

- Palpate the chest for tenderness and deformities, thoracic expansion, and tactile fremitus.
- Percuss the chest with the patient seated (toddlers and older). Gently percuss the anterior chest, lateral chest/axilla, and posterior chest.
- Auscultate the chest and always place your stethoscope directly on the patient's skin, never over their clothes. You should listen for cardiac and pulmonary sounds on the anterior chest, lateral chest/axilla, posterior chest, and perform bronchophony and egophony on anterior and posterior surfaces.

> **CLINICAL PEARL:** Consider performing auscultation of the heart and lungs at the beginning of the exam if you think the other examinations may cause the child to cry.

The most common diagnoses are listed in Table 1.7 along with the potential physical exam findings.

TABLE 1.7 Common Exam Findings for Acute and Chronic Cough in Pediatric Patients

Clinical Condition	Physical Exam Findings
Asthma	Pursed lips, tripod position, increased respiratory rate, audible wheezing, tight breath sounds, and wheezing on auscultation; the patient may have respiratory distress
Bronchiolitis	Low-grade fever, cough, increased respiratory rate, retractions, increased work of breathing, wheezing, and crackles along with symptoms of upper respiratory infection (nasal drainage, congestion)
Pneumonia	Fever, tachypnea, increased work of breathing, retractions, crackles, decreased breath sounds on auscultation, bronchophony, and dullness to percussion
Sinusitis	Wet or dry cough, nasopharyngeal and oropharyngeal erythema, fever, halitosis, and normal exam on auscultation; patient may have mucopurulent drainage in oropharynx
Whooping cough	Paroxysms of coughing, possible inspiratory whoop with other symptoms of URI, such as nasal drainage and congestion; patient may have posttussive vomiting, increased work of breathing, and prolonged coughing spells
Airway foreign body	Patient may present with a wide range of symptoms such as inspiratory wheezing, obstruction, and/or dyspnea; symptoms may be prolonged but of reduced severity; suspicion for airway obstruction should increase if patient has cyanotic spells, stridor on auscultation, and unilaterally diminished breath sounds; chest x-ray may be done but with any clinical suspicion of foreign body aspiration, the patient should undergo CT or bronchoscopy
Croup	Barking cough, nasal discharge, fever, hoarseness, and stridor; patient may have respiratory distress and may have worsening symptoms when presenting at night

URI, upper respiratory infection.

Diagnostic Plan

- Development of your differential diagnosis usually begins when you ask whether the patient has an acute or chronic cough. The 2017 CHEST Guideline and Expert Panel Report defines chronic cough as longer than 4 weeks for patients ≤14 years old.[10]
- Pulmonary function tests (PFTs) can be done using a variety of methods. The simplest way of assessing vital capacity and expiratory flow rates can be done with a spirometer. Most children over the age of 6 years will be able to perform these tests but they may need training and coaching during the assessment. PFTs may be useful to help determine whether a patient has obstructive or restrictive disease and are often used in the diagnosis and management of asthma.

- Diagnostic testing is variable depending on the differential diagnoses you are considering. See Table 1.8 for the best diagnostic tool to diagnose a specific condition.

TABLE 1.8 Evaluation Method for Chronic Cough Causes in Children

Pulmonary Causes	Evaluation Method
Asthma	Pulmonary lung function
Aspiration	Swallowing assessment
Chronic endobronchial suppurative disease (cystic fibrosis, bronchiectasis, chronic lung disease)	Sweat test, genetic screening, evaluation of immune function, cilia biopsy
Chronic pneumonia	Chest CT, bronchoscopy, relevant microbial assessment
Eosinophilic lung disease	Blood work and bronchoalveolar lavage
Inhaled retained foreign body	Bronchoscopy
Interstitial lung disease	Genetic testing, autoimmune testing, +/- lung biopsy
Mechanical inefficiency (tracheobronchomalacia or vascular rings)	Bronchoscopy, chest CT w/contrast, chest MRI
Noninfective bronchitis (environmental pollutant exposure)	Remove trigger
Post-infection (self-resolving viral infections)	PCR and/or serology
Space-occupying lesions (cysts, tumors)	Chest CT or MRI
Extra pulmonary Causes	
Cardiac	EKG
Ear disease	Examination of ear canal and removal of object or treatment of disease
Esophageal disorders (GERD)	pH monitoring or endoscopy
Medications (ACE-inhibitors, PPIs, inhaled medications, cytotoxic drugs)	D/C medication or evaluate for interstitial lung disease (cytotoxic drugs)
Tic Cough (habit cough)	Behavioral therapy
Somatic cough disorder (psychogenic cough)	Psychotherapy
Upper airway pathology (sinusitis, OSA)	CT, nasal endoscopy, polysomnography

ACE, angiotensin-converting enzyme; D/C, discontinue; GERD, gastroesophageal reflux disease; OSA, obstructive sleep apnea; PCR, polymerase chain reaction; PPIs, proton-pump inhibitors.
Source: Adapted from Kliegman R, ed. *Nelson Textbook of Pediatrics.* 20th ed. Philadelphia, PA: W. B. Saunders; 2016:2090.

Initial Management

- Most cases of acute cough in children are associated with respiratory infections and can be managed with conservative, comfort measures unless symptoms are progressively increasing in severity over 2 to 3 weeks.

- If a patient presents with cough and shortness of breath and pulse oximetry below 90% (depending on your elevation), they should be assessed in an ED setting.
- Patients who present with cough, fever, and crackles on auscultation should be treated for PNA. PNA is suggested by fever for 2 to 5 days, localized signs (crackles, dull percussion), tachypnea, and absence of stridor or wheeze. A CXR is not always needed for this diagnosis.
- Bronchiolitis is suggested by patient age (<2 years old) presenting during RSV season (December to March in North America) with cough, wheezing, rhinorrhea, tachypnea, crackles, and increased respiratory effort.[11]
- Most recurrent or persistent wheezing in children is the result of airway reactivity. While viral respiratory infections, including bronchitis, are important triggers for asthma exacerbations, they should not be treated with antibiotics.
- Not all that wheezes is asthma. There is a long list of asthma masqueraders but the more common diagnoses are gastroesophageal reflex, sinusitis, viral bronchiolitis, and vocal cord dysfunction.
- Consider a CXR for severe cases of PNA, lower respiratory tract infections, true hemoptysis (not nosebleeds), recurrent fever, increasing frequency/severity >2 to 3 weeks, or signs of chronic lung disease.
- A missed FB can lead to prolonged acute or chronic cough. A CXR may be normal so suspect FB if a patient presents with sudden onset, progressive cough, hemoptysis, and/or asymmetric wheeze/breath sounds/hyperinflation. These patients should have an urgent CT or bronchoscopy.
- Paroxysmal cough suggests pertussis.[12] A review of the patient's immunization records can usually help move this diagnosis up or down on your differential list.
- Do not use cough suppressants or OTC cough meds in pediatric patients.[10] OTC medications are as effective as placebo for acute cough with head colds in children.[9]
- Do not use narcotic cough suppressants with pediatric patients.[13]

Key Points

- Most cases of acute cough in children are associated with viral respiratory infections and can be managed with conservative, comfort measures unless symptoms progressively increase in severity over 2 to 3 weeks.
- Most recurrent or persistent wheezing in children is the result of airway reactivity. However, not all that wheezes is asthma.
- Children in whom an inhaled FB is a likely cause of cough should undergo urgent bronchoscopy.

Fever

Children mount a strong immunologic response, so it is no surprise that a large proportion of ED and ambulatory pediatric office visits involve fever (temperature greater than 100.4°F). Nearly one third of all pediatric visits present with fever, and fever is one of the top 10 concerns addressed via parental advice lines.[14] The evaluation of fever is particularly difficult due to the wide variety of potential etiologies, ranging from self-limited to life-threatening.

Differential Diagnosis

The initial evaluation and assessment of the patient with fever must involve a stratification of the patient by appearance, followed by history and physical exam, as the combination of appearance with history and physical exam has great value for identifying those patients with serious bacterial infections (SBIs) from those with milder illnesses.[15] The differential diagnosis of fever includes the following:

- Bacterial infections such as acute otitis media (AOM), bacteremia, cellulitis, endocarditis, meningitis, osteomyelitis, pneumonia (PNA), septic arthritis, sepsis, skin infections, sinusitis, pharyngitis/tonsillitis, urinary tract infection (UTI)/pyelonephritis, and whooping cough
- Viral infections such as the common cold or an upper respiratory infection (URI), croup, gastroenteritis, herpangina, influenza, viral enanthems (a rash on the mucous membranes), and exanthems (a rash on the skin)
- Rheumatologic conditions
- Malignancy

History

When taking the history of a patient with fever, one of your goals is to evaluate the pretest probability of an SBI. SBIs include meningitis, bacteremia, sepsis, PNA, and UTI. There are certain factors that carry a higher probability of this:

1. Children with no or incomplete immunizations
2. Children younger than 2 years of age
3. Children who are ill appearing[16]

Meeting all three of these criteria places a child at higher risk for SBI, whereas meeting one or less significantly lowers the probability. The presence of additional risk factors, such as those listed in Table 1.9, help further define a child's risk for localized or systemic bacterial infection.

- Onset, duration, timing: Ask about when the fever started, how the family collected the temperature (e.g., tactile vs. oral thermometer vs. ear thermometer), how quickly it has risen and the highest temperature (T_{max}) reached. In addition, although not a true predictor of illness, the T_{max} may help stratify the youngest patients (0–3 months) into risk groups for SBI.

TABLE **1.9** Factors That Increase a Child's Risk for Febrile Infections

Age	Risk Factors
Neonates	Prematurity
	Prolonged rupture of membranes
	Maternal fever
	Maternal group B *Streptococcus* infection with less than recommended treatment protocol
Children	Close-contact exposure
	Day-care attendance
	Indwelling medical devices (ports, shunts, catheters)
	Recent travel
	School-aged siblings
	Secondhand smoke exposure
	Uncircumcised males younger than 12 months of age
Adolescents	Close-contact exposures
	Contact sports
	High-risk behaviors

- Provocation/alleviating factors: With a plethora of over-the-counter (OTC) remedies readily available to parents, it is imperative that you ask parents what they have tried for symptom relief. Nonpharmaceutical treatments are an important piece of information because some practices may actually be exacerbating the problem. For example, using rubbing alcohol or cold baths causes vasoconstriction of peripheral vasculature, which can in turn signal the need to increase the body temperature further.
- Quality: Ask about fever patterns and intermittent periods of defervescence. A low-grade fever that suddenly increases may indicate a superimposed bacterial-on-viral illness, whereas a relapsing–remitting fever could indicate a tick-borne, zoonotic, or parasitic disease.
- Symptoms associated with the fever: Fever is not a disease itself, but merely an indicator of thermoregulation dysfunction, so uncovering other symptoms may help you find the underlying disease.
  - Associated symptoms that may indicate a more serious etiology include poor appetite, a change in type of cry, irritability, and lethargy.
  - Inquire about systemic complaints specific to the differential diagnosis. Cough and tachypnea can signal PNA, whereas pain with urination may indicate occult UTI. Nasal congestion and sore throat may indicate URI, whereas headache and sore throat may lead you toward a strep pharyngitis diagnosis. Ear pain, flank pain, or joint pain would indicate a localized infection, whereas constitutional symptoms of weight loss, night sweats, and bone pain may suggest a noninfectious etiology.

Other Medical History Specific to Complaint

- Collecting a past medical history of similar febrile episodes, previously diagnosed infections, and chronic illnesses is important.

- Family history of febrile seizures increases a child's risk of having a febrile seizure, although the pathophysiology of febrile seizures has not yet been clearly elucidated.[17]
- Social history should include child-care details, contact with ill individuals, passive smoke exposure, and parental health literacy level.
- Immunization status should be reviewed to identify patients at risk of infections that can be prevented by a vaccine, especially pneumococcal infections.

Physical Examination

General assessment should be a systematic means of determining whether the child is toxic, ill, or well appearing. The following factors can all be used, in addition to observation and response to exam, to determine the status of the child's condition:

- Signs of dehydration should be noted such as capillary refill longer than 2 seconds, scant or no tears, sunken fontanelle, decreased urine output, dry skin and lips, and tacky or dry mucous membranes.[18]
- Note the quality of the cry, the child's response to parental stimulation, and the child's state (alert, sleepy, difficult to arouse, etc.).
- "Red flags" for a toxic-appearing child include, but are not limited to, lethargy (or submissiveness), capillary refill time longer than 2 seconds, tachypnea/bradycardia, cyanosis, poor perfusion, inconsolability, petechiae/purpura, changes in work of breathing, and occasionally hypothermia.

> **CLINICAL PEARL:** An infant who smiles has a very low likelihood of having meningitis.[18]

- A focused, yet thorough exam, may reveal the cause of the fever. Several physical exam findings and their associated etiology are listed in Table 1.10.[16,19]

TABLE 1.10 Physical Exam Findings Suggestive of Fever Etiology

Physical Exam Finding	Possible Etiology
Bulging fontanelle	Meningitis, encephalitis
Loss of extraocular movements (in a child with developmental ability for coordinated eye movements)	Orbital cellulitis
TMs with erythema and minimal mobility	AOM
Pinna of ear has forward displacement	Mastoiditis
Clear nasal discharge	URI
Purulent nasal drainage	Sinusitis
Nasal flaring	Lower respiratory tract infection
Vesicular lesions on lips/vermillion border	HSV

(continued)

TABLE **1.10** Physical Exam Findings Suggestive of Fever Etiology (*continued*)

Physical Exam Finding	Possible Etiology
Vesicular lesions on gingiva	Gingivostomatitis
Vesicular lesions on posterior O/P	Hand–foot–mouth disease or herpangina
Palatal petechial with tonsillar enlargement and exudate	Strep pharyngitis or mononucleosis
Lymphadenopathy	Anterior→strep Posterior→viral
Nuchal rigidity/(+) Kernig or Brudzinski	Meningitis, CNS infection
Lungs with crackles	Pneumonia
Lungs with wheezes	Bronchitis or bronchiolitis
New murmur	Rheumatic fever or endocarditis
Flank pain	Pyelonephritis
Diffuse abdominal discomfort	Gastroenteritis
Localized abdominal pain (McBurney's point)	Appendicitis, mesenteric lymphadenitis
Suprapubic tenderness	UTI
Joint pain or swelling	Septic arthritis
Bone pain	Osteomyelitis, malignancy
Skin with erythema, warmth, tenderness	Abscess, cellulitis
Skin with vesicles	Possible viral exanthem (varicella, hand–foot–mouth disease, bullous impetigo)
Skin with honey-colored crusting	Impetigo
Skin with sandpapery rash	Scarlet fever, possibly measles
Skin with petechiae or purpura	Meningococcemia, RMSF

AOM, acute otitis media; CNS, central nervous system; HSV, herpes simplex virus; O/P, oropharyngeal; RMSF, Rocky Mountain Spotted Fever; TM, tympanic membrane; URI, upper respiratory infection, UTI, urinary tract infection.

Diagnostic Plan

- Repeat temperature: Identifying accurate temperature measurements are critical to ensure that the child is truly febrile by medical definition and to monitor response over time.
- Point-of-care testing such as rapid flu, rapid strep and/or UA may be useful to confirm or rule down your suspected diagnoses.
- Laboratory investigation:
  - Depending on the age of the child and the length of fever, if a source for the fever is not readily apparent, you may need to collect a CBC, urine sample (via catheterized or suprapubic sample) for UA/urine culture, stool cultures, and/or viral tests (respiratory syncytial virus [RSV], influenza, etc.).
- Other studies: Always remember that the initial diagnostic and management plan should center on stabilizing the patient as you arrive at a diagnosis. Infants and children who are critically ill will require timely and

highly invasive stabilization methods. Table 1.11 gives a broad overview of how you should approach the stabilization of patients depending on their presentation.

TABLE 1.11 Signs and Symptoms of a Pediatric Patient and Stabilization Techniques to Consider

Assessment	Think of ...	What to do to stabilize ...
Normal appearance, but increased work of breathing	Respiratory distress	Apply oxygen Keep child calm Place in position of comfort that minimizes the respiratory effort
Normal appearance with signs of poor perfusion	Hypothermia Mild to moderate dehydration Congenital heart defect Compensatory shock	Warm patient IV access and IV fluids Apply oxygen Call EMS
Abnormal appearance with increased work of breathing	Early respiratory failure	Call EMS Apply oxygen and/or consider intubation
Abnormal appearance with decreased work of breathing	Late respiratory failure	Call EMS Intubation Pediatric advanced life support
Abnormal appearance and poor perfusion	Shock	Call EMS IV access and IV fluids Pediatric advanced life support
Abnormal appearance, but normal respiratory effort and circulation	Neurologic insult Electrolyte abnormality	Call EMS IV access and IV fluids

EMS, emergency medical services; IV, intravenous.
Source: Dieckmann RA, Brownstein D, Gausche-Hill M. The pediatric assessment triangle: a novel approach for the rapid evaluation of children. Pediatr Emerg Care. 2010;26(4):312-315. doi:10.1097/PEC.0b013e3181d6db37.

  ○ Specific studies may be performed if the clinical suspicion is high for potentially life-threatening conditions. These include a lumbar puncture to evaluate for meningitis, blood cultures for bacteremia/sepsis, chest x-ray (CXR) for respiratory complaints, and US for appendicitis or pyelonephritis.

Initial Management

- Initial management depends on the age of the patient, the child's appearance, and the history and physical findings. An algorithmic approach to pediatric fever management is outlined in Figures 1.2, 1.3, 1.4, and 1.5.
- Neonates (<28 days) with rectal temperature greater than 100.4°F should be sent to the ED for evaluation. History and physical exam cannot differentiate minor illness from SBI in a neonate, so the newborn will need evaluation with access to immediate labs and imaging.

- Infants 28 to 90 days old should receive a full sepsis workup, but appearance of the child will determine whether this can be done in an inpatient or outpatient setting.
- Children 3 to 36 months old with a temperature higher than 102.2°F should be stratified by appearance. Any child who appears toxic or ill should be admitted to the hospital for further workup and treatment, whereas well-appearing infants and toddlers with a temperature >102.2 F will likely need a UA at a minimum and possibly a CXR.
- Children older than 36 months with no source for a fever identified after 8 days now have a fever of unknown origin (FUO). FUO comes with its own algorithms that are outside the scope of this book.
- Supportive measures for fever include acetaminophen or ibuprofen as an antipyretic, with ibuprofen having a longer lasting, more robust antipyretic effect.[20]
- Reassurance is sometimes the most effective treatment for families.
- According to the American Academy of Pediatrics' (AAP) policy statement on fevers and antipyretic use, "the primary goal of treating the febrile child should be to improve the child's overall comfort rather than focus on the normalization of body temperature. When counseling the parents or caregivers of a febrile child, the general well-being of the child, the importance of monitoring activity, observing for signs of serious illness, encouraging appropriate fluid intake, and the safe storage of antipyretics should be emphasized".[21]

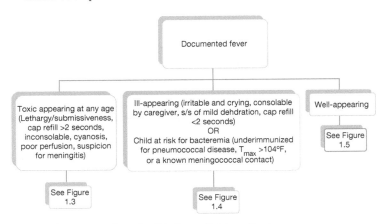

FIGURE 1.2 Approach to the febrile pediatric patient.

s/s, signs and symptoms.

Source: Adapted from Baraff, LJ. Management of fever without source in infants and children. *Ann Emerg Med.* 2000;36(6):602–614. doi:10.1067/mem.2000.110820; Avner JR. Acute fever. *Pediat Rev.* 2009;30(1):5–13. doi:10.1542/pir.30-1-5.

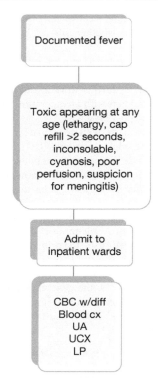

Figure 1.3 Approach to toxic-appearing, febrile child.
Blood cx, blood culture; CBC, complete blood count; LP, lumbar puncture; UA, urinalysis; UCX, urine culture.
Source: Adapted from Baraff, LJ. Management of fever without source in infants and children. *Ann of Emerg Med.* 2000;36(6):602–614. doi:10.1067/mem.2000.110820; Avner JR. Acute fever. *Pediat Rev.* 2009;30(1):5–13. doi:10.1542/pir.30-1-5

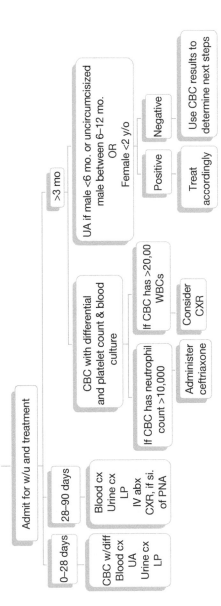
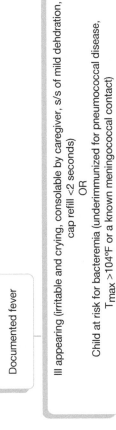

FIGURE 1.4 Approach to ill appearing, febrile child.

abx, antibiotics; CBC, complete blood count; cx, culture; CXR, chest xray; CXR, if si. of PNA, chest x-ray if there are signs of pneumonia; IV, intravenous; LP, lumbar puncture; PNA, pneumonia; s/s, signs and symptoms; UA, urinalysis; WBC, white blood cell; w/u, workup. *Source:* Adapted from Baraff, LJ. Management of fever without source in infants and children. *Ann Emerg Med.* 2000;36(6):602–614. doi:10.1067/mem.2000.110820; Avner JR. Acute fever. *Pediat Rev.* 2009;30(1):5–13. doi:10.1542/pir.30-1-5

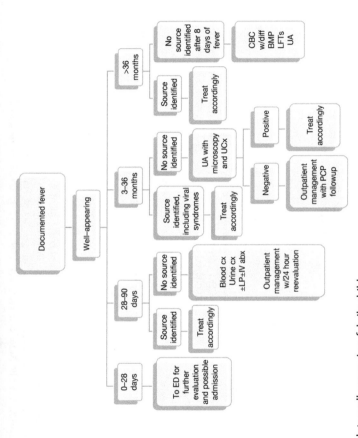

FIGURE 1.5 Approach to well-appearing, febrile child.

BMP, basic metabolic panel; CBC, complete blood count; cx, culture; IV abx, intravenous antibiotics; LFTs, liver function tests; LP, lumbar puncture; PCP, primary care provider; UA, urinalysis; UCx, urine culture.

Source: Adapted from Baraff, LJ. Management of fever without source in infants and children. *AnnEmerg Med.* 2000;36(6):602–614. doi:10.1067/mem.2000.110820; Avner JR. Acute fever. *Pediat Rev.* 2009;30(1):5–13. doi:10.1542/pir.30-1-5

Key Points

- Fever has a varied differential diagnosis; therefore, making an overall assessment of the child's appearance and conducting a focused history and physical examination are the most important tasks needed to diagnose a pediatric patient.
- Assessing appearance can be done with a variety of observation scales, but in general, assessing the child's hydration status, cry, social interactions, state change, color, and response to stimuli together are good predictors of well versus ill appearance.
- Be sure to consider "red-flag symptoms" when assessing a fever, such as ill or toxic appearance of the child, other abnormal vital signs, dehydration, and lethargy, as they may indicate an SBI. Fevers without these red-flag symptoms are associated with diseases that have a lower mortality risk.
- The primary initial treatment goal is to stabilize the patient.

GROWTH AND DEVELOPMENT

Because a large majority of outpatient, community-based pediatrics focuses on measuring and monitoring growth and development via the well-child exam, the approach to the well-child visit, including normal growth and development, is presented separately in Chapter 4, The Well-Child Check and Preventative Care Guidelines.

When a child presents with his or her caregivers with growth or developmental concerns, it is important to identify the factors that contribute to abnormal growth or development. Environmental, social, genetic, medical, and nutritional factors can individually (or cumulatively) contribute to abnormalities in growth or development. Many growth and developmental concerns are actually recognized or identified during routine well-child visits; however, astute parents may bring a child in for a concern in the interim period between well visits, especially after the age of 2 when well-visit spacing increases.

GROWTH & DEVELOPMENT CONCERNS

Many times parental concerns around growth are determined to be unfounded given the child's genetic potential, but they may also be early indicators of a deeper social, medical, or nutritional problem. The most common growth concerns identified in pediatric practices are associated with stature, weight, and pubertal development. The concerns typically fall on the extremes, such as short or tall stature, under- or overweight, early or late pubertal development.

When a developmental concern is noted via a routine screening tool or during a surveillance visit, it is important to recognize that it is merely one point in time and may not accurately reflect the dynamic nature of child development. Engaging the family in a discussion about the findings may reveal unspoken parental concerns about a single domain or several domains of development. The most common isolated developmental concerns are centered on language acquisition and communication or failure to perform basic gross motor skills. Concerns in two or more domains open up a larger differential with poorer prognoses and the need for multimodal interventions.

Differential Diagnosis

The differential for growth and developmental concerns includes the following:

- Normal growth or normal development
- Constitutional growth delay or constitutional growth advancement
- Familial short or tall stature
- Inadequate nutrition
- Failure to thrive (FTT)
- Obesity
- Precocious puberty
- Delayed puberty
- Child abuse/neglect
- Chromosomal syndromes
- Hypothyroidism
- Isolated developmental delay (such as developmental language delays or cerebral palsy)
- Global developmental delay (GDD)
- Autism spectrum disorder (ASD)
- Learning issues/school problems (such as learning disability, attention deficit hyperactivity disorder [ADHD], depression, or anxiety)
- Systemic illness like celiac disease, Crohn's disease, cystic fibrosis, congenital heart defects, chronic renal disease, and chronic steroid use

History

The history for both growth and development concerns should delve into birth and development history, assess nutritional status and environmental exposures (e.g., lead, phytoestrogens), evaluate growth velocity, calculate the child's growth potential, review psychosocial risk factors, and identify signs/symptoms of a systemic illness.

- Onset, duration, and timing: Elicit a birth and development history, paying particular attention to risk factors that might place the child at increased risk for growth or developmental problems. Some of the risk factors to consider when taking your history can be found in Table 1.12.
  - ○ The development history should include the age at which the child met developmentalmilestones. The development history can identify where development of a particular domain stalled, but can also help differentiate genetic syndromes associated with short stature (Prader–Willi syndrome) or delayed puberty (Turner syndrome) from other causes.

TABLE **1.12** Key History Items That May Increase a Child's Risk for Growth or Developmental Problems

History	Conditions to Consider	Possible Effects on Growth	Possible Effects on Development
Prematurity	Cerebral palsy Short stature	FTT Short stature	Cognitive and behavioral deficits
Late-preterm birth		Growth faltering <2 years old	
Low birth weight	Cerebral palsy	FTT Short stature	Motor delays Cognitive and behavioral issues
Perinatal hypoxia (including history of breech presentation, traumatic delivery, perinatal intubation, low Apgar scores)	Cerebral palsy GH deficiency, Hypopituitarism, Hypothyroidism	Short stature (GH deficiency, hypothyroidism)	Intellectual disability (hypopituitarism) Motor delays (CP)
IUGR	TORCH infections	FTT Short stature	Developmental delays
Maternal infections	CMV, HIV, rubella, syphilis, toxoplasmosis, Zika	FTT Microcephaly Short stature	Developmental delays
Maternal chronic disease (DM, HTN, CKD, autoimmune diseases, malnutrition)	GDM associated with macrosomia	Obesity	
Feeding difficulty in infancy	Turner syndrome	Short stature	
Lack of prenatal care	Social and environmental factors		Language delays
Food and shelter insecurity	Environmental exposures Malnutrition Neglect	FTT Short stature	Developmental delays
Exposure to toxins (lead, mercury, etc.)			Intellectual/cognitive delays
Neonatal CNS infection	CP (increased inflammation could contribute to this); Meningitis (poses a risk for damage to the pituitary gland)	Short stature (CNS insult)	Motor delays (CP)

CKD, chronic kidney disease; CMV, cytomegalovirus; CNS, central nervous system; CP, cerebral palsy; DM, diabetes mellitus; FTT, failure to thrive; GDM, gestational diabetes mellitus; GH, growth hormone; HTN, hypertension; IUGR, intrauterine growth restriction; TORCH, toxoplasmosis, other, rubella, cytomegalovirus, herpes.

○ The development history is important as a developmental delay may trumpet a deeper problem, such as ASD, or may herald possible learning disabilities in the future.

○ A history of regression of milestones should warrant an urgent workup or referral.

• Provocation/risk factors: Growth is highly affected by intake and output, so these are important factors to discuss in an interview regarding growth or development. A dietary history is essential in order to differentiate inadequate calorie consumption from adequate calorie consumption with a disruption in the absorption/metabolism of the nutrients (celiac disease, cystic fibrosis, or Crohn's disease). This history can also identify potential environmental contributors to growth/developmental concerns (e.g., type and amount of liquid used to mix formula [malnutrition], exposure to lead in cookware [cognitive delay], and exposure to phytoestrogens [precocious puberty]).

• Quality: Understanding the quality or character of the concern is also important, as it can help you determine the workup you perform or the referrals you make. In addition, it can help you understand how concerning the problem is to the family. Does the child make certain syllables, but struggles with others? Has the growth velocity changed slowly over time or was there a rapid change at a particular point in time? Did the pubertal development follow a predictable pattern with appropriate intervals between milestones?

> **CLINICAL PEARL:** Precocious puberty is most commonly idiopathic in girls, but the majority of boys with precocious puberty are noted to have an identified central nervous system (CNS) lesion.[22]

• Radiation: Ascertain whether the growth or developmental concern is localized to a particular developmental domain or body region.

○ Macro- and microcephaly could indicate the need for a deeper investigation of development parameters, whereas faltering weight with normal height and head circumference may be an early indicator of malnutrition or a systemic illness, such as cystic fibrosis or kidney disease.

○ An isolated speech delay would drive a different workup than a motor delay.

○ Thelarche without menarche may indicate an anatomic issue, whereas complete lack of pubertal development may indicate a hormonal or pituitary etiology.

• Severity/Associated Symptoms: Finally, a review of systemic symptoms that might indicate an underlying cause for the growth concern is reasonable.

Other Medical History Specific to Complaint

- Family history is vital to assessing a child with growth or developmental concerns, as genetics play a large role in stature, onset of puberty, and development. Only 5% to 15% of stature, pubertal, and weight concerns are of a medical nature. Family history of delayed growth spurt (constitutional growth delay), early thelarche/menarche (precocious puberty), or siblings with school difficulties (learning disability) may direct investigations around growth and development.
- Family/social history can help identify cultural beliefs, poverty, parental educational level, and family dynamics. Many times family dynamics can be intimated by watching parent–child interactions.

> **CLINICAL PEARL:** Poverty and parental educational level have a more significant effect on a child's long-term development than even highly correlated birth events like prematurity and birth weight.[23]

Figures 1.6a and 1.6b show an algorithmic approach to narrowing the differential diagnosis when evaluating a patient for a growth or developmental concern.

> **CLINICAL PEARL:** Familial short stature, followed by constitutional growth delay, are the most common causes of short stature. Cerebral palsy is the most common cause of motor delays; however, language delays are the most common developmental delay.

Physical Examination

- Calculating growth potential is mandatory for any growth concerns, as understanding whether a child is appropriate for his or her genetic potential can differentiate genetics from medical or social issues.
  - Calculating a midparental target height depends on gender
  - Boys: [(Father's height in cm) + (Mother's height in cm) +13 cm] / 2
  - Girls: [Father's height in cm) + (Mother's height in cm) – 13 cm] / 2
- Once a midparental target height is calculated, it is important to review the child's growth chart in detail, looking for growth that has followed its trajectory, dropped over time, increased over time, or plateaued. Having a keen eye on the growth charts helps to detect these changes early.
  - A height trajectory less than the 5th percentile in the first 2 years of life (short stature), especially when not associated with a premature infant, may indicate an underlying endocrine disorder, whereas significant drops in weight trajectory may indicate the need for further evaluation surrounding FTT due to organic and nonorganic etiologies.

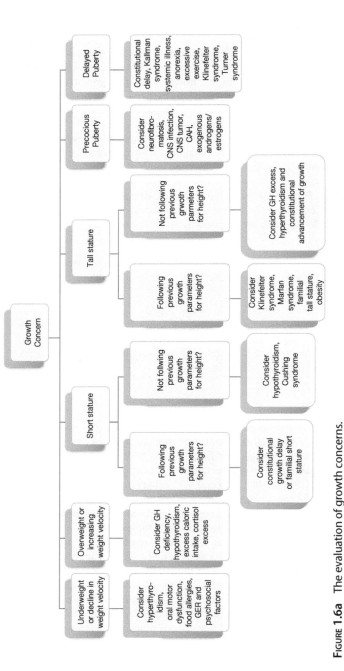

FIGURE 1.6a The evaluation of growth concerns.
CAH, congenital adrenal hyperplasia; CNS, central nervous system; GER, gastroesophageal reflux; GH, growth hormone.

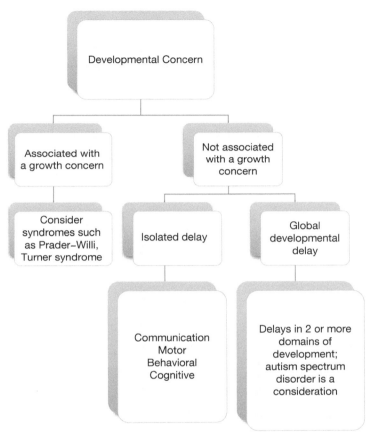

FIGURE **1.6b** The evaluation of growth concerns.

○ Head circumference below the 5th percentile (microcephaly) or above the 95th percentile (macrocephaly) could be indicative of an undetected perinatal infection, hydrocephalus, intracranial mass, or craniosynostosis, all of which can be related to poorer developmental outcomes.[24]

CLINICAL PEARL: An increase or decrease that crosses two (2) major percentile lines on the growth chart should trigger further investigation.

● A complete physical exam is usually warranted when evaluating a child with a growth or developmental concern, including a thorough fundoscopic exam, skin exam, and Tanner staging. Table 1.13 notes the physical exam findings that could provide clues to the etiology of a growth or developmental concern.

TABLE 1.13 Exam Findings That May Correlate to Growth or Developmental Concerns

Finding	Etiology to Consider	Growth Correlate	Developmental Correlate
Dysmorphic features	Multiple chromosomal abnormalities	Turner syndrome (delayed puberty and short stature) Klinefelter syndrome (delayed puberty and tall stature)	
Macrocephaly	Increased ICP		Cognitive deficits Motor deficits
Microcephaly	Congenital viral infection Craniosynostosis FAS Fetal drug exposure Hypoxic–ischemic encephalopathy Meningitis	Short stature	Cognitive deficits
Papilledema	Increased ICP	Delayed puberty or precocious puberty	
Ear malformations			Cognitive impairments Hearing impairment Language delay
Goiter	Hypothyroidism	Short stature	Cognitive impairments
Midline defects	Hypopituitarism		
Webbed neck	Turner syndrome	Short stature	
High-pitched voice	GH deficiency	Short stature	
Abdominal mass	Ovarian mass/tumor	Precocious puberty	
Central adiposity and a chubby face	GH deficiency Prader–Willi syndrome	Short stature (GH)	Developmental delays (Prader–Willi)
Bruising and signs of injury that are not well explained by the mechanism	Abuse or neglect	FTT Short stature	Developmental delays
Café-au-lait spots	Neurofibromatosis	Precocious puberty	
Disproportionate arm:torso ratio	Achondroplasia Marfan syndrome	Short stature Tall stature	
Dystonia, spasticity, or ataxia	Cerebral palsy		Motor delays
Micropenis	Hypopituitarism		
Ambiguous genitalia	CAH	Precocious puberty	

CAH, congenital adrenal hyperplasia; FAS, fetal alcohol syndrome; FTT, failure to thrive; GH, growth hormone; ICP, intracranial pressure.

Diagnostic Plan

The diagnostic plan will vary depending on whether the concern is developmental, pubertal, or growth in nature.

- Developmental concerns
  - Hearing and vision screen
  - Hemoglobin level
  - Lead level
  - Screening evaluation
- Pubertal concerns
  - Luteinizing hormone (LH) and follicle-stimulating hormone (FSH)
  - Serum testosterone
  - Serum estradiol
  - Bone age
  - Pelvic ultrasound (US) for girls
  - Imaging, if brain or abdominal pathology is suspected (endocrine tumors, brain trauma, ovarian or uterine enlargement)
- Growth concerns
  - Bone age to assess skeletal maturity
  - Complete blood count (CBC) with differential to investigate for anemia and neoplasms
  - Thyroid-stimulating hormone (TSH), free T4 (FT4), total T3 to rule out hypothyroidism
  - Serum tissue transglutaminase immunoglobulin A (tTG IgA) to evaluate for celiac disease
  - Serum insulin-like growth factor-1 (IGF1) to determine if there is an underlying growth hormone (GH) deficiency
  - Fecal fat will help assess for malabsorption
  - Urinalysis (UA) to quickly evaluate for signs of chronic kidney disease (CKD), renal tubular acidosis, and/or diabetes

Initial Management

The initial management depends on the underlying etiology.

- If weight concerns are primary, you may require that the family keep a food diary for 3 to 7 days to identify inadequate or excess caloric intake.
- If familial short stature or constitutional growth delay is suspected, you can provide reassurance and continued monitoring.
- If the child appears to be an early or late bloomer, you should discuss therapeutic hormonal injections (to affect the hypothalamic–pituitary gonadal [HPG] axis and subsequently delay or jump start puberty) and counseling options, if the child is significantly impacted by the pubertal timing.
- If a developmental delay is noted, early intervention can help connect the family with the appropriate resource(s), such as a speech–language

pathologist, physical therapist, behavioral therapist, occupational therapist, and so on.

Key Points

- Only a small proportion of children will have a true underlying medical problem that affects growth; therefore, understanding normal growth and developmental patterns is essential in pediatrics.
- Detecting a growth or developmental problem and intervening early has the greatest impact on long-term outcomes.
- Identifying and treating a child with faltering weight or height may prevent developmental delays and vice versa, so it is important to track growth and development at every visit.

REFUSAL TO USE LIMB

Common to pediatrics, a child refusing to use a limb conjures up a litany of differentials with a host of etiologies. A child who refuses to use a limb can mean that there is complete nonuse or the child may use the limb in an abnormal manner secondary to pain or neuromuscular dysfunction. In children, refusal to use a limb is commonly noted after trauma, but it may also be noted more insidiously with no landmark event to herald its onset. Either way, refusal to use is quite bothersome for parents and is one of the top 10 reasons for an urgent care or ED visit.[25]

Differential Diagnosis

Ranging from traumatic or infectious to inflammatory or neoplastic, many of the differentials for children who refuse to use a limb can be narrowed by area of the body involved; however, you should always consider trauma, child abuse, infection, and inflammatory diseases regardless of the site. Table 1.14 provides a brief overview of differential diagnoses to consider by etiology, whereas Table 1.15 narrows the differential diagnosis anatomically.

TABLE **1.14** Common Diagnoses for Refusal to Use by Etiology

Etiology	Common Conditions
Infectious	Osteomyelitis
	Septic arthritis
	Transient synovitis
Rheumatologic	Juvenile idiopathic arthritis
	Reactive arthritis
	Systemic lupus erythematosus
	Ankylosing spondylitis
Traumatic	Dislocation (shoulder, nursemaid's elbow)
	Fracture (FOOSH, Toddler's fracture, stress fracture)

(continued)

TABLE **1.14** Common Diagnoses for Refusal to Use by Etiology (*continued*)

Etiology	Common Conditions
	NAT
	Overuse disorders (Swimmer's shoulder, Little Leaguer's elbow, Osgood–Schlatter, condromalacia patella, stress fractures)
	Sprain or strain
	Torticollis
Bony pathology	DDH
	LCPD
	Malignant and benign bone tumors
	SCFE
Neuromuscular	Cerebral palsy
	Muscular dystrophy
	Myopathy
	Myositis

DDH, developmental dysplasia of the hip; FOOSH, fall onto outstretched hand; LCPD, Legg–Calve–Perthes disease; NAT, nonaccidental trauma; SCFE, slipped capital femoral epiphysis.

TABLE **1.15** Common Diagnoses for Refusal to Use by Anatomic Region

Anatomic Region	Common Diagnoses
Neck	Poor posture
	Trauma such as sprain or strain
	Torticollis
Shoulder	Fracture (long bones or clavicle)
	Overuse disorders (Little Leaguer's shoulder)
	Trauma (sprain, strain or dislocation)
Elbow	Fracture (supracondylar fracture)
	Overuse disorders (Little Leaguer's elbow)
	Trauma (Nursemaid elbow)
Forearm/Wrist/Hand	Cerebral palsy
	Fractures (FOOSH)
	NAT
	Soft tissue injury
Hip	LCPD
	DDH
	SCFE
Knee	Condromalacia patellae
	Osgood–Schlatter
	Sprain/Strain
Lower leg	Cerebral palsy
	Fracture (Toddler's fracture)
	Growing pains
	Muscular dystrophy
	Soft-tissue injury

(*continued*)

TABLE **1.15** Common Diagnoses for Refusal to Use by Anatomic Region
(*continued*)

Anatomic Region	Common Diagnoses
Ankle/Foot	Fractures
	Overuse disorders
	Sprain/Strain
Variable locations	JIA
	Myopathies
	Neoplastic conditions with Neoplasms (malignant and benign bone and soft tissue tumors)
	NAT
	Osteomyelitis
	Reactive arthritis
	Septic arthritis
	SLE
	Transient synovitis

DDH, developmental dysplasia of the hip; FOOSH, fall onto out stretched hand; JIA, juvenile idiopathic arthritis; LCPD, Legg–Calve–Perthes disease; NAT, nonaccidental trauma; SCFE, slipped capital femoral epiphysis; SLE, systemic lupus erythematosus.

History

One of the first questions that you should think about when a pediatric patient presents with refusal to use a limb is whether there is pain associated with the refusal. Although nonpainful causes of refusal to use a limb do occur, they are less frequent and represent mostly a mechanical or neuromuscular etiology.[26]

- Onset, duration, timing: Knowing the onset, duration, and timing of the refusal is useful in understanding possible etiologies. Refusing to use a limb involving acutely painful symptoms points toward traumatic or infectious etiologies, whereas a gradual refusal to use more often indicates an inflammatory or mechanical cause. Duration and timing of pain also provides useful information toward narrowing the differential. Pain that is worse in the morning and improves with activity or throughout the day may point toward an underlying inflammatory condition, whereas constant severe pain that is unchanged by activity may indicate an infectious, oncologic, or traumatic source.

> **CLINICAL PEARL:** Remember that osteomyelitis is often associated with a minor trauma, but typically has a gradual onset over days to weeks.

- Provocation/alleviating factors: A detailed history of any preceding trauma can help you move fractures, soft tissue injuries, and child abuse up or down on your differential diagnosis list. If there is an unwitnessed history of trauma, delay in seeking care, an inconsistent history for the child's development, or the mechanism does not suit the extent of the injury, you should suspect nonaccidental trauma (NAT)/child abuse.

> **CLINICAL PEARL:** Always have a high suspicion for physical abuse for those children with a developmental disability or an emotional/behavioral problem, as well as any children in foster care who present refusing to use a limb.

Asking about what improves or aggravates the symptoms is another useful clue. Identifying the position of comfort (hip that is flexed and externally rotated should bring septic arthritis and transient arthritis higher on the differential, whereas a knee that is swollen and flexed should make you think of JIA), movements that increase pain (flexion at the shoulder with a clavicular fracture), supportive measures that decrease pain (massage may improve growing pains, whereas ice or heat helps with trauma).

> **CLINICAL PEARL:** A hip that is flexed and externally rotated minimizes the stretch on the joint capsule, so consider intra-articular pathologies if a child preferentially positions the hip in this manner.

- Quality: Characterizing the refusal allows you to better understand the acute versus chronic nature and whether there is pain or not. Also, elucidating whether the refusal is complete nonuse or an abnormal use of the limb helps identify possible causes and may direct your initial workup.
- Radiation: Location of the pain is an essential clue in the mystery of a refusal-to-use patient, as locating the source of the pain is helpful in sorting out different infectious causes from traumatic or oncologic causes. Pain noted in the joint may point you toward an inflammatory arthritis, whereas bone pain might suggest osteomyelitis, leukemia, or bone tumors. Ligamentous or muscular pain points toward growing pains, trauma, or myopathies.[27] Because young children may not be able to verbalize or locate their pain, your history, physical exam findings, and observation of the child during the visit are integral to sorting through the differential diagnosis possibilities.
- Symptoms: Associated symptoms may provide some of the largest clues about the nonuse of a limb. Fever may point toward infectious or oncologic diseases, whereas a malar rash may increase your suspicion for systemic lupus erythematosus and a migratory salmon-pink rash should make you think of JIA. Abdominal pain or back pain may indicate an intra-abdominal or vertebral pathology with referred pain.

Other Medical History Specific to Complaint
- Past medical history is important for some autoimmune and inflammatory conditions, as a history of similar "episodes" may help identify a subtle pattern of recurrent joint pain or an infectious insult that may have precipitated a reactive arthritis. Understanding the birth history and risk factors

that could participate in a neuromuscular disorder, like CP, or in DDH are also important to capture in the history of a younger patient. A family history of autoimmune disease may increase the probability of considering these diagnoses on your differential; whereas a parent with a history of SCFE increases the likelihood that the child might also have this diagnosis.

- A thorough social history is quite important in a refusal to use situation, as understanding more about the child's social situation, caretakers, activities, and risk factors can help narrow down the etiology of problem and makes honing in on a diagnosis much easier.
- A thorough review of systems is obligatory for a refusal to use a limb complaint, as so many of these diagnoses are also accompanied by other constitutional and dermatologic findings.

Physical Examination

As is the case with other clinical presentations, making an assessment of the child's overall appearance and determining well versus ill are critical first steps when examining a patient who is refusing to use a limb.

- If the refusal is related to the lower extremity, an assessment of gait should be done before other aspects of the exam, as the type of gait will help to narrow the differential. For example, an antalgic gait is more commonly associated with pain and/or swelling, whereas the steppage and equinus gaits are typically associated with neuromuscular disease.[28]
- Asking the patient to identify the painful area is more accurate in older patients, but may help to lateralize the pain in younger patients.

> **CLINICAL PEARL:** Contrary to popular belief, true hip pathology causes pain in the groin, and gluteal or back pain causes pain at the area lateral to the iliac crest.

- Inspection of the limb or joint suspected of causing the refusal is essential, but so, too, is a thorough evaluation of the joint above and below the suspected area. If the refusal appears to be coming from the hip, you should consider genitourinary, back, and abdominal pathology in your differential, as pain from any of these areas can refer to the groin/hip.

> **CLINICAL PEARL:** In children, knee pain is often referred pain secondary to ankle, lower leg, thigh, hip, or back conditions.[29]

- Inspection for signs of trauma (bruising, deformity) and inflammation (swelling, redness, edema) can help to localize the condition and identify referred versus localized pain.

> **CLINICAL PEARL:** Bruises should be appropriate to the developmental level of the child (e.g., a 2-year-old walker may have shin bruises), so bruising in a nonambulating child without a clear history for the cause should raise suspicion for NAT.

- ○ You should carefully palpate the area of concern for swelling, warmth, pain, crepitus (fracture), laxity (trauma), step-offs (trauma/fracture), and masses (tumors).
- ○ Inspecting muscle bulk and tone can help to identify a neuromuscular disorder by identifying an area of increased tone, hypertrophy, or wasting. In muscular dystrophy, some patients have the appearance of hypertrophy at the calf and wasting at the thigh.
- ○ Localizing pain to the joint space or the bone can differentiate a septic arthritis from an osteomyelitis and a sprain from a fracture.
- Passive and active range of motion (ROM) are essential to determine the extent to which the refusal is the result of pain versus a mechanical cause and can sometimes distinguish similar disease states. For example, if you suspect an osteomyelitis, but need to differentiate it from a septic arthritis, knowing that osteomyelitis will typically allow for passive ROM, but septic arthritis will not, can help you make this differentiation.
  - ○ A modified logroll test can help identify the degree of passive ROM. While the child is lying supine, gently hold the big toe and pretend to examine the foot from different angles, shifting the foot (and subsequently the hip) internally and externally. If you can rotate the hip >30° on internal and external rotation without pain, transient synovitis is more likely than septic arthritis.
- Strength testing is important as well, especially if there is no pain and muscle weakness is suspected. Dystrophic myopathies commonly first present with weakness of the neck flexors and normal strength in the neck extensors. Gowers's sign, the use of hands and arms to walk the body to a standing position, is an indication of proximal muscle weakness, which can be seen in neuromuscular diseases such as Duchenne muscular dystrophy, dermatomyositis, and polymyositis. Distal weakness can be assessed by toe walking, grip strength, and finger adduction/abduction.

Diagnostic Plan

The next steps for diagnosis will depend highly on what is found on the history and physical exam. For most conditions, a baseline CBC with differential and inflammatory markers (e.g., an ESR or C-reactive protein [CRP]) are a good place to start.

- If you suspect infection, you should also order a blood culture, joint aspiration, and possibly a bone scan.

- If your history and physical exam findings point to the diagnostic criteria for a rheumatologic condition, an antinuclear antibody (ANA) profile (including double-stranded DNA, Smith, ribonucleic protein, and Sjogren-specific antibodies) will help diagnose and characterize lupus, whereas antiphospholipid antibodies can help to detect those patients at risk for thrombosis with their lupus.[30] An HLA-B27 antigen can help identify ankylosing spondylitis.[22]
- If you suspect trauma, ordering x-rays or US can identify fluid, swelling, and fractures.
- If you suspect bony pathology, such as a tumor or leukemia, you should start your workup with x-rays (if you suspect a solid tumor), a CBC with peripheral smear and serum chemistries with potassium, calcium, phosphorus. Uric acid and lactate dehydrogenase (LDH) levels will help to identify tumor lysis level.
- If you suspect a neuromuscular disease, a creatinine kinase (CK) would be an initial laboratory test.

Initial Management

- Many refusal-to-use-a-limb scenarios can be managed in the outpatient or urgent care setting; however, infections of the bone, joint, or muscle require hospitalization. These serious infections can affect long-term outcomes, destabilize bone and joint integrity, cause pain, and possibly result in deformity. Involving a pediatric surgeon and an infectious disease specialist is imperative at this point.
  - ○ Septic arthritis: Emergent decompression of the joint capsule via joint aspiration or surgical incision and drainage (I&D) to decompress the joint will try to prevent avascular necrosis and the use of IV antibiotics.
  - ○ Osteomyelitis: Surgical debridement of abscess, if present, and IV antibiotics are warranted.
- Trauma: External support, such as a brace or a splint, is appropriate, with casting for fractures when the initial swelling has decreased.
- Nursemaid's elbow can usually be easily reduced in the office, but shoulder dislocations may require conscious sedation for relocation of the bone in the joint.
- Overuse injuries typically respond well to rest and supportive measures with a slow return to activities, but physical therapy may be indicated for return to pain-free activities.

Key Points

- A patient who is refusing to use a limb in its intended manner, whether that be complete nonuse, partial use, or modified use, is best stratified by age and anatomic location, as the differential becomes much more manageable.
- The most common cause of refusal to use a limb is trauma in all areas except the hip. Here the issues are more deeply seated and involve primarily a vascular insult that allows for hematogenous spread of infection or necrosis

of the femoral head. Anatomic abnormalities are also to blame for refusal to use the hip.

- Although the majority of problems associated with refusal to use a limb can be managed in the outpatient setting with minor management and supportive care, any child who is ill appearing should be evaluated for more serious, life-threatening etiologies such as infectious, inflammatory, neoplastic, and abusive causes.

SKIN CHANGES

Skin changes are one of the biggest concerns for parents and caregivers alike. As the skin is the largest organ in the body, it is no wonder that the differential for changes in the skin run the gamut from mild, benign problems to life-threatening. Understanding these changes and their significance will be a huge boon for your pediatrics rotation.

Medical providers have their own dermatological terminology to describe skin lesions and changes to the skin and this will be valuable when you are asked to write a SOAP note or discuss the patient with other medical providers. This nomenclature can be separated by primary and secondary lesions, which are noted in Tables 1.16 and 1.17.

TABLE 1.16 Primary Lesion Descriptions

Lesion Type	Description
Macule	Flat, well-circumscribed lesion with color, measuring up to 1 cm in diameter
Papule	Circumscribed, elevated, solid lesion, <1 cm in diameter
Patch	Similar to a macule, but large (>1 cm)
Nodule	Elevated, solid lesion with depth up to 2 cm
Tumor	Large circumscribed lesion with depth >2 cm
Plaque	Elevated lesion >2 cm in size
Pustule	Papule that contains purulent exudate, <1 cm
Vesicle	Circumscribed, elevated, fluid filled, <1 cm
Bulla	Fluid-filled lesion >1 cm
Wheal	Rounded or flat-topped edematous plaque that is transient; size varies greatly

Source: Adapted from Paller AS, Mancini, A. *Hurwitz Clinical Pediatric Dermatology: A Textbook of Skin Disorders of Childhood and Adolescence.* 5th ed. Toronto, Ontario, Canada: Elsevier; 2015.

TABLE 1.17 Causes of Secondary Lesions

Lesion Type	Cause
Scale	Results from abnormal keratinization; may be fine or sheet like
Crust	Dried collection of serum and cellular debris

(continued)

TABLE **1.17** Causes of Secondary Lesions (*continued*)

Lesion Type	Cause
Erosion	Caused by loss of the epidermis; moist, shallow lesion
Ulcer	Circumscribed, depressed, focal loss of entire epidermis into dermis
Atrophy	A shallow depression; results from thinning of epidermis or dermis
Scar	Thickened, firm, and discolored collection of connective tissue; the result of dermal damage; initially pink and lightens with time
Sclerosis	Circumscribed or diffuse hardening of skin, usually forms in a plaque
Lichenification	Accentuated skin lines or markings; results from thickening of the epidermis
Excoriation	Superficial erosion, linear, caused by scratching
Fissures	Linear breaks within the skin surface; usually painful

Source: Adapted from Paller AS, Mancini, A. *Hurwitz Clinical Pediatric Dermatology: A Textbook of Skin Disorders of Childhood and Adolescence.* 5th ed. Toronto, Ontario, Canada: Elsevier; 2015.

Differential Diagnosis

When patients present with skin changes, eruptions, or lesions, these can be categorized in a number of ways and, by virtue of the description or category, you will be able to narrow your differential diagnosis list. You should consider using the following categories:

- Eczematous
- Papulosquamous
- Vesiculobullous
- Pustular
- Reactive

The medical diagnoses included in Table 1.18 are nonexhaustive and you should consider purchasing and using a dermatology atlas or use the electronic resources listed at the end of this chapter.

TABLE **1.18** Common Descriptive Categories and Associated Diseases

Lesion Category	Disease
Eczematous	Atopic dermatitis
	Nummular dermatitis
	Seborrheic dermatitis
	Stasis dermatitis
	Dyshidrotic eczema
	Contact dermatitis *
	Lichen simplex chronicus
	Tinea corporis
Papulosquamous	Psoriasis
	Lichen planus
	Pityriasis rosea

(*continued*)

TABLE **1.18** Common Descriptive Categories and Associated Diseases (*continued*)

Lesion Category	Disease
	Tinea versicolor/corporis
	Secondary syphilis
	Discoid lupus erythematous
	Infestation (e.g., lice, scabies)
	Ecchymosis/petechiae
Vesiculobullous	Pemphigus
	Varicella
	Herpes zoster
	Bullous impetigo
	Contact dermatitis *
	Phototoxic drug reaction
	Second-degree burns
Pustular	Acne vulgaris
	Perioral dermatitis
	Folliculitis
	Impetigo
	Hidradenitis suppurativa
	Candidiasis
	Tinea corporis
Reactive	Urticaria
	Erythema nodosum
	Erythema multiforme

*Contact dermatitis and tinea corporis may present with different characteristics and are listed more than once.

History

When a patient presents with a skin complaint, it is important to consider demographic data, morphology of the lesion(s), chronologic course, distribution, associated symptoms, and any treatments utilized. Including a review of previous medical issues, immunization status, and family and social history is also important.[31]

- Onset, duration, timing: The patient or family should be asked when the skin change first appeared, its timing related to other symptoms, and how long it has been present. The timing of the skin changes may be one of the key features to probe when taking a history. Knowing whether the skin changes developed before, during, or after a fever can help in your differential decision-making.
  - For example, a childhood exanthem, roseola, typically appears once the child has defervesced, but the rash of meningococcemia occurs during the febrile period.

- Provocation/alleviating factors: Any inciting factors, such as preceding trauma; travel; or a change in soap, lotion, or detergent may provide key clues to the diagnosis. In addition, understanding what helps to relieve any pain or pruritus associated with the skin changes could help determine the underlying etiology and can be incorporated into your initial management of the condition.
- Quality: Understanding how the lesion or skin change first appeared, what changes it has undergone, and how it may change throughout the day can provide differentiating clues.
  - ○ Tinea corporis (ringworm) may begin as a small erythematous patch that enlarges over time to an annular appearance with fine scale, whereas nummular eczema typically retains its round appearance, but does not develop the ring appearance and scale.
  - ○ Knowing whether a skin change has spread or migrated can help differentiate lesions as well. For example, urticaria notoriously has a migratory pattern, whereas a phytoreaction may remain localized.
  - ○ Differentiating painful from nonpainful and itching from burning can also help narrow the differential diagnosis for skin lesions.
- Radiation: Location of lesions can be diagnostic, as some are classic for a particular disease.
  - ○ Henoch–Schonlein purpura (HSP) is classically noted to cause purpuric lesions on the buttocks.
  - ○ Fifth's disease (a childhood exanthem caused by parvovirus) classically appears as a slapped cheek.
  - ○ The classic head-to-toe presentation of neonatal jaundice can help you determine the severity of the illness, depending on how far down the body the jaundice is noted.
- Symptoms: Many skin changes in pediatrics are related to infectious, inflammatory, and systemic illness, so associated symptoms, such as pain, pruritus, and fevers, are key.

Other Medical History Specific to Complaint

- Past medical history is important for some skin diagnoses, as a history of similar lesions helps to distinguish reactivated infections, such as herpes simplex virus (HSV), from those that create lifelong immunity. Lesions that appear at a similar time of year can point you in a differential direction that is focused on environmental triggers (dyshidrotic eczema).
- Family history of atopy can provide evidence to support an eczema diagnosis, whereas knowing whether there are other contacts in the house or community with similar lesions can point toward an infectious agent.
- A thorough review of systems is obligatory for skin changes, as many of them have a systemic component that can be correlated with other symptoms.
  - ○ A history of joint pain, morning stiffness, and a migratory salmon-pink rash may point you toward juvenile idiopathic arthritis (JIA),

whereas Janeway lesions and splinter hemorrhages associated with fatigue, weight loss, and myalgias should make you suspect subacute infective endocarditis.

Physical Examination

A patient presenting with skin changes, eruptions, or lesions should have a comprehensive exam as an essential component of developing a differential diagnosis.

- The body parts affected must be carefully examined with both a visual and tactile assessment. You should document the appearance, size, shape, color, texture, configuration, and distribution of the lesion.
  - ○ Inspect for color, uniform appearance, and any secondary lesions.
  - ○ Assess temperature by placing the back of the hand on the patient's arms, assess moisture and texture using the fingertips, and assess hydration by examining skin turgor.[32]

> **CLINICAL PEARL:** Gently pinch a small section of skin on the forearm (not on the back of the hand) and release. The skin should move back into place immediately upon release. Decreased turgor will result in "tenting" of the skin.

  - ○ Lesions should be palpated with a gloved hand. There are circumstances when texture of the lesion can be better assessed without gloves but universal precautions should be used in most instances. Oral lesions or lesions within mucous membranes should always be palpated with a gloved hand.
  - ○ Assess condition and hygiene of fingernails for color, shape, and for structural irregularities such as ridging or bands.
- The patient's skin should be completely exposed and examined, including scalp, posterior surfaces, diaper area, palms, and soles, although this should be performed with the patient's modesty in mind.
- Common tools and equipment necessary for a general dermatological exam will include a centimeter ruler (flexible, clear), handheld magnifying lens, good lighting, a Wood's lamp, KOH (potassium hydroxide) for slide preparations, and proper draping.
  - ○ Lesions should be measured and reported in millimeters or centimeters.
  - ○ Describe the lesion characteristics. These may include the following:
    - Size, shape, color, and texture
    - Elevation/depression
    - Grouped or linear
    - Location and distribution
    - Generalized or localized
    - Region of body
    - Diffuse or confluent

- Complete a cardiovascular, pulmonary, and abdominal exam in all cases, paying special attention to possible systemic clues.
- When suspecting a skin change that may have enanthems, such as hand, foot, and mouth disease (HFMD) or measles, a keen view of the oropharynx and buccal mucosa is important.

> **CLINICAL PEARL:** An exanthem is an eruption on the skin occurring as a symptom of a disease or infection, whereas an enanthem is a rash or eruption on mucous membranes usually due to an acute infection. Many infections, such as measles, can cause both exanthems and enanthems.

Diagnostic Plan

Developing the differential diagnosis can usually be completed with only the patient's history and physical exam findings, but some diagnostics may be indicated depending on the differentials you entertain.

- Point-of-care testing may include KOH or saline preparations, using either clippings or scrapings of the patient's skin, hair, or nails. These preparations would be viewed under the microscope in the office.
- Samples sent to the laboratory include bacterial culture swabs, viral culture swabs, fungal culture specimens, and excisional biopsies.
- Occasionally, bloodwork may be indicated for hematologic, autoimmune, or infectious differentials.

> **CLINICAL PEARL:** If you suspect a hypersensitivity reaction, such as urticaria, you can perform a test called "dermatographism." Using moderate pressure with a short fingernail, draw a line along the inside of the patient's forearm. If an erythematous, slightly raised line persists for more than 2 to 3 minutes, this is consistent with dermatographia.

Initial Management

After a differential diagnosis has been generated, treatment may begin immediately or the provider may wait until diagnostic testing results are known.

- Treatment for common childhood viral exanthems may include a watchful-waiting approach along with symptomatic care.
- Prescription medications for dermatological conditions may include topical and/or oral antibiotics, antifungals, antihistamines, and glucocorticoids; oral antivirals; or surgical excision.

CLINICAL PEARL: When patients are diagnosed with atopic dermatitis, it is essential to send them home with written instructions for treatment as there can be multiple topical agents prescribed and the regimen for their use can be complicated.

- Prescriptions for topical steroids should usually be written for small-sized tubes and topical emollients should be written for larger quantities. This helps the parent to remember that steroids should be used sparingly and only as needed for acute flares, whereas emollients may be used liberally two to three times per day.
- Impetigo treatment includes topical antibiotics and the patient should refrain from any close contact with playmates or athletic competitors. Suspension of play should persist until lesions are dry and fully crusted over. Patients diagnosed with other "wet" wounds, such as varicella zoster, herpes zoster, and tinea corporis, should refrain from competition or close play until the lesions are dry or treatment has been in place for a predetermined length of time.
- *Tinea* is a generic term for a type of fungal infection that many people refer to as "ringworm." There is not a worm associated with this infection but there can be a ring-shaped lesion with raised borders and central clearing. The color can vary from salmon pink to brightly erythematous. Treatment will vary depending on the location of the infection and may vary from OTC topical antifungals used daily for 1 to 2 weeks for body lesions to oral medications taken for 2 to 3 months for scalp lesions.
- Diaper rash is usually the result of irritant contact dermatitis. As babies wear occlusive diapers their skin comes into contact with enzymes, urine, and feces, creating by-products that raise the pH, which further breaks down the first skin layers. This provides a prime environment for organisms to grow, most commonly *Candida*. First-line therapy should include a topical barrier ointment and good diaper hygiene (e.g., frequent changing, "air time," gentle cleansing). Topical OTC antifungals should be second-line treatment and should be used three times a day for 3 days after the rash clears. In severe cases, a low-potency topical corticosteroid may be used for 3 to 10 days only in combination with a topical antimicrobial.
- Scabies, lice, and other infestations require strict treatment for complete resolution of symptoms. All family members should be treated; all bedding and clothing washed in hot water and all floors should be vacuumed. Patient and parents should be reassured that the pruritus that is associated with these parasites can persist for 1 to 2 weeks after treatment and this can be helped with oral antihistamines. Parents can be advised to complete a second, and final, treatment 2 weeks after the first course to be sure all nits and eggs are killed.

- Acne vulgaris can often be treated with OTC benzoyl peroxide, the first-line treatment. If symptoms are severe or not responding to OTC products, patients can consider prescription medications such as topical retinoids, topical or oral antibiotics, oral retinoids, or oral corticosteroids.
- Acute onset urticaria is often allergy related and culprits can be determined with a careful history. Clinicians should focus on foods eaten close to the start of the urticaria as well as any possible environmental contacts. Food ingredients should be studied for a common agent present at the time of eruptions and a food diary may be helpful. Drug reactions, insect bites, and viral exanthems can present as similar eruptions and the history should help differentiate the etiologies. Treatment for urticaria can range from oral antihistamines to oral corticosteroids. If symptoms are not improving with these medications, a comprehensive workup is required.[33]

Key Points

- Treatment for common childhood viral exanthems may include a watchful-waiting approach along with symptomatic care.
- Patients diagnosed with "wet" wounds, such as impetigo, varicella zoster, herpes zoster, and tinea pedis, should refrain from competition or close play until the lesions are dry.
- First-line therapy for diaper dermatitis should include a topical barrier ointment and good diaper hygiene.
- Scabies, lice, and other infestations require strict treatment for complete resolution of symptoms and all family members should be treated.

REFERENCES

1. Chinai S, Guth T, Lovell E, Epter M. Taking advantage of the teachable moment: a review of learner-centered clinical teaching models. *West J Emerg Med.* 2018;19(1):28–34. doi:10.5811/westjem.2017.8.35277
2. American Academy of Pediatrics. Top 25 pediatric diagnoses revisited. *AAP Pediat Coding Newsl.* 2013;8(11). https://coding.solutions.aap.org/article.aspx?articleid=1901421.
3. Tsao K, Anderson KT. Evaluation of abdominal pain in children. *BMJ Best Practice.* http://bestpractice.bmj.com/topics/en-us/787. Updated June 2018.
4. Sherman R. Abdominal pain. In: Walker WK, Hall WD, Hurst JW, eds. *Clinical Methods: The History, Physical, and Laboratory Examinations* [online]. 3rd ed. Boston, MA: Butterworths; 1990:444. https://www.ncbi.nlm.nih.gov/books/NBK412/
5. Appendicitis in children. Cleveland Clinic website. https://my.clevelandclinic.org/health/diseases/10792-appendicitis-in-children
6. Benabbas R, Hanna M, Shah J, Sinert R. Diagnostic accuracy of history, physical examination, laboratory tests, and point-of-care ultrasound for pediatric acute appendicitis in the emergency department: a systematic review and meta-analysis. *Acad Emerg Med.* 2017;24(5):523–551. doi:10.1111/acem.13181
7. Reynolds SL, Jaffe DM. Children with abdominal pain: evaluation in the pediatric emergency department. *Pediat Emerg Care.* 1990;6(1):8–12. doi:10.1097/00006565-199003000-00004

8. Kliegman R., ed *Nelson Textbook of Pediatrics.* 20th ed. Philadelphia, PA: W. B. Saunders; 2016:2090.

9. Shields MD, Bush A, Everard ML, et al. BTS guidelines: recommendations for the assessment and management of cough in children. *Thorax.* 2008;63(suppl 3):iii1–iii15. doi:10.1136/thx.2007.077370

10. Chang AB, Oppenheimer JJ, Weinberger MM, et al. Use of management pathways or algorithms in children with chronic cough. *Chest.* 2017;151(4):875–883. doi:10.1016/j.chest.2016.12.025

11. Ralston SL, Lieberthal AS, Meissner HC, et al. Clinical practice guideline: the diagnosis, management, and prevention of bronchiolitis. *Pediatrics.* 2014;134(5):e1474–e1502. doi:10.1542/peds.2014-2742

12. Cherry JD, Tan T, Wirsing von König C-H, et al. Clinical definitions of pertusis: summary of a global pertussis initiative roundtable meeting, February 2011. *Clin Infect Dis.* 2012;54(12):1756–1764. doi:10.1093/cid/cis302

13. Gibson PG, Chang AB, Glasgow NJ, et al. CICADA: cough in children and adults: diagnosis and assessment. Australian cough guidelines summary statement. *Med J Aust.* 2010;192:265–71. https://www.mja.com.au/journal/2010/192/5/cicada-cough-children-and-adults-diagnosis-and-assessment-australian-cough

14. Belman S, Chandramouli V, Schmitt BD, et al. An assessment of pediatric after-hours telephone care: a 1-year experience. *Arch Pediatr Adolesc Med.* 2005;159(2):145–149. doi:10.1001/archpedi.159.2.145

15. McCarthy PL, Lembo RM, Baron MA, et al. Predictive value of abnormal physical examination findings in ill-appearing and well-appearing febrile children. *Pediatrics.* 1985;76(2):167–171. https://pediatrics.aappublications.org/content/76/2/167

16. Consolini DM, Kimmel S. Fevers in infants and children. *Merck Manual Professional Version* [online]. https://www.merckmanuals.com/professional/pediatrics/symptoms-in-infants-and-children/fever-in-infants-and-children

17. Shinnar RC, Shinnar S. Febrile seizures. Child Neurology Foundation website. http://www.childneurologyfoundation.org/disorders/febrile-seizures

18. McCarthy PL, Sharpe MR, Spiesel SZ, et al. Observation scales to identify serious illness in febrile children. *Pediatrics.* 1982;70(25):802–809. https://pediatrics.aappublications.org/content/70/5/802

19. Hay WW Jr, Levin MJ, Deterding RR, Abzug MJ, eds. *Current Diagnosis & Treatment Pediatrics.* 24th ed. New York, NY: McGraw Hill Education; 2018.

20. Crocetti M, Moghbeli N, Serwint J. Fever phobia revisted: have parental misconceptions about fever changed in 20 years? *Pediatrics.* 2001;107(6):1241–1246. doi:10.1542/peds.107.6.1241

21. Sullivan JE, Farrar HC, Section on Clinical Pharmacology and Therapeutics, Committee on Drugs. Fever and antipyretic use in children. *Pediatrics.* 2011;127(3):580–587. doi:10.1542/peds.2010-3852

22. Shah SS, Ronan JC, Alverson B. *Step-up to Pediatrics.* Philadelphia, PA: Wolters Kluwer Health/Lippincott Williams & Wilkins; 2014:162.

23. Resnick MB, Gueorguieva RV, Carter RL, et al. The impact of low birth weight, perinatal conditions, and sociodemographic factors on educational outcome in kindergarten. *Pediatrics.* 1999;104(6):e74. doi:10.1542/peds.104.6.e74

24. Hay WW Jr, Levin MJ, Deterding RR, Abzug MJ, eds. *Current Diagnosis & Treatment Pediatrics.* 24th ed. New York, NY: McGraw-Hill; 2018:785–787.

25. Leonard K. Top reasons children end up in the hospital. *US News and World Report.* https://health.usnews.com/health-news/best-childrens-hospitals/slideshows/top-reasons-children-end-up-in-the-hospital?slide=11. Published June 10, 2014.

26. Naranje S, Kelly DM, Sawyer JR. A systematic approach to the evaluation of a limping child. *Am Fam Physician.* 2015;92(10):908–918. https://www.aafp.org/afp/2015/1115/p908.html

27. Tse SML, Laxer RM. Approach to acute limb pain in childhood. *Pediat Rev.* 2006; 27(5):170–180. doi:10.1542/pir.27-5-170

28. Gait abnormalities. Stanford Medicine website. https://stanfordmedicine25.stanford.edu/the25/gait.html.

29. Hill D, Whiteside J. Limp in children: differentiating benign from dire causes. *J Fam Pract.* 2011;60(4):193–197. https://www.mdedge.com/familymedicine/article/64261/pediatrics/limp-children-differentiating-benign-dire-causes

30. Soep JB. Rheumatic diseases. In: Hay WW Jr Levin MJ, Deterding RR, Abzug MJ, eds. *Current Diagnosis & Treatment Pediatrics.* 24th ed. New York, NY: McGraw-Hill Education; 2018:889–897

31. Kliegman R, ed. Nelson. *Textbook of Pediatrics.* 20th ed. Philadelphia, PA: W. B. Saunders; 2016:3105.

32. Paller AS, Mancini, A. *Hurwitz Clinical Pediatric Dermatology: A Textbook of Skin Disorders of Childhood and Adolescence.* 5th ed. Toronto, Ontario, Canada: Elsevier; 2015.

33. Guldbakke KK, Khachemoune A. Etiology, classification and treatment of urticaria. *Cutis.* 2007;79:41–49. https://www.mdedge.com/dermatology/article/67464/urticaria/etiology-classification-and-treatment-urticaria

ELECTRONIC RESOURCES

Alvarado Score:

https://www.mdcalc.com/alvarado-score-acute-appendicitis

Online Dermatology Atlas:

https://www.dermnetnz.org/glossary

Pediatric Appendicitis Score:

https://www.mdcalc.com/pediatric-appendicitis-score-pas

Pediatric Dermatology Learning Module:

https://www.aad.org/education/basic-derm-curriculum

Urticaria and angioedema:

https://www.dermnetnz.org/topics/urticaria-an-overview/?utm_source =TrendMD&utm_medium=cpc&utm_campaign=DermNet_NZ_TrendMD_0

2

Common Disease Entities in Pediatrics

Introduction

Although many of the diagnoses you will come across in medicine may appear similar whether in young adults, middle-aged, and geriatric patients, pediatrics has unique disease entities that do not manifest in older populations or that manifest differently. This chapter offers a brief introduction to some of the most common pediatric diseases, their etiology, clinical presentation, and how to diagnose and manage them. Organized by body systems, it is important to recognize that some of these diseases may present with various appearances and that the diseases may overlap with several body systems.

CARDIOVASCULAR SYSTEM

Cardiovascular diseases in newborns, infants, and children are undeniably stressful, especially because of the vital nature of the the cardiovascular system. Diagnosing cardiovascular problems promptly and with acumen can have long-standing effects. The most common cardiovascular issues in pediatrics include congenital heart defects, viral infections, murmurs, and hypertension. Syncope is included in the cardiovascular section, but in pediatrics syncope can also be a manifestation of an underlying neurologic, vestibular, or volume disturbance.

CONGENITAL HEART DEFECTS: CYANOTIC AND ACYANOTIC LESIONS

Etiology

As the name implies, congenital heart defects occur during fetal formation and can include abnormal anatomic development of the heart walls, valves, or vessels. Risk factors for a congenital heart defect include genetics, prescription medication or illicit substance use during pregnancy, infections during pregnancy, and gestatational diabetes. These congenital problems are divided into two categories: cyanotic and acyanotic lesions. Classically, cyanotic lesions create hypoxia with oxygenated blood mixing with deoxygenated blood. The five most common cyanotic lesions are listed as the five T's—*t*etralogy of Fallot (ToF), *t*ransposition of the great arteries (TGA), *T*otal anomalous pulmonary venous return (TAPVR), *t*runcus arteriosus, and *t*ricuspid valve abnormalities (tricuspid atresia and stenosis).

- ToF: This congenital heart defect (CHD) involves right ventricular hypertrophy, ventral septal defect (VSD), overriding aorta, and pulmonary stenosis (PS). In this condition, blood flows from the right atrium to the right ventricle, but instead of being pumped out to the lungs (due to the PS), the majority of the blood is shunted through a VSD to the left ventricle. Here it mixes with oxygenated blood and is pumped out the aorta.

> **CLINICAL PEARL:** To remember the components of tetralogy of Fallot (ToF), think PROVe (**P**ulmonary stenosis, **R**ight ventricular hypertrophy, **O**verriding aorta, **V**entricular septal defect).

- TGA: The aorta arises from the right ventricle rather than the left ventricle and pulmonary arteries arise from the left ventricle rather than the right. This creates a parallel circuit with deoxygenated blood returning to the right heart and being pumped out to the body without oxygenation. Often combined with a VSD, there is mixing of the oxygenated blood from the left parallel circuit, but there is still a relative hypoxemia.
- TAPVR: In this condition, pulmonary veins do not drain into the left atrium, but instead follow an anomalous pathway (supracardiac, infracardiac, directly into the right atrium, or a combination of anomalous pathways) to the systemic venous return system. The oxygenated blood eventually drains back to the right heart.
- Truncus arteriosus: Children with this defect have a single arterial trunk that arises at the ventral septum and receives blood from both the right and left ventricles (causing mixing of oxygenated with deoxygenated blood) and supplies the pulmonary and systemic circulation simultaneously with mixed blood.
- Tricuspid valve abnormalities: This defect is caused by a failure to form a tricuspid value or the valve leaflets are fused together. This defect limits the movement of blood from the right atrium to the right ventricle (stenosis) or fails to connect the atrium to the ventricle and requires a VSD to be compatible with life.

> **CLINICAL PEARL:** A great way to remember the five congenital cyanotic heart lesions is one, two, three, four, and five. One trunk (*truncus arteriosus*), two interchanged vessels (*transposition of the great arteries*), three leaflets (*tricuspid valve abnormalities*), four cardiac abnormalities (*tetralogy of Fallot*), and five words (*total anomalous pulmonary venous return*).

Acyanotic heart defects are typically described as left-to-right shunts or outflow obstructions. The most common left-to-right acyanotic shunts are atrial septal defect (ASD), VSD, and patent ductus arteriosus (PDA), whereas PS, aortic stenosis (AS), and coarctation of the aorta (CoA) represent outflow obstructions.

- ASD: This septal defect occurs between the left and right atria, and as blood moves down a pressure gradient it is shunted from the left atrium into the right atrium. This creates right heart overload and can eventually lead to congestive heart failure (CHF).
- VSD: A VSD creates an abnormal communication between the right and left ventricles. A higher pressure in the left ventricle causes blood to shunt to the right ventricle. This increases pulmonary flow and congestion.
- PDA: This is a persistent opening between the pulmonary artery and the aorta. Pressure in the aorta shunts blood to the pulmonary artery and increases pulmonary artery pressure.
- PS: PS is most commonly due to valve stenosis, but can also be caused by supra- or subvalvular obstruction. This limits blood flow to the lungs and creates right ventricular hypertrophy with decreased cardiac output.
- AS: Usually caused by an abnormality of the valve (bicuspid) or vessel stenosis before or after the aortic valve. This limits cardiac output and can lead to left ventricular hypertrophy with or without dysfunction.
- CoA: A narrowing of the aorta creates an obstruction that in time can lead to left ventricular hypertrophy and hypertension. It is most commonly noted as juxtaductal; however, aortic coarctations can occur supraductally and intraductally as well. Severity of the obstruction, age of the child, and the location of the obstruction along the aorta determine the severity of the symptoms and the age of presentation.

It is important to recognize that structural heart and valve defects create an environment in which there may be mixing of oxygenated and deoxygenated blood, which causes a problem with circulation overload. An overload on the pump can eventually lead to a pump failure, which can manifest as poor feeding, diaphoresis with feeding, poor growth, and easy fatigue. Heart failure can also mimic respiratory or gastrointestinal (GI) problems such as colic, pneumonia, or other respiratory infections.

Epidemiology

About 40,000 births per year are affected by CHDs, or 1% of the population, with the most common CHD being a ventricular septal defect.[1] Overall, congenital heart defects tend to be slightly more prevalent in males than females with the exception of ASD.[2] The epidemiology of specific diseases are noted in Table 2.1.

TABLE 2.1. Congenital Heart Defects Epidemiology

CHD		Prevalence	Significant Differences
Cyanotic	Tetralogy of Fallot	1 in every 2,518	Males > Females
	Transposition of the great arteries	1 in every 3,300	Males > Females No racial disparity
	TAPVR	1 in every 10,000	3:1 male: female predominance
	Truncus arteriosus	<1 in every 10,000 (300 per year)	No gender or racial disparity
	Tricuspid atresia	1 in every 10,000	No gender or racial disparity
Acyanotic	ASD	1 in every 770	2:1 female: male predominance
	VSD	1 in every 240	No gender or racial disparity
	PDA	1 in every 2,000 with increased rates among premature infants[1]	No gender or racial disparity
	PS	1 in every 7,700 for pulmonary atresia	Slight female predominance[3]
	AS	<1 in every 1,000	White > Black/Hispanic 4:1 male: female predominance[2]
	CoA	1 in every 2,500	Males > Females

AS, aortic stenosis; ASD, atrial septal defect; CHD, congenital heart disease/defect; CoA, coarctation of the aorta; PDA, patent ductus arteriosus; PS, pulmonary stenosis; TAPVR, total anomalous pulmonary venous return; VSD, ventral septal defect.

Sources: Data taken from Centers for Disease Control and Prevention. Congenital heart defects: data and statistics on congenital heart defects. CDC website. https://www.cdc.gov/ncbddd/heartdefects/data.html; 1. Dice JE, Bhatia J. Patent ductus arteriosus: an overview. *J Pediatr Pharmacol Ther.* 2007;12(3):138–146. doi:10.5863/1551-6776 -12.3.138; 2. Weber HS. Pediatric valvar aortic stenosis. In: Patnana SR, ed. Medscape. https://emedicine. medscape.com/article/894095-overview#a6. Updated July 25, 2018; 3. Ren X. Pulmonic stenosis. In: Lange RA, ed. Medscape. https://emedicine.medscape.com/article/157737-overview#a6. Updated December 22, 2014.

Clinical Presentation

Newborns with a cyanotic heart defect may present with central cyanosis, respiratory distress, feeding difficulties, and signs of CHF (tachycardia, hepatomegaly, edema). Infants with any type of congenital heart defect tend to grow poorly and may present with a heart murmur. Determining the side of the heart on which the murmur is originating can be done by paying attention to the intensity of the murmur during the respiratory cycle. Right-sided heart murmurs get louder on inspiration and left-sided heart murmurs get louder on expiration.[4] The murmurs classically associated with the defect are listed in Table 2.2.

TABLE 2.2. Congenital Heart Defects and Associated Heart Murmurs

CHD		How It May Present	Heart Murmur
Cyanotic	ToF	Central cyanosis Clubbing	Grade 3–4 long systolic ejection murmur heard at ULSB; may have holosystolic murmur at LLSB
	TGA	Cyanosis in first week of life Clubbing Signs of CHF	Murmur may be absent or a grade 3–4 holosystolic murmur at LLSB and mid-diastolic murmur at apex
	TAPVR	Signs of CHF at 1–2 months of life	Grade 2–3 systolic ejection murmur at ULSB with a grade 1–2 mid-diastolic flow rumble at LLSB
	Truncus arteriosus	Signs of CHF with minimal cyanosis	Holosystolic murmur (ventricular septal defect) with a mid-diastolic rumble
	Tricuspid atresia	Cyanosis in first few days/weeks of life Clubbing Signs of CHF before 1 month of life	Holosystolic murmur at LLSB or midsternal border
Acyanotic	ASD	Usually asymptomatic and found incidentally, but could present with signs of CHF	Usually grade 2–3 systolic ejection murmur best heard at ULSB; **wide split fixed S_2**; may have a diastolic flow rumble at LLSB
	VSD	Asymptomatic to signs of CHF	Grade typically depends on size of the defect with small defects having a louder murmur; grade 2–5 holosystolic murmur at LLSB without radiation; may also hear a mid-diastolic rumble
	PDA	Easy fatigue Fatigues with feeding	Grade 1–5 continuous, crescendo–decrescendo murmur in ULSB
	PS	Usually asymptomatic, but may have respiratory symptoms secondary to the pulmonary congestion	Grade 2–5 systolic ejection murmur heard best at ULSB radiating to infraclavicular regions, axillae, and back; may hear ejection click

(continued)

TABLE 2.2. Congenital Heart Defects and Associated Heart Murmurs (*continued*)

CHD		How It May Present	Heart Murmur
	AS	Newborns may present with CHF Usually asymptomatic, but may present with dyspnea, easy fatigue, or syncope	Grade 2–5 systolic ejection murmur heard best at URSB with radiation to carotid arteries; left ventricular heave; thrill at ULSB or suprasternal notch
	CoA	In older children, presents with hypertension and decreased femoral pulses Fatigue Leg claudication	Heart murmur may or may not be present. If heard, it is a systolic ejection murmur heard best over the interscapular region secondary to collateral vasculature.

AS, aortic stenosis; ASD, atrial septal defect; CHD, congenital heart disease/defect; CHF, congestive heart failure; CoA, coarctation of the aorta; LLSB, lower left sternal border; PDA, patent ductus arteriosus; PS, pulmonary stenosis; TAPVR, total anomalous pulmonary venous return; TGA, transposition of the great arteries; ToF, tetralogy of Fallot; ULSB, upper left sternal border; URSB, upper right sternal border; VSD, ventral septal defect.

Sources: Adapted from Frank JE, Jacobe KM. Evaluation and management of heart murmurs in children. *Am Fam Physician*. 2011;84(7):793–800. https://www.aafp.org/afp/2011/1001/p793.html; Biancaniello T. Innocent murmurs. *Circulation*. 2005;111:e20–e22. doi: 10.1161/01.CIR.0000153388.41229.CB

Diagnosis

Congenital heart defects are often found prenatally on ultra sound (US) and are known at the time of delivery; however, if not detected prenatally, but noted in the transition period, further investigation with echocardiogram is typically done. For asymptomatic newborns, pulse oximetry in the first 24 hours of life has become a standard component of the clinical exam, as the use of pulse oximetry in combination with the clinical exam increases sensitivity of detecting a CHD.[3] If heart failure is suspected, a chest x-ray, EKG, and echocardiogram are typically ordered to evaluate for heart enlargement, structure, and function.

Management

Management in the immediate newborn period should include a consultation with a pediatric cardiologist. Depending on the type of defect, treatments may include serial exams, watchful waiting, medications, and/or more invasive cardiac treatments.

ENDOCARDITIS: ACUTE AND SUBACUTE BACTERIAL ENDOCARDITIS

Etiology

Transient bacteremia coupled with turbulent blood flow causes localized infection of the endocardium and valves. The infection can be acute or subacute and is more common in children with congenital heart disease or risk factors for infection, such as an indwelling catheter.

Epidemiology

Any patients found to have bacteremia with *Haemophilus parainfluenzae, Aggregatibacter, Cardiobacterium hominis, Eikenella corrodens,* and *Kingella kingae* should be evaluated for infective endocarditis. However, as most infections are secondary to Gram-positive cocci, it is important not to forget about *Staphylococcus aureus, Streptococcus viridans,* enterococcus, and pneumococcus.

Clinical Presentation

Clinical presentation will vary depending on the acuity of the infective endocarditis. Patients with acute bacterial endocarditis will typically present as ill appearing with high fevers or have a septic clinical picture. Subacute endocarditis can include prolonged low-grade fever with weight loss, fatigue, abdominal pain, and nausea and vomiting. Most patients will have a new-onset heart murmur and can present with some of the classic findings such as Janeway lesions, Roth's spots, Osler's nodes, splinter hemorrhages, petechiae, and/or splenomegaly.

Diagnosis

As Duke criteria are used to determine a definite diagnosis of infective endocarditis, repeat blood cultures, echocardiogram, and rheumatoid factor are needed for diagnosis. Patients must have two of the three major criteria *or* five of the six minor criteria *or* one major criterion with three minor criteria. Point-of-care decision tools, such as MDCalc, can help you determine whether your patient meets the Duke criteria (www.mdcalc.com/duke-criteria-infective-endocarditis).

Management

Empiric therapy with vancomycin until culture and sensitivity return is standard protocol. The patient will require 4 to 6 weeks of intravenous (IV) antibiotics.

Heart Murmur: Innocent Versus Pathologic

Etiology

Heart murmurs are merely sounds heard during the pumping or filling phases of the heart cycle. The majority of heart murmurs in children are innocent and represent turbulent blood flow within the heart or vessels. Fever, anemia, physical activity, and rapid growth can all be associated with innocent murmurs. A pathologic heart murmur in children is almost always related to a congenital heart defect.

Epidemiology

The risk for a structural defect associated with a heart murmur decreases by seven fold with increasing age in the first year of life.[5] Because of a wide range of prevalence, innocent heart murmurs are thought to occur in all children at some point during childhood.

Clinical Presentation

Patients with an innocent heart murmur are usually asymptomatic and the murmur is noted incidentally on auscultation. Differentiating an innocent from pathologic murmur is important and you can use the five S's to delineate an innocent murmur from one that would require referral. Innocent murmurs are typically heard only in *s*ystole, are *s*hort in duration, are *s*oft, *s*ound musical and change when the child is *s*upine.

Diagnosis

Heart murmurs are typically first detected on auscultation, with definitive diagnosis of the structural or turbulent causes of murmur diagnosed with echocardiogram. Often, further evaluation is not necessary when the murmur is described as innocent, as listed in Table 2.3.

TABLE 2.3. Innocent Heart Murmur Characteristics

Murmur	Sound	Heard Best	Most Common Age Range	Often Confused With/ Differentiated by
Still's murmur	Low pitched Musical/ squeaky	With bell at the LLSB	2–7 years old	VSD, but VSD is typically holosystolic and does not change with Valsalva maneuver
Pulmonary flow murmur	High pitched	With diaphragm at ULSB; may radiate to back and axilla	Adolescents and children with pectus excavatum	ASD, but ASD is associated with a wide, fixed, split S_2 rather than a normal second heart sound
Systemic flow murmurs	High pitched Harsh	With diaphragm in carotid arteries		PS, but PS has an ejection click and pulmonary and systemic flow murmurs do not
Venous hum	Low pitched Continuous, but louder in diastole and on the right	Bell in the neck area	3–8 years old	PDA, but a PDA does not change with changes in posture/neck position

(continued)

Tᴀʙʟᴇ **2.3.** Innocent Heart Murmur Characteristics (*continued*)

Murmur	Sound	Heard Best	Most Common Age Range	Often Confused With/ Differentiated by
Physiologic peripheral pulmonary stenosis	Low pitched Soft and blowing systolic ejection murmur, but can be continuous	With bell at left infraclavicular area with radiation to bilateral axilla and back	Birth to 6 months	PS, but PS is a louder, harsher murmur, associated with ejection click or thrill VSD, but VSD does not radiate to axilla PDA, but PDA is machine-like and lower pitched Pathologic PPS, but pathologic murmur is seen in older children and is longer in duration and higher in pitch

ASD, atrial septal defect; LLSB, lower left sternal border; PDA, patent ductus arteriosus; PPS, peripheral pulmonic stenosis; PS, pulmonary stenosis; ULSB, upper left sternal border; VSD, ventral septal defect.
Source: Adapted from information from Biancaniello T. Innocent murmurs. *Circulation*. 2005;111:e20–e22. doi:10.1161/01.CIR.0000153388.41229.CB

> **Cʟɪɴɪᴄᴀʟ Pᴇᴀʀʟ:** Red-flag characteristics that should make you consider congenital heart defects include a holosystolic murmur; a decrease in intensity when moving from standing to squatting; systolic click, grade 3 or higher; maximal intensity at the upper left sternal border (ULSB), an abnormal S_2, and/or a harsh quality.[3]

Management

Innocent heart murmurs can be managed with parental education and reassurance, once a structurally normal heart is confirmed. Pathologic heart murmurs will require a pediatric cardiology referral and interventions as determined by the cardiology evaluation.

Hʏᴘᴇʀᴛᴇɴsɪᴏɴ

Etiology

Causes of hypertension vary depending on the age of the patient, with younger children more likely to have an underlying renal, cardiovascular, or endocrine disorder, whereas older patients with obesity and/or a strong family history of hypertension are more apt to have essential hypertension.[6]

Epidemiology

The prevalence of elevated blood pressure (BP) and hypertension has been increasing since 1988 and is noted to be more common in males, Hispanics, African Americans, adolescents, and patients with chronic diseases such as obesity, sleep-disordered breathing, and chronic kidney disease.[6] Elevated BP in childhood is associated with higher rates of hypertension in adulthood.

Clinical Presentation

Patients with hypertension are typically asymptomatic and are noted to have a BP >95th percentile for age, gender, and height on three or more separate occasions. Although patients may not identify specific symptoms of their hypertension, physical exam can provide some clues to possible secondary causes of hypertension. Table 2.4 provides a brief synopsis of the physical exam findings with etiologies to consider.

TABLE 2.4. History and Physical Exam Findings and Possible Etiologies for Hypertension in Children

History or Physical Exam Finding	Possible Etiology
History of snoring	Sleep-disordered breathing
Use of pharmacologic agents	Herbal and over-the-counter agents (cough and cold medications, antihistamines)
	Prescription medications (oral contraceptives, ADHD treatments, corticosteroids)
	Illicit drugs
Family history of early- onset hypertension	Renal
Decreased LE pulses or a decreased BP in LE compared to UE	CoA
Proptosis	Hyperthyroidism
Adenotonsillar hypertrophy	Sleep-disordered breathing
Obesity	Cushing syndrome
	Insulin resistance
Goiter	Hyperthyroidism
Acne, hirsutism, striae	Cushing syndrome
Acanthosis nigricans	Insulin resistance and type 2 diabetes
Palpable kidneys	Polycystic kidney disease
Joint swelling	Rheumatologic disorders such as SLE

BP, blood pressure; CoA, coarctation of the aorta; LE, lower extremity; SLE, systemic lupus erythematosus; UE, upper extremity.

Source: Adapted from Flynn JT, Kaelber DC, Baker-Smith CM, et al. Clinical practice guideline for screening and management of high blood pressure in children and adolescents. *Pediatrics.* 2017;140(3):e20171904. doi:10.1542/peds.2017-1904

CLINICAL PEARL: Suspect coarctation of the aorta (CoA) in an older child or teen with hypertension, progressive fatigue, and lower leg cramps.

Diagnosis

Initial screening for hypertension should occur annually after the age of 3 years and an initial screening can be done as part of the routine healthcare needs of children. Table 2.5 provides the guidelines from the 2017 updated American Academy of Pediatrics (AAP) guidelines.[6]

TABLE 2.5. AAP Guidelines for Blood Pressure Screening in Pediatric Patients

Boys			Girls		
Age in Years	Systolic BP	Diastolic BP	Age in Years	Systolic BP	Diastolic BP
1	98	52	1	98	54
2	100	55	2	101	58
3	101	58	3	102	60
4	102	60	4	103	62
5	103	63	5	104	64
6	105	66	6	105	67
7	106	68	7	106	68
8	107	69	8	107	69
9	107	70	9	108	71
10	108	72	10	109	72
11	110	74	11	111	74
12	113	75	12	114	75
≥13	120	80	≥13	120	80

AAP, American Academy of Pediatrics; BP, blood pressure.
Source: Adapted from Flynn JT, Kaelber DC, Baker-Smith CM, et al. Clinical practice guideline for screening and management of high blood pressure in children and adolescents. *Pediatrics.* 2017;140(3):e20171904. doi:10.1542/peds.2017-1904

Children and adolescents with BP measurements, in either systolic or diastolic, above those listed in the table should be further evaluated with a repeat BP measurement that is then compared to the values for age, gender, and height in the standardized pediatric BP tables.

Management

With the introduction of new AAP guidelines, management of hypertension in primary care pediatrics has become a focus for routine well-visit care, as well as follow-up care. Figure 2.1 shows an algorithm of blood pressure management in pediatric patients.

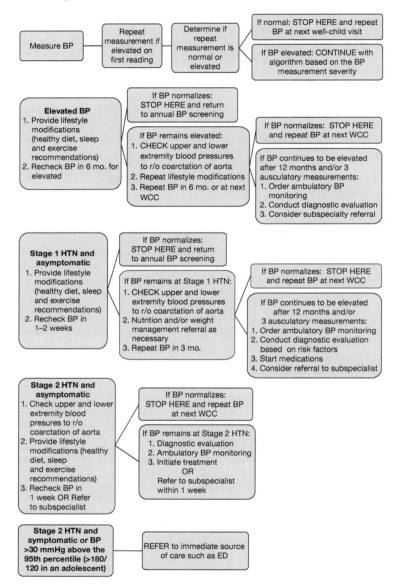

FIGURE 2.1. Algorithm for blood pressure management in pediatric patients.

BP, blood pressure; HTN, hypertension; r/o, rule out; WCC, well-child check.

Source: Adapted from Flynn JT, Kaelber DC, Baker-Smith CM, et al. Clinical practice guideline for screening and management of high blood pressure in children and adolescents. *Pediatric*s. 2017;140(3):e20171904. doi:10.1542/peds.2017-1904

SYNCOPE

Etiology

When cardiogenic in origin, the abrupt, yet transient, loss of consciousness is typically related to structural, functional, or electrical diseases of the heart or main vessels. A problem with the pump causes a compromise in cerebral blood flow, which then results in the transient loss of consciousness.

In contrast, neurally mediated syncope (often referred to as "vasovagal syncope") is caused by a change in the sympathetic tone, which in turn affects vascular tone or heart rate. This causes BP and heart rate to drop, affecting oxygen delivery to the brain, and the presyncopal or syncopal events.[5]

Epidemiology

Beginning in the toddler years with "breath-holding spells," the incidence of syncope increases throughout childhood and peaks in adolescents, with girls affected more often than boys. Although the majority of syncopal episodes are by definition transient and do not represent serious cardiovascular disease, it is important to recognize that syncope in a patient with known cardiac disease or with exertion is at increased risk for sudden, premature death.

Clinical Presentation

Because syncope can result from various physiologic mechanisms, the presentation and recovery of each mechanism can help distinguish between underlying etiologies and will help direct your evaluation.

- Breath-holding spells: Normally occurring in patients between 6 months and 3 years of age, breath-holding spells with syncope are usually precipitated by an emotional or physical trigger that causes the child to cry with poor oxygen exchange. Marked by cyanosis and a visible episode of breath-holding, young children typically stop crying, become pale, and have opisthotonia. The symptoms generally resolve over about a minute and children appear tired and sleepy afterward. Breath-holding spells as a toddler are associated with adolescent syncopal events in about one in five children.[5]
- Cardiogenic syncope: Nearly 5% of patients referred to a pediatric cardiologist will have a primary concern of syncope.[5] Most of these patients will present with a recent history of sudden, unanticipated collapse and loss of consciousness with no warning signs. The loss of consciousness occurs for only a few seconds and recovery is equally as rapid with few to no residual symptoms.
- Neurally mediated syncope: Patients with vasovagal syncope typically present with a history of standing for a prolonged period of time; being overheated; feeling dizzy, nauseated, and having darkening or loss of the peripheral visual fields. Bystanders will describe the patient as appearing pale and then collapsing. Recovery is prolonged compared to cardiogenic syncope and is typically associated with dizziness, fatigue, and headache.

> **CLINICAL PEARL:** Prodromal symptoms are most commonly associated with benign syncope.

Diagnosis

Diagnosis is typically made via a detailed history and physical exam; however, as your role is to mitigate risk for serious adverse outcomes, an EKG is routinely recommended. Female patients should also be evaluated with a pregnancy test. "Unless supported by the history and exam, other tests are expensive, invasive, and may cause false positives that can lead to further unnecessary testing and caregiver anxiety".[7] The use of orthostatic BP measurements has not been proven to be effective in determining the type of syncope,[8] but if you are considering postural orthostatic tachycardia syndrome (POTS), "use of supine and 3-minute standing HR [heart rate] measurements (without obtaining blood pressure) is reasonable with a cutoff of a 40 bpm increase and a standing HR of >115 to 120 at 3 minutes distinguishing a normal versus exaggerated response to orthostatic pulse in an office setting". [8]

Management

Management of syncope depends on the underlying cause. If symptoms are thought to be cardiogenic, a patient should be referred to a pediatric cardiologist for further evaluation, which may include a tilt-table test, echocardiogram, Holter monitor, and so on. Patients with vasovagal syncope can usually be managed with reassurance, by encouraging hydration, and a slight increase in dietary salt and slow transition in position changes. Reassurance can be given to parents with children who have breath-holding spells, as these typically resolve by the age of 5 years old.

ELECTRONIC RESOURCES

Pediatric Heart Murmurs

http://www.murmurlab.com/card6/website/index.cfm?fuseaction=create MainMenuFrames

Blood Pressure Tables

https://www.nhlbi.nih.gov/files/docs/guidelines/child_tbl.pdf

DERMATOLOGIC SYSTEM

The pediatric medical team will assess skin conditions on a daily basis. One of the most common complaints is dermatitis, but acne vulgaris, eczema, viral exanthems, and diaper rash are also very common. Many rashes and lesions can be difficult to differentiate and so it is wise to first determine how to appropriately describe a lesion. Learning the correct medical terminology for dermatological conditions is vital to be able to document and discuss the patient's condition. Are there blisters? Is it itchy? Has the rash developed slowly over the past few weeks or did it erupt spontaneously over night? After a management plan has been developed by the medical team, consider the information you want to give the patient and family. Many dermatological conditions can be quite stressful for the patient and his or her family due to the appearance of a lesion or the associated dermatological symptoms, such as itch or discomfort.

ACANTHOSIS NIGRICANS

Etiology

The skin lesions of acanthosis nigricans (AN) may be genetic due to mutations in the fibroblast growth factor receptor gene or acquired as a manifestation of insulin resistance. Insulin resistance with compensatory hyperinsulinism may lead to insulin binding to and activating insulin-like growth factor (IGF) receptors, which ultimately promotes epidermal growth. Common causes of insulin resistance in children are obesity and diabetes mellitus, with AN seen in more than 60% of children with a body mass index (BMI) >98%.[9]

Epidemiology

AN is found more commonly in African American, Hispanic, and Native American children. The clinical severity and histopathologic features of AN correlate positively with the degree of hyperinsulinism and with the degree of obesity.

Clinical Presentation

AN is characterized by symmetric, hyperpigmented, velvety, hyperkeratotic plaques usually located in intertriginous areas. The most common locations are the posterior neck and axillae, but it is also seen in the inframammary areas, groin, inner thighs, and anogenital region. Prior to plaque development, parents notice a "dirty" appearance of affected skin that does not wash clean.

Diagnosis

AN is easily diagnosed on exam and rarely will biopsies or further testing be necessary. Blood tests should be considered to rule out diabetes mellitus or insulin resistance.

Management

Treatment is aimed at resolution of the underlying disorder. AN in the obese child is associated with risk factors for diabetes, and counseling families on its causes and consequences may motivate them to make healthy lifestyle changes that can decrease the risk for development of cardiac and diabetic complications. In children with obesity-related AN, weight loss should be the primary goal.

ACNE

Etiology

The primary pathophysiologic alterations in acne during the preteen and teen years are abnormal keratinization of the follicular epithelium, resulting in impaction of keratinized cells within the follicular lumen, increased production of sebum by the sebaceous gland, proliferation of *Propionibacterium acnes* within the follicle, and inflammation.[10] Acne vulgaris, particularly of the central face, is frequently the first sign of pubertal maturation. At puberty, the sebaceous gland enlarges and sebum production increases in response to the increased activities of androgens of primarily adrenal origin. The cause or causes of neonatal and infantile acne are not fully understood.

The prevailing theory for neonatal acne is it may be an inflammatory response to Pityrosporum species rather than true acne. Other theories include a placental transfer of maternal androgens or a hypersensitivity response to androgenic hormones. A child with refractory infantile acne warrants a search for an abnormal source of androgens, such as a virilizing tumor or congenital adrenal hyperplasia.[10]

Epidemiology

Acne vulgaris occurs in approximately 80% of adolescents. It affects males and females equally although female adolescents report a flare in their acne the week before menstruation. Neonatal acne affects 20% of neonates in the first month of life, whereas infantile acne begins between 3 months to 2 years of age and affects boys more than girls. Infantile acne usually resolves before 4 years of age. Acne in all age groups effects all ethnicities equally.

Clinical Presentation

Adolescents present with myriad symptoms, including occasional, scattered microcomedones to inflammatory nodular-cystic, scarring acne. The pathogenesis of acne is obstruction of the sebaceous follicles, but the underlying etiology of inflammatory acne is less well known.

Diagnosis

The diagnosis of acne vulgaris, neonatal acne, and infantile acne can be made clinically. If there are any signs of virilization, such as hirsutism, further workup should be initiated.

Management

The mainstay of acne management includes topical keratolytic agents such as retinoic acid cream or benzoyl peroxide gel. These topical agents are used for mild to moderate symptoms. Oral medications are considered when topical medications are not adequate and these include oral antibiotics and oral retinoids. Female patients who consider taking oral retinoids, such as isotretinoin, should have an initial pregnancy test, ongoing monthly pregnancy tests, and contraceptive counseling as these medications can result in teratogenic malformations in a fetus.

Atopic Dermatitis/Eczema

Etiology

"Atopic dermatitis" (AD) and "eczema" are terms that are used interchangeably. AD is a hereditary disorder often denoted by a triad of symptoms: asthma, allergic rhinitis, and AD. Rarely do patients suffer from all three, but up to 50% of patients with AD have either allergic rhinitis or asthma.

Epidemiology

AD usually begins by 4 months of age and the usual distribution of signs and symptoms is on the cheeks, face, trunk, and extensor surfaces of upper and lower extremities. Most patients who have symptoms in infancy or childhood will no longer have symptoms in adolescence or adulthood.

Clinical Presentation

Patients may present with a variety of symptoms in various stages of development. Patients may have very dry skin to cracked, severely erythematous macules with lichenification from prolonged scratching or fissures and breaks in the skin with secondary bacterial infection. In some cases, patients can present with a vesicular weepy rash. In infantile eczema, eruptions occur mainly on the cheeks, face, trunk, and extensor surfaces, whereas the childhood stage evolves to lesions on the feet and flexural areas such as antecubital fossa, popliteal fossa, and neck. Examples of common eczema presentations are seen in Figures 2.2 through 2.4.

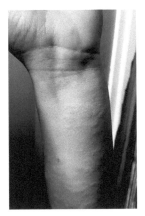

Figure 2.2. Eczema on palmar surface of the forearm with mild plaque-like lesions with erythema.
Photo courtesy of Tanya Fernandez, PA-C.

Diagnosis

Diagnosis is often made through clinical judgment, but clinicians may also add allergy testing as immunoglobulin E (IgE) levels may be elevated. Allergy

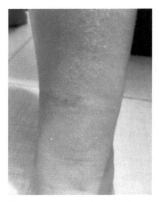

Figure 2.3.   Excoriated eczematous lesion on the posterior lower leg.
Photo courtesy of Tanya Fernandez, PA-C.

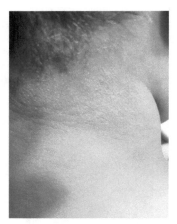

Figure 2.4.   Mild scaling on the posterior neck in a child with atopy.
Photo courtesy of Tanya Fernandez, PA-C.

testing is usually included in a workup to guide the patient and family to avoid certain foods, animals, or products or be prepared for flares during different seasons of the year.

Management

There are short-term and long-term management options for patients with AD. For acute flares of symptoms, use of mild- to moderate-potency topical steroid creams or ointments as well as wet dressings may reduce inflammation. These measures are used for 1 to 2 weeks along with frequent use of emollients and soap substitute (e.g., Cetaphil). Once these patches improve, the patient or family will reduce or stop the use of the topical steroids and continue frequent emollient application, soap substitutes, wear loose-fitting cotton clothing, and avoid overheating. Patients may also find that taking a daily oral antihistamine reduces itching.

If patients are found to be allergic to environmental allergens, immunotherapy may be prescribed to desensitize the patient to the allergen. Immunotherapy may be administered through weekly to monthly injections or daily sublingual drops.

BACTERIAL AND SPIROCHETAL INFECTIONS

Etiology

Bacterial and spirochetal infections infect the host and begin replication. The replication and shedding of the organism can precipitate the signs and symptoms seen.

Epidemiology

The epidemiology of bacterial and spirochetal infections are discussed in Table 2.6.

Clinical Presentation

Of the numerous bacterial and spirochetal infections, each has its own "classic" presentation, which can be found in Table 2.6.

TABLE 2.6. Bacterial and Spirochetal Infections of the Skin

Clinical Presentation	Epidemiology	Classic Signs and Symptoms
Cellulitis	All ages	Cellulitis can occur anywhere and appears as warm, tender, erythematous plaques with ill-defined borders. Associated findings may include fever, regional lymphadenopathy, and/or possible preceding abrasions, punctures, or cuts.
Ecthyma	All ages	Lesions are usually firm, dry, dark crusts with surrounding erythema and induration. With direct pressure on the crusts, purulent material can be expressed from beneath the crust.
Impetigo	All ages	Erosive, honey-colored lesions can occur anywhere but classically appear around the mouth or nose. Lesions begin as small vesicles with a fragile roof that can quickly be lost to expose a moist crust.
Scarlet fever	All ages	Associated with streptococcal pharyngitis, the scarlet fever exanthem appears 24–48 hours after the start of the infection. Erythematous macules and papules appear on the neck or upper chest and spread downward over the thorax and across the extremities.

(*continued*)

TABLE 2.6. Bacterial and Spirochetal Infections of the Skin (*continued*)

Clinical Presentation	Epidemiology	Classic Signs and Symptoms
Lyme disease	All ages; geographic and seasonal variation	A unique skin eruption called *erythema chronicum migrans* may occur with Lyme disease that begins 4–20 days after a tick bite. A red papule emerges over the tick bite and then slowly enlarges to form an annular ring with an erythematous macular plaque. A secondary annular ring may form creating a "target" lesion. Associated symptoms may include fever, joint pain, myalgias, headache, and fatigue.
RMSF	All ages; geographic and seasonal variation	The skin eruptions associated with RMSF can be non-specific, but the classical appearance is a blanching erythematous macular plaque that becomes petechial over 3–5 days. The lesions characteristically appear on the ankles and wrist and spread to the thorax and in later stages appear on palms and soles. Associated symptoms include fever, headache, myalgias, arthralgias, and malaise.

RMSF, Rocky Mountain spotted fever.
Source: Adapted from information from Weston W, Lane A. *Color Textbook of Pediatric Dermatology.* 3rd ed. St. Louis, MO: Mosby; 2002:89–118.

Diagnosis

Most skin changes are diagnosed by history and physical exam. Table 2.7 lists the most common causative organisms, diagnosis, and treatment.

Management

Bacterial and spirochetal skin diseases are treated with antibiotics, but the route of administration depends on whether the infection is localized, systemic, and/or severe. For ecthyma and impetigo, oral antibiotics are recommended if the infection is extensive or proves slow to respond to topical antibiotics. Table 2.7 lists the usual route of treatment.

TABLE 2.7. Common Clinical Skin Presentations, Causative Organism, Diagnosis, and Treatment

Clinical Presentation	Common Causative Organisms	How Is It Diagnosed?	How Is It Treated?
Cellulitis	Pathogenic *Streptococcus*, *Haemophilus influenzae*, and *Staphylococcal aureus*	Clinical	Oral antibiotics
Ecthyma	*S. aureus* or pathogenic *Streptococcus*	Clinical	Topical/oral antibiotics

(*continued*)

TABLE **2.7.** Common Clinical Skin Presentations, Causative Organism, Diagnosis, and Treatment (*continued*)

Clinical Presentation	Common Causative Organisms	How Is It Diagnosed?	How Is It Treated?
Impetigo	*S.aureus* or pathogenic *Streptococcus*	Clinical	Topical/oral antibiotics
Scarlet fever	Group A *Streptococcus*	Clinical	Oral antibiotics
Lyme disease	*Borrelia burgdorferi*	Clinical/serology	Oral antibiotics
Rocky Mountain spotted fever	*Rickettsia rickettsia*	Clinical/serology	Oral antibiotics

Source: Adapted from Weston W, Lane A. *Color Textbook of Pediatric Dermatology.* 3rd ed. St. Louis, MO: Mosby; 2002:89–118.

CONTACT DERMATITIS

Etiology

Contact dermatitis results from substances coming into direct contact with the skin and is divided into two subtypes: primary irritant contact dermatitis and allergic contact dermatitis. Table 2.8 outlines the etiology, epidemiology, clinical presentation, diagnosis, and management of the contact dermatitis lesions.

TABLE **2.8.** Epidemiology, Etiology, Clinical Presentation, and Diagnosis and Management of Contact Dermatoses

Contact Dermatitis	Epidemiology/ Etiology	Clinical Presentation	Diagnosis/Management
Primary Irritant Contact Dermatitis			
Diaper dermatitis	Occurs in ~7% of all infants <2 years. Symptoms begin when there is prolonged contact of urine and feces with perineal skin.	Symptoms vary from mild erythematous, chafing skin in the diaper area to ulcerative lesions, and beefy, red spreading lesions with concomitant *Candida albicans* infection.	Dx: Use clinical judgment. Management can vary from removing the wet diaper from the skin and keeping the skin dry to application of topical hydrocortisone 1% and nystatin cream. Parent education is vital as this condition may recur until the child achieves toilet training.
Dry skin dermatitis	Environmental humidity <30% is the most significant factor along with frequent use of soap.	Chief complaint is dry, itchy skin with or without scale, papules, or erythema.	Dx: Use clinical judgment. Improving moisture balance in the skin is preeminent therapy. Liberal use of emollients 3–4 times daily. May consider use of humidifier and reduced use of soap.

(*continued*)

TABLE 2.8. Epidemiology, Etiology, Clinical Presentation, and Diagnosis and Management of Contact Dermatoses (*continued*)

Contact Dermatitis	Epidemiology/ Etiology	Clinical Presentation	Diagnosis/Management
Allergic Dermatitis			
Allergic contact dermatitis	Occurs in 5%–10% of all dermatitis. Symptoms are usually limited to area of contact with the external substance. Common agents are poison ivy, nickel (jewelry/clothing), cosmetics, and topical neomycin.	Acute erythema of affected skin is often accompanied by vesicles and oozing. Location of eruption may help with diagnosis.	Dx: Use clinical judgment. Removal of the offending agent is paramount and then topical steroid creams or ointments of mild to moderate potency will reduce inflammation within 1–3 weeks. Topical steroids should be used for the shortest possible time. For larger surface areas, consider oral glucocorticoid use for 7–14 days and taper doses greater than 10 days.

Dx, diagnosis.
Source: Adapted from Weston W, Lane A. *Color Textbook of Pediatric Dermatology.* 3rd ed. St. Louis, MO: Mosby; 2002:89–118.

HIVES/URTICARIA

Etiology

Urticaria is a spectrum of disease characterized by vascular insult and complex interaction among chemical mediators such as histamine, complement, and IgE-mediated allergens. Transient urticaria (96% of cases) is caused by bites and stings, oral medications, foods, infection, heat, cold, exercise, and inflammatory systemic disease.

Epidemiology

It is suspected that 3% of preschoolers and 5% to 10% of school-aged children have had some type of urticaria or angioedema. The face, hands, and feet are involved in 85% of cases.

Clinical Presentation

Patients may present with a sudden onset of pruritic, erythematous raised wheals anywhere on the body. Some lesions may have erythematous borders with pale centers. Angioedema, or subcutaneous swelling, may occur and can cause a severe appearance when affecting the lips or skin around the eyes. Symptoms of angioedema can be life-threatening if they cause oral, tongue, or pharyngeal swelling.

Diagnosis

Diagnosis may be obtained through clinical judgment but discovering the causative agent may be a challenge. Dermatographism is usually present in the physical urticarias and can be diagnostic for that type of urticaria. Serology and immune function workup may be considered for recurrent or persistent symptoms.

Management
Oral, over-the-counter antihistamines may be helpful in symptomatic control of mild forms of urticaria, whereas others may require hydroxyzine or oral glucocorticoids. Avoidance of triggers may be the best therapy for some patients.

IDIOPATHIC THROMBOCYTOPENIA PURPURA

Etiology
Immune-mediated thrombocytopenia purpura (ITP) commonly follows a viral illness or vaccinations. Both are thought to stimulate the immune system, which subsequently develops antibodies against platelet glycoproteins. These antibodies bind to the platelets and trigger macrophages to clear circulating platelets. This eventually results in thrombocytopenia.

Epidemiology
ITP occurs more frequently in females and is predominantly seen in children younger than 10 years old. There is commonly an associated antecedent illness. Breastfeeding infants are at slightly increased risk for ITP-associated platelet counts below $20,000/mm^3$, as breast milk is low in vitamin K.

Clinical Presentation
Patients typically present as afebrile and well appearing with a history of sudden onset of a petechial rash, bruising, bleeding gums, or nosebleeds. The exam is virtually normal with the exception of the hemorrhagic symptoms.

Diagnosis
As ITP is a diagnosis of exclusion, it is essential that you rule out the other items on your differential, such as acute lymphoblastic leukemia, infection, platelet function disorders, and marrow production defects. A well-appearing child with only a petechial rash and history of preceeding viral illness is usually sufficient to make the diagnosis; however, to confirm your diagnosis a complete blood count (CBC) will typically show an isolated thrombocytopenia without anemia. The peripheral smear should have normal to slightly enlarged platelets and no blasts should be seen. The patient's prothrombin time (PT) and activated partial thromboplastin time (aPTT) are normal.

Management
Management of ITP is based on severity of the disease, which is graded from I to IV; risk factors for bleeding complications; and active versus inactive bleeding. Management of ITP based on these criteria are outlined in Table 2.9.

All patients should be educated on activity restriction, avoidance of antiplatelet and anticoagulant medications, regular monitoring of platelet count, and monitoring for clinical bleeding.[11]

TABLE 2.9. Severity Grading of Immune-Mediated Thrombocytopenia Purpura Symptoms and Management Options

Bleeding Severity Based on Clinical Symptoms	Grade	Risk of Bleeding Complications	Management
Minor: Few petechiae (≤100) and/or ≤5 bruises <3 cm in diameter	I	Low risk	Watchful waiting
Mild: >100 petechiae and/or bruises >3 cm in diameter	II	Low risk	Watchful waiting
Moderate: Brief epistaxis, intermittent gum bleeding, menorrhagia	III	Medium-risk Platelet count <30,000/mm^3 plus one or more of the following risk factors: Use of antiplatelet or anticoagulants Concomitant bleeding disorder Very active lifestyle subjecting the patient to frequent trauma Follow-up, parental supervision or access to medical care are limited	Oral glucocorticoids Alternatives may include IVIG, anti-D immunoglobulin or IV steroids
Severe: Mucosal bleeding or internal hemorrhage that requires immediate medical attention	IV	High risk	IV methylprednisolone AND Anti-D immunoglobulin ± IVIG
Life-threatening: Documented intracranial hemorrhage or life-threatening hemorrhage	IV	High risk	Platelet transfusion AND IV methylprednisolone AND anti-D immunoglobulin ± IVIG

IV, intravenous; IVIG, intravenous immunoglobulin.

Source: Adapted from Provan D, Stasi R, Newland AC, et al. International consensus report on the investigation and management of primary immune thrombocytopenia. *Blood.* 2010;115:168–186. doi:10.1182/blood-2009-06-225565

LICE

Etiology

A louse infestation can progress rapidly over the course of a single week, as the louse, *Pediculus humanus capitis,* lays nits that hatch within 1 week and develop into adults over the next week. While the louse only lives about 2 weeks and can only live for a few hours off the human scalp (as it needs to eat every 4–6 hours), lice are transmitted by sharing hats, caps, brushes, and combs. The louse grasps the hair near the scalp and lays eggs as it moves along the hair shaft.

Epidemiology

Most common in 3- to 11-year-olds, but can occur at any age. Girls are more affected than boys and lice infestations tend to occur more commonly in the spring and summer months. White children are more affected than Black children, secondary to the louse's claws gripping cylindrical hair better than non-cylindrical hair.

Clinical Presentation

Patients may present for evaluation secondary to a school outbreak or they may present with a complaint of "dandruff" in the hair. Lice can be visualized with the naked eye, but it is more common to see the grayish-white oval nits adhering to the hair shaft. Typically noted as itching on the back of the scalp or behind the ears, eczematous lesions or a hypersensitivity rash may precipitate. Occipital and posterior cervical lymphadenopathy is a common sign with pediculosis capitis.

Diagnosis

Diagnosed clinically by observing live lice or nits within 4 mm of the scalp. Nits alone are not diagnostic.[12]

Management

Pediculocides are the mainstay of treatment, along with environmental controls and complete nit removal. Permethrin 1% or 5% shampoos are available over-the-counter and are applied to the hair, left on for 10 minutes and then rinsed off. As these products are not ovicidal, a repeat treatment is necessary in 7 to 14 days.[12]

> **CLINICAL PEARL:** Items like plush toys, baseball caps, or those that cannot be washed should be sealed in a plastic bag for 2 weeks.

PITYRIASIS ROSEA

Etiology

The most likely etiology of pityriasis rosea is viral as it often occurs in small case clusters, but no exact virus or other microbial agent has been implicated. Because patients and parents report a prodrome of viral symptoms, it has been hypothesized that one of the human herpesviruses (HHVs) is the culprit.

Epidemiology

Pityriasis rosea usually occurs in children and adolescents. There are no differences in occurrences among races and genders.

Clinical Presentation

Patients or parents may report a prodrome of pharyngitis, headache, malaise, or lymphadenopathy before an annular, scaly, erythematous lesion, called the "herald patch," appears. Additional, smaller, patches appear 1 to 30 days later and can persist for 4 to 8 weeks. These macular oval patches usually appear on the trunk and can have a thin scale in the center of the lesions. They are occasionally pruritic and the herald patch can be misdiagnosed as tinea. Once the generalized eruption appears, it may be confused with urticaria, viral exanthem, drug reaction, or guttate psoriasis.

Diagnosis

Diagnosis is usually made by clinical judgment. The presence of the herald patch is a useful feature to help make the appropriate diagnosis.

Management

Most patients will not need any treatment and lesions will resolve with time. The symptoms may persist for 4 to 8 weeks so appropriate family education is necessary to reassure that lesions will disappear and leave normal-appearing skin.

SCABIES

Etiology

The mite *Sarcoptes scabiei hominis* burrows under the epidermis in human hosts and begins tunneling and depositing feces and laying eggs in the tunnels, which hatch after 3 to 4 days. The burrowing itself can create itching, but hypersensitivity to the mites and their by-products is a large component of the pruritus classic with this infection.[12] With a first infestation, sensitization takes several weeks, but once sensitized the pruritus begins. Although mostly transmitted by skin-to-skin contact, scabies can remain alive for 48 hours on clothing or bedding, so this mite can pose a risk for outbreaks in facilities that do not wash sheets regularly.

Epidemiology

In children, nodular scabies is more common than crusted scabies. Most cases of scabies occur in children under the age of 5 years old, but you should consider genital infestation on your differential for an adolescent with pruritus.

Clinical Presentation

Patients often present with intense pruritus that is worse at night and may be localized to the hands, feet, knees, buttocks, waist, and/or axilla. Mites tend to migrate to areas with thinner skin and fewer hair follicles, so interdigital web spaces of the hands or feet are classic areas to find burrow lines. There may or may not be a rash associated with the itching, but if it is present, the rash may have crusted, excoriated, papular lesions. However, in some children, the lesions may appear more vesicular or pustular and may appear in common eczematous sites. Burrow lines may appear as skin-colored serpiginous lesions with a faint papule at the end of the burrow. Some families may return several times prior to diagnosis, as scabies is commonly misdiagnosed as eczema and treated with oral or topical steroids, which mask the infestation until discontinued.

Diagnosis

Having a high level of suspicion is important with this disease, as visualization of the mites is not always possible. If burrows are noted, placing a drop of mineral oil over the burrow and then scraping the burrow off with a scalpel will allow for microscopy. Seeing mites, eggs, or scybala (feces) is diagnostic.

Management

Scabicides are the principal treatment regimen, including permethrin 5% cream. This regimen is applied to all areas of the body from the neck down and left on for 8 to 12 hours before washing. All household members and close contacts should be treated simultaneously. Topical emollients and antihistamines can be used to help calm the itching associated with the infestation.

TINEA: CORPORIS, CRURIS, CAPITUS, PEDIS, VERSICOLOR

Etiology

Dermatophyte infection by *Microsporum canis, Trichophyton tonsurans, Trichophyton mentagrophytes, Trichophyton rubrum, Trichophyton verrucosum, Malassezia furfur,* and *Pityrosporum orbiculare* are the most common organisms that cause tinea corporis, tinea capitus, tinea pedis, and tinea versicolor, respectively.

Epidemiology

Tinea often affects children and adolescents equally except tinea pedis and tinea versicolor tend to affect postpubertal adolescents.

Clinical Presentation

An erythematous, scaly area with irregular but well-defined borders is seen. Oftentimes these erythematous patches will have central clearing and give rise to the nickname "ringworm." Tinea corporis lesions can appear on the trunk or extremities; tinea capitis occurs on the scalp; tinea cruris appears on the inner thighs and perineal area; tinea pedis occurs on the feet and ankles; and tinea versicolor can be found on the neck, chest, upper back, shoulders, and upper arms. The color of tinea versicolor lesions can vary depending on pigmentation of the patient. Light-skinned patients will have darker macular patches and dark-skinned patients will have hypopigmented lesions that may appear tan or dark brown in the winter months as the surrounding skin color fades. Tinea pedis may cause interdigital maceration with peeling of skin. Infection can spread to the nailbeds causing onychomycosis.

Diagnosis

Most cases of tinea will be diagnosed clinically. Skin scrapings with KOH (potassium hydroxide) examination under a microscope can help to identify hyphae and/or budding.

Management

Topical medications are the therapeutic mainstay, including clotrimazole and miconazole. These can be applied twice daily for 10 to 14 days. Patients with tinea pedis should be educated to change their socks several times per day to keep their feet dry and they should be informed to wear shoes that allow their feet to "breathe." Families of children treated for tinea corporis and capitis should be advised to keep any pet dogs out of the children's room and to limit how much the child carries the pet as symptoms are often caused by an organism that is found on dogs. The dog should be treated for this infection as well.

VIRAL EXANTHEMS

Etiology

The etiology of most viral exanthems occurs via respiratory droplet transmission, inoculation of the mucous membranes, and then viral replication and disease manifestations.

Epidemiology

Young children are the most susceptible to viral exanthems with most children having been exposed by the age of 5.

Clinical Presentation

Table 2.10 shows the most common viral exanthems in childhood with the most common causative virus along with their classic signs and symptoms. All of these exanthems could have secondary complications, such as a bacterial super infection, or systemic complications, such as dehydration or febrile seizures, although most patients will present as described within the table.

TABLE 2.10. Common Childhood Viral Exanthems

Clinical Presentation	Most Common Causative Organism	Classic Signs and Symptoms
Hand-foot-and-mouth disease	Coxsackievirus group	Scattered papules on palms, fingertips, interdigital spaces, and soles appear suddenly. Occasional oral lesions can be seen but lesions are not usually painful. Patients are rarely febrile and do not have associated symptoms.

(continued)

TABLE **2.10.** Common Childhood Viral Exanthems (*continued*)

Clinical Presentation	Most Common Causative Organism	Classic Signs and Symptoms
Erythema infectiosum	Parvovirus B19	Classically begins with confluent erythema of both cheeks, hence the name "slapped-cheek syndrome." The pink to erythematous eruption may then spread to extremities, chest, and abdomen and appears as a lacy, salmon-colored cutaneous plaque that lasts 3–5 days. A minority of patients will have associated fever or joint pain.
Roseola	HHV-6	Usually a benign illness in children, it generally affects those under 4 years of age. It begins as a 3-day fever and as this wanes, a pink, morbilliform eruption appears across the thorax, extremities, and face and fades within 24–48 hours. Slight edema of the eyelids and posterior cervical lymphadenopathy occasionally occurs.
Varicella	VZV or HHV-3	Characterized by crops of papules that appear abruptly and progress to vesicles and then crust over across 48 hours with new crops of lesions developing over 2–5 days so lesions are present in various stages of development. Fever is usually low grade and associated symptoms are mild. The outbreak is usually contagious for 2 days before symptoms onset and for 5–6 days after the start, usually as the final lesions have crusted over.
Warts	HPV group	These virus-induced epidermal tumors are caused by HPV and can arise anywhere on the body. Most are nontender and appear in various sizes and shapes due to epidermal proliferation, including a solitary papule with scaly texture to filiform, pedunculated structures that project from the surface of the skin. In addition, lesions can be flat or multiple, confluent papules with an irregular surface. Most spontaneously resolve in 12–24 months.
Cold sores or fever blisters	HSV-1 or HSV-2	Seen as grouped vesicles on an erythematous base regardless of location. Lesions on mucous membranes can easily lose their blister roof and appear as erosions. HSV infections can be primary or recurrent. Associated symptoms include pruritis, pain, and underlying neuropathic pain.
Molluscum contagiosum		These flesh-colored, dome-shaped papules are typically nontender with an umbilicated center and are most often found in elementary school-aged children. Children with underlying atopic dermatitis (AD) are at higher risk for having more molluscum contagiosum lesions and a concominant dermatitis. Lesions can last 6-12 months before they completely resolve without intervention with the face, hands, axilla and arms most commonly affected.

HHV, human herpesvirus; HPV, human papillomavirus; HSV, herpes simplex virus.
Source: Adapted from Weston W, Lane A. *Color Textbook of Pediatric Dermatology.* 3rd ed. St. Louis, MO: Mosby; 2002:89–118.

Diagnosis

The diagnosis of most viral exanthems occurs based on history and physical exam findings. Confirmation of the diagnosis may be done by serology or culture, but this is rarely indicated.

Management

The majority of viral illnesses can be managed with conservative, comfort measures. Table 2.11 demonstrates the most common viral exanthems and their treatment.

TABLE 2.11. Common Viral Exanthems and Their Clinical Management

Clinical Presentation	Diagnosis	Management
Hand-foot-and-mouth disease	Clinical	None in mild cases; in severe cases or immunocompromised patients: IVIG or antiviral pleconaril
Erythema infectiosum	Clinical/ serology	Conservative treatment only
Roseola	Clinical	Conservative treatment only
Varicella	Clinical	Conservative treatment/may consider oral antiviral medications
Molluscum contagiosum (Figure 2.5)	Clinical	None in mild cases; use sharp curette to remove papules or cantharidin may be applied
Warts	Clinical/ aceto-whitening	Cryotherapy, occlusive dressing (duct tape), salicyclic acid, lasers, cantharidin, surgery, immunologic medications, podophyllin, retinoic acid, or nothing
HSV	Clinical/viral culture	IV or oral antiviral medications

HHV, human herpesvirus; HPV, human papillomavirus; HSV, herpes simplex virus; IV, intravenous; IVIG, intravenous immunoglobulin.

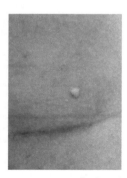

FIGURE 2.5. Molluscum contagiosum: a flesh-colored papule noted on the popliteal fossa.

Photo courtesy of Tanya Fernandez, PA-C.

ENDOCRINE SYSTEM

Endocrine disorders are a common and challenging area of medicine for primary care pediatric providers. This section provides a brief overview of the most common endocrine diseases in pediatrics and offers clinical pearls that can help in the management of these disorders. However, as endocrinology is complicated by high growth states, puberty, and environmental conditions, involving an endocrinologist in the treatment of these diseases may be beneficial for your patients and families.

DIABETES: TYPE 1 AND TYPE 2

Etiology

Characterized by a decrease in insulin production secondary to autoimmune destruction of beta cells in the pancreas, type 1 diabetes is essentially a low-insulin state of starvation. Insulin normally promotes the synthesis and storage (while simultaneously inhibiting the degradation) of macronutrients, but in a low insulin state these normal physiologic processes do not occur, even in the presence of food. This sends the body into alternative pathways for energy, such as lipolysis and proteolysis. These alternative energy-producing pathways, along with decreased glucose utilization, effectively increase circulating glucose and create a hyperosmolar environment with subsequent disturbances in electrolytes and fluids.[13] The use of alternative pathways is not without a price, however. Metabolic derangements are directly implicated in the long-term complications seen with diabetes, such as weight loss, muscle wasting, small vessel damage, and renal dysfunction.

In type 2 diabetes, there is a two-part problem. First, there is a relative insensitivity to insulin at the target cells, which causes decreased glucose utilization at the cellular level. This insensitivity is thought to occur as a result of increased numbers of fat cells that produce the hormones adiponectin, leptin, and resistin. These hormones antagonize insulin, creating a relationship between obesity and type 2 diabetes. Second, the normal pancreatic response to hyperglycemia is unresponsive. Normally, elevated circulating glucose signals increased insulin production; however, in type 2 diabetes, the pancreas cannot increase insulin secretion, resulting in a relative insulin deficiency.

Epidemiology

Diabetes mellitus are the most common pediatric endocrine disorders with no gender inequality noted. Historically, type 1 diabetes was found to affect Whites significantly more than Blacks; however, there have been increasing diagnoses in African Americans over the last decade. Showing some seasonality (fall and winter), type 1 diabetes peaks between 5 and 7 years old and again in puberty. The presentation at age of onset tends to be more abrupt the younger the child.[13]

Type 2 diabetes is highly correlated with childhood obesity and is more prevalent in Native Americans, African Americans, Mexican Americans, and Southeast Asians. There is a strong family history, suggesting a genetic component to type 2 diabetes, but increased sedentary lifestyle and high-calorie, carbohydrate-based diets have been linked as well. Girls are more afflicted with type 2 diabetes than boys.

Clinical Presentation

Classically noted for a relatively rapid onset of polyuria, polyphagia, polydipsia, and weight loss or failure to gain weight despite a healthy intake of food, type 1 diabetes, if not recognized, can manifest as diabetic ketoacidosis (DKA). DKA may go unrecognized and misdiagnosed as it can present similarly to gastroenteritis (with vomiting, polyuria, and dehydration), an acute abdomen (abdominal pain and rigidity), or bronchiolitis or asthma (Kussmaul respirations). Altered mental status and ultimately coma ensue secondary to hyperosmolarity.

Type 2 diabetes may be relatively asymptomatic and may be found only with targeted screening. On some occasions, type 2 diabetes is suspected based on the presence of AN or recurrent vaginal or fungal skin infections.[14] In about 6% of type 2 diabetes, the primary presentation is DKA; however, after recovery, type 2 diabetics will continue to have some insulin production with insulin levels incompatible with type 1 diabetes.

Diagnosis

Both type I and type 2 diabetes present with laboratory findings of glucosuria and hyperglycemia, with or without ketonuria, or metabolic acidosis. Biochemical parameters are essential for the diagnosis and can be collected with a fasting glucose level, oral glucose tolerance test, or hemoglobin A1C (HgbA1C). Diabetes mellitus can be confirmed with:

- Fasting plasma glucose measurement of $\geq$126 mg/dL
- Random glucose measurement of $\geq$200 mg/dL and symptoms of hyperglycemia
- 2-hour glucose measurement of $\geq$200 mg/dL during an oral glucose tolerance test
- HgbA1C measurement of $\geq$6.5%[14]

Differentiating between type 1 and 2 diabetes is not easily done, but measuring fasting C-peptide levels and islet cell and glutamic acid decarboxylase autoantibodies can help support a diagnostic decision.

Management

Type 1 diabetes presenting with DKA requires hospitalization, careful fluid resuscitation, and the initiation of exogenous insulin. Insulin, both short-acting and long-acting, is the mainstay of type 1 treatment and is most often managed by a pediatric endocrinologist. For more information on the management of DKA, see Chapter 5, Urgent Management in Pediatrics.

The goal of treatment for type 2 diabetes is managing glycemia with the objective of getting fasting blood glucose levels to 70 to 130 mg/dL, 2-hour postprandial measurement to less than 180 mg/dL and/or HgbA1C measurement less than 7%.[14] Lifestyle interventions, such as weight reduction, dietary modifications, and exercise, should be reinforced throughout treatment, but typically is not sufficient to reach goal levels. See Table 2.12 for recommended treatment options depending on random blood glucose levels.

TABLE 2.12. Type 2 Diabetes Treatment Options for Children Older Than10 Years Based on Random Blood Glucose Levels

Random Blood Glucose Level	Treatment Options
<200 mg/dL	Metformin
200–249 mg/dL	Insulin alone, metformin alone, or metformin with insulin
>250 mg/dL	Start insulin therapy if there is ketonuria or DKA, HgbA1C >9%

DKA, diabetic ketoacidosis; HgbA1C, hemoglobin A1C.

FAILURE TO THRIVE

Etiology

The etiology of failure to thrive (FTT) is broad and multifactorial in many cases. FTT can occur with dysfunctions in nearly every organ system, as well as secondary to infection, genetics, metabolism, and psychological issues. FTT can be classified into three categories: inadequate intake/absorption, inefficient use of calories, and excessive metabolic demands.[15]

Epidemiology

The rate of FTT in the United States can range from 5% to 10% of children in a primary care setting,[16] but there are no robust studies to define whether there are race, gender, or socioeconomic differences in children with faltering growth.

Clinical Presentation

The classic presentation for FTT is typically not found on the physical exam, but is seen on evaluation of the child's growth chart. It can present as 2 or more points on the growth chart in which weight is below the second percentile for age and gender, weight is less than 80% of the ideal weight for age, or weight velocity crosses two major percentile lines (e.g. weight was initially at the 75th percentile, but now is at the 20th percentile, having crossed the 50th and 25th percentile) after 6 months of age.

Diagnosis

The work up of an FTT child should focus on the findings from the history and physical exam. Very infrequently laboratory tests have a diagnostic significance; however, you may see that laboratory tests were ordered. These could include a CBC where you would be looking for anemia; a comprehensive metabolic panel that includes tests to search for hepatic or renal dysfunction;

a urinalysis (UA) and urine culture (UCx) that would help investigate for a kidney infection or renal tubular acidosis; an erythrocyte sedimentation rate (ESR) and a C-reactive protien (CRP), both of which might help determine if there is an underlying inflammatory disorder such as irritable bowel disease; tissue transglutaminase immunoglobulin A (TTG IgA) and total IgA, which could signal celiac disease.

Management

FTT can usually be successfully managed in the primary care setting and rarely requires hospitalization. After the underlying cause of the FTT is identified, management should focus on treatment of the underlying cause. Because FTT is multifactorial, family support, psychological support, education, and frequent follow-up are critical for success. As the most common etiology of FTT is inadequate caloric intake, the main goal of management is to increase caloric intake to maximize catch-up growth. For infants this may include supplementing expressed breast milk or formula after breastfeeding, using a human-milk fortifier with expressed breast milk or a change to a more calorie-dense formula. For children taking in solids, catch-up growth should be encouraged via three meals and three snacks a day of high-quality foods.

OBESITY

Etiology

With an interplay of genetics, epigenetics, and environment, obesity is a multifactorial disease with an increase in adipose tissue at the core of the disease. Changes in socioeconomic and environmental factors have increased the consumption of energy-dense foods and sugar-sweetened beverages, amplified portion sizes, created food desert in lower socioeconomic areas, and reduced physical activity for both adults and children.[17] Because children often model behaviors seen in adults, they are likely to follow eating habits similar to their parents.

Epidemiology

More than 20% of children are considered overweight or obese, with girls faring worse than boys. As in adults, obesity is higher among non-Hispanic Blacks and Hispanics compared to non-Hispanic Whites and Asians. Although some children will "outgrow" or change their lifestyles to lower their body mass index (BMI), approximately 80% of obese children will continue into adulthood as obese.[18] Of children entering kindergarten, 12.4% are obese, and another 14.9% are overweight.[19]

Clinical Presentation

Pediatric obesity has the hallmark of increased waist circumference and abdominal fat,[20] but may also present with comorbidities such as slipped capital femoral epiphysis (SCFE), psychosocial problems, type 2 diabetes mellitus, hyperlipidemia, elevated liver function levels, cholelithiasis, obstructive sleep apnea, and high BP.

It is important that you remember to consider endocrine-induced obesity on your differential, such as growth hormone (GH) deficiency, hypothyroidism, or Cushing disease.[18] These can be distinguished from non-endocrine-induced obesity as the patient will likely have decreased stature and height velocities; potentially earlier thelarche, pubarche, and menarche in girls; and delayed testicular development, but advanced skeletal development in boys.[18]

Diagnosis

Calculating a BMI and plotting it on a growth chart will diagnose overweight and obesity. The BMI is an indirect measure of fat in children and is closely correlated to risk for comorbidities. Unlike adults, BMI cutoffs are not a standardized number, but rather a plotted point on a growth curve for BMI. Table 2.13 shows medical categories as they relate to the BMI percentile.

TABLE 2.13. BMI Percentile and Corresponding Medical Category for Pediatric Patients

Category	BMI Percentile
Normal	5th to 85th percentile for age and gender
Overweight	85th to 94th percentile for age and gender
Class 1 obesity	≥95th percentile for age and gender
Class 2 obesity	120% of the 95th percentile for age and gender OR BMI of 35–39
Class 3 obesity	140% of the 95th percentile for age and gender OR BMI ≥40

BMI, body mass index.

Should a pediatric patient fall in the overweight or obese BMI categories, the AAP and The Task Force for Pediatric Obesity of the Endocrine Society recommend that you perform screening laboratory tests to evaluate for comorbidities.[18,21] The laboratory studies recommended are noted in Table 2.14.

TABLE 2.14. Laboratory Screening Exams for Overweight and Obese Pediatric Patients

Exam	Evaluating For
Fasting glucose and HgbA1C	Diabetes
Liver function studies	Steatohepatitis
Thyroid function studies	Hypothyroidism
Fasting lipid panel	Hyperlipidemia
Blood pressure	Hypertension
Free and total testosterone	PCOS
Nocturnal polysomnography	Sleep apnea[a]

[a] If there is a family history.

HgbA1C, hemoglobin A1C; PCOS, polycystic ovarian syndrome

Management

Even though a huge focus in the United States has been on diagnosing and managing the complications of obesity, very few interventional programs have demonstrated efficacy in changing attitudes and behavior around childhood obesity. Prevention and management programs should start in utero and extend throughout childhood, adolescence, and adulthood, with a major focus geared toward family support and role-modeling of behaviors. A model that has had some success with changing pediatric behaviors is the 5-2-1-0 initiative. Started in Maine, the *Let's Go! 5-2-1-0* program focuses on promoting five servings of fruits and vegetables per day, 2 hours or less of screen time a day, 1 hour of physical activity a day, and zero sugar-sweetened beverages. Maine's comprehensive program has had success in increasing awareness of good dietary principles, increasing fruit and vegetable intake, lowering sugar-sweetened beverage intake, and showing a stabilization of obesity rates in girls ages 3 to 18 years old;[22] however, adoption of other aspects, especially physical activity, has been less successful.[23]

With 80% of overweight and obese children continuing this pattern into adulthood, obesity is clearly a progressive disease. Despite this, there are very few nonoperative treatments for children. The only Food and Drug Administration (FDA)-approved medication for pediatric patients with obesity is orlistat and its efficacy is moderate for weight loss and decreases in waist circumference; however, weight gain is noted at discontinuation.[24] That being said, bariatric surgery has emerged as a treatment modality in recent years for many individuals. A graduated algorithm for obesity management has been created by the AAP Institute for Healthy Childhood Weight (ihcw.aap.org/Pages/Resources_ClinicalSupports.aspx).

> **CLINICAL PEARL:** Teaching children to "eat a rainbow" of fruits of vegetables each day, can make the five servings of fruits and vegetables a day more tangible, increase variety, and engage children in healthy habits.

SHORT STATURE

Etiology

Short stature is a common parental concern, but it represents a symptom rather than a specific disease. The majority of patients are noted to have a normal variant of growth such as familial short stature or constitutional growth delay; however, pathologic causes, such as GH deficiency, hypothyroidism, and celiac disease, are important to keep on your differential list as you are working through possible diagnoses for a patient with short stature.

Epidemiology

Familial short stature, followed by constitutional growth delay, are the most common diagnoses associated with short stature. Males have traditionally been referred for evaluation of short stature more frequently than females. When females are referred they tend to be referred at an older age and have an almost threefold increase in pathologic diagnoses.[25]

Clinical Presentation

Short stature is typically noted when a child's height is 2 or more standard deviations below the mean height for the child's age and gender. Children with underlying medical conditions that contribute to the short stature may have physical exam findings that can provide evidence toward a diagnosis of the underlying condition. These may include a goiter (hypothyroidism); webbed neck and shield-shaped chest (Turner syndrome); midline defects, including a micropenis (hypopituitarism); or increased central adiposity with a chubby appearance (GH deficiency).

Diagnosis

Calculating a midparental height is extremely important when evaluating the child with short stature, so you have an idea of the genetic potential for the child. If your exam reveals clues that point toward an underlying medical issue, the workup should be tailored for that specific issue; however, if there are no physical exam findings that make you suspect an underlying medical condition, the first step in evaluating short stature is obtaining a bone-age x-ray (a single view of the left hand, fingers, and wrist). Using standardized comparisons, radiologists are able to compare epiphyseal maturation to determine whether the child's skeletal maturity matches the child's chronologic age. A child with constitutional delay will typically have skeletal maturity 2 to 3 years behind the child's chronologic age, whereas familial short-stature patients typically have a bone age similar to the chronologic age. Pathologic causes of short stature will usually present with a bone age more than 2 to 3 years behind the chronologic age.

A thorough evaluation of short stature should also include some basic laboratory tests to rule out pathologic causes. These include electrolytes and CBC with differential (systemic disorders), ESR (inflammatory disease), thyroid-stimulating hormone (TSH) with free T4 (thyroid dysfunction), TTG IgA (celiac), and an insulin-like growth factor 1 (IGF-1) and IGF-binding protein-3 (GH deficiency).[26]

Management

As constitutional growth delay and familial short stature are the most common diagnoses associated with short stature, the main management plan typically includes education and reassurance. Children with thyroid dysfunction, diabetes, and GH deficiency should be referred to a pediatric endocrinologist for further management.[26]

THYROID DYSFUNCTION

Etiology

Thyroid dysfunctions can be congenital or acquired and may cause overactive or underactive thyroid function. Congenital hypothyroidism is most often secondary to thyroid dysgenesis, whereas acquired thyroid diseases are primarily autoimmune in nature. Autoimmune hyperthyroidism (often referred to as "Graves' disease") usually develops when antibodies bind to and mimic thyrotropin, which cause increased thyroid hormone production and secretion. The unregulated stimulation of the thyroid gland causes it to increase in size as well. Acquired hypothyroidism (often referred to as "Hashimoto's thyroditis") occurs when antibodies (most notablyy anti-thyroid peroxidase) damage the thyroid gland and decrease its ability to produce thyroid hormone. As thyroid hormone is a key component in growth and development, inadequate or excessive levels can disrupt normal growth and development patterns in pediatric patients.

Epidemiology

Found more often in females than males, both acquired hypothyroidism and hyperthyroidism are noted to have a family history of autoimmune disease. Congenital hypothyroidism has also been found to have a genetic basis, but familial inheritance is not clear.

Clinical Presentation

Congenital hypothyroidism typically presents asymptomatically at birth and is detected on newborn metabolic screening. If left untreated, infants can develop unspecific symptoms that can be easily mistaken for other conditions, such as jaundice, poor feeding, constipation, and a hoarse cry. The classically described findings are umbilical herniation, enlarged posterior and anterior fontanelles, coarse features, hypotonia, delayed reflexes, and macroglossia.[27,28] Acquired hypothyroidism presents with some of the same signs, symptoms, and findings as congenital hypothyroidism, including fatigue, constipation, enlarged fontanelles with delayed closure. With older children, it can present as cold intolerance, slowed mentation, goiter, and linear growth decelerations. The diagnosis of acquired hyperthyroidism is often delayed, as the signs and symptoms may lead practitioners down a different diagnostic pathway, such as behavioral disorders, neuromuscular disease, and cardiopulmonary disease. Children and adolescents with Graves' disease may present with anxiety or inattention, hyperactivity or fidgeting, hand tremors, proximal muscle weakness, shortness of breath, or palpitations. On physical exam, many are noted to have a growth acceleration with delayed puberty and a goiter.[27] Approximately one third will have findings consistent with exophthalmos.[27]

Diagnosis

Primary thyroxine (T4) testing via newborn metabolic screening with heel-prick samples obtained between 2 and 5 days of life identifies those infants who require confirmatory serum thyroid hormone samples. Both acquired hypo- and hyperthyroidism can be detected using serum thyrotropin (also known as "TSH") and free T4 samples, but the addition of T3 is useful in making the diagnosis of Graves' disease. Table 2.15 shows the trends in laboratory values depending on the diagnosis.

TABLE 2.15. Laboratory Values for Hypothyroid and Hyperthyroid Diagnosis

Laboratory Value	Hashimoto's Thyroiditis	Subclinical Hypothyroidism	Central Hypothyroidism	Graves' Disease
Thyrotropin/ TSH	↑	↑	Normal to low	↓
Free T4	↓	Normal	↓	↑
T3	–	–	–	↑ T3:T4 ratio
Follow-up testing	Antithyroid peroxidase	Most will convert to normal with observation	MRI to evaluate for mass lesions	Thyroid-stimulating immunoglobulin antibody or thyrotropin receptor antibody

TSH, thyroid-stimulating hormone.

Management

Management of thyroid dysfunction is dependent on the diagnosis. Table 2.16 shows the various treatment options for the primary thyroid dysfunctions.

TABLE 2.16. Treatment and Monitoring Recommendations for Common Thyroid Dysfunctions

Disease	First-Line Treatment	Goal	Monitoring
Congenital hypothyroidism	Levothyroxine 10–15 mcg/kg once daily (crushed and administered with breast milk, water, or formula)	Normalize total T4 levels in 2 weeks → maintain in upper half of normal range Normalize TSH in 1 month	Every 2 weeks until TSH is normal Every 3 months until child is 3 years old Every 6 months after the age of 3 years old[29]

(continued)

TABLE 2.16. Treatment and Monitoring Recommendations for Common Thyroid Dysfunctions (*continued*)

Disease	First-Line Treatment	Goal	Monitoring
Hashimoto thyroiditis	Levothyroxine 3–6 months (8–10 mcg/kg/d) 6–12 months (6–8 mcg/kg/d) 1–5 years (5–6 mcg/kg/d) 6–12 years (4–5 mcg/kg/d) >12 years (2–3 mcg/kg/d)	Normalization of T4 and TSH and restore normal function	Recheck TSH level 1–2 months after starting levothyroxine or with dose change Every 3 months until child is 3 years old Every 6 months after the age of 3 years old[29] until finished growing and going through puberty After puberty, monitor annually[30]
Graves' disease	Methimazole 0.2–0.5 mg/kg/d once daily Cardioselective beta-blocker for significant signs and symptoms	Normalization of T3 and T4 levels	Monitor T3 and T4 levels every month until euthyroid, then annually until discontinuation recommended Every 3 months for the first year after discontinuation, then annually[30]

TSH, thyroid-stimulating hormone.

ELECTRONIC RESOURCES

Provider Resources for Childhood Obesity:
https://ihcw.aap.org/Pages/Resources_ClinicalSupports.aspx
https://ihcw.aap.org/Pages/EFHALF_parents.aspx

GASTROINTESTINAL SYSTEM

The GI system is essential for the digestion, absorption, excretion, and elimination of energy sources, and as such can be one of the most intimidating organ systems to approach in pediatrics. The number of items on the differential is typically quite extensive and many of the conditions present with overlapping symptoms or similar presentations.

ALLERGIES: MILK PROTEIN ALLERGY, FOOD ALLERGIES, AND LACTOSE INTOLERANCE

Etiology

In milk protein allergy, the casein and whey in cow's milk trigger a cell-mediated immune response with inflammation occurring anywhere along the small intestine, large intestine, colon, or rectum. Patients with enteropathy (small intestine involvement only) and enterocolitis (involvement of the small and large intestines) have more severe symptoms than those with proctocolitis (involvement of the distal colon and rectum). Although other food allergies can present with symptoms similar to milk protein allergies, these typically present later in life with the addition of complementary feedings and may present as vomiting, diarrhea, or even anaphylaxis secondary to an IgE-mediated hypersensitivity reaction to a component of the trigger food. The most serious allergic reactions reported include eggs, peanuts, tree nuts, and seafood.[31] Lactose intolerance is not an allergy, but a deficiency in the digestive enzyme lactase, which is found on the tip of the villi in the small intestines.

Epidemiology

Lactose intolerance is very common with 70% of the world's population demonstrating some form of lactose intolerance; however, intolerance is highly variable depending on ethnicity. Blacks, Asians, Hispanics, and Native Americans have the highest prevalence at 60% to 100%, whereas Northern Europeans and Indian children have a 2% to 30% prevalence.[32] Age of onset is also variable with Hispanic children displaying symptoms more often before the age of 5 and Caucasian children well after the age of 5.

Clinical Presentation

Clinical presentation of food allergies and intolerances is quite variable depending on the degree of intestinal involvement and sometimes the quantity of food ingested. With mild milk protein allergies, such as proctocolitis, an infant will usually present with flecks of blood in the stool, but is otherwise healthy and well appearing. Milk protein–induced enterocolitis may present as a septic newborn provided cow's milk formula. Milk protein allergies tend to present with vomiting, heme-positive diarrhea, and abdominal distension, whereas IgE-mediated food allergies can present with:

- Skin reactions, such as swelling, rash, hives, or eczema
- Wheezing or difficulty breathing
- Runny nose and sneezing
- Red or watery eyes
- Stomach pain, nausea, vomiting, or diarrhea
- Anaphylaxis (less common)

Lactose intolerance tends to develop over time and typically presents as abdominal distension, flatulence, abdominal cramping, and diarrhea.

Diagnosis

The medical history for any food allergies and intolerances is really the key to determining the patient's pretest probability and helps identify whether the reaction is IgE-mediated or non-IgE-mediated. There is no one laboratory test to diagnose a food allergy; rather patients may need to undergo a diagnostic elimination diet, skin-prick test with follow-up IgE-blood tests, and an oral food challenge. The double-blind oral food challenge is considered the gold standard for diagnosis and should be done under the supervision of a pediatric specialist. An elimination diet for lactose intolerance followed by a lactose challenge is an easy method to make a lactose intolerance diagnosis, but a hydrogen breath test can also be used to make the diagnosis.

Management

Food avoidance/elimination is the mainstay of management of food allergies and intolerances, but it is important that you consider whether the elimination of a dietary component may have unintended consequences, such as a vitamin or mineral deficiency. Supplementing possible deficiency is an important part of the management. In addition, if an IgE-mediated food allergy is present, education on the importance and use of an epinephrine autoinjector is essential.

APPENDICITIS

Etiology

As the name implies, appendicitis occurs when the appendix, anatomically located in the right lower quadrant (RLQ), becomes inflamed secondary to a fecalith or food particle obstruction at the cecal outpouch.

Epidemiology

Most common in the second decade of life and with a slightly higher male-to-female incidence, appendicitis is the most common reason for emergent pediatric surgery.

Clinical Presentation

Children with an appendicitis classically present with a low-grade fever, anorexia, and diffuse periumbilical discomfort that migrates to the RLQ. The pain usually precedes any vomiting that the child may demonstrate. On exam, the patient usually guards the abdomen by splinting and lying completely still. Pain may be generated with walking or bed movement. Tenderness at McBurney's point can help to identify an appendicitis, but a positive psoas sign or obturator sign may be present without pain at McBurney's point if the appendix is retrocecal or pelvic. Gynecologic, testicular, and rectal exams can help differentiate ovarian, adnexal, and testicular pathology from abdominal pathology in adolescents.

> **CLINICAL PEARL:** To remember the maneuvers for detecting an appendicitis in children, think of *OH MY!* (**o**bturator, **h**eel jar, **M**cBurney's, and **y**oungster less than 2 years old are more likely to have diffuse tenderness!)

Diagnosis

Clinical suspicion can be supported by clinical decision rules such as calculating an Alvarado score or the Pediatric Appendicitis Score, and those children determined to be at a moderate- or high-risk stratification can be confirmed with laboratory and/or imaging studies. Labs that would suggest an acute inflammatory process with possible infection would include a CBC that shows an elevated white blood cell (WBC) count with a left shift, elevated CRP, and/or sterile pyuria. Dehydration secondary to the anorexia and/or vomiting might manifest as electrolyte abnormalities or urine with a high specific gravity or ketones. In many institutions, the first line for pediatric patients with suspected appendicitis is ultrasonography, although it is less accurate than CT scan.[33]

Management

Definitive treatment of appendicitis continues to be appendectomy; however, broad-spectrum, preoperative antibiotics, such as ceftriaxone and metronidazole, are routinely administered as bridge therapy prior to surgery.[34] In addition, IV hydration and pain control are critical in the pre- and postoperative periods.

COLIC

Etiology

As colic is not well understood and is a diagnosis of exclusion, no clear etiology has been identified. It is sometimes defined as crying that lasts 3 or more hours/day occurring more than 3 days a week for at least 3 weeks. Hypotheses propose that it may be a combination of an immature nervous system, GI discomfort, and psychosocial factors. Some of the most commonly associated GI issues include gas, gastroesophageal reflux (GER), and milk protein intolerance. Neurologic immaturity may contribute to overly sensitive pain receptors or an immature ability to self-soothe. Overstimulation, parental coping skills, and parental anxiety may also contribute to colic symptoms.

Epidemiology

We know that all babies cry and that there is a documented pattern of crying that is associated with normal development between 2 weeks and 4 months of age.[35] The pattern of crying typically ramps up and peaks at 2 months of age, but will continue on (in decreasing intensity) until 4 months of age. Babies with colic may be resistant to soothing; can cry unexpectedly, but typically more often in the evening; appear to be in pain while crying; and cry for long periods of time.[35] Some estimates list the incidence of colic in infants at 40%.[36]

Clinical Presentation

Typically, infants with excessive crying present to the pediatric office happy and calm. The history is consistent with crying that is resistant to soothing or the types of soothing that have worked in the past are not calming the child now. There is a history of crying more often in the early evenings that may or may not respond to low lighting and quiet environments. These infants are rarely afflicted with an underlying medical issue, so the exam is typically quite normal.

Diagnosis

This is a diagnosis of exclusion, so a careful history, careful growth chart evaluation, and physical exam are needed to identify whether there are underlying medical or psychosocial components. The physical exam should pay particular attention to signs of infection or trauma, the abdominal exam, and close evaluation of the genitalia and the digits, as identifying a testicular torsion, or a hair or string tourniquet can save the infants from vascular compromise and may improve the colic symptoms. Corneal abrasions and hunger can cause prolonged crying in infants as well.

Management

The most beneficial management you can provide for a family with this concern is to acknowledge how stressful a crying infant can be and present some techniques that might help with GI discomfort (e.g., feeding in upright position to minimize GER, abdominal massage, feeding smaller amounts more frequently) and augment the infant's self-soothing abilities with dimmed lights, minimal stimulation, soothing music, swaddling, and nursing or use of a pacifier. Educating families about the normalcy of this developmental stage, acknowledging that things that have worked in the past may or may not soothe the baby over time, and creating a safety plan with families around what they will do when frustrated/overwhelmed by a crying infant to avoid the potential for child abuse or shaken baby syndrome should be top priority for families with a "colicky" infant.

CONSTIPATION

Etiology

Constipation is a common complaint throughout the pediatric ages, with the majority of constipation issues arising from retentive behaviors; however, a lack of fiber, dehydration, or excessive milk intake can also be implicated. Less common, but important to consider in the differential for constipation, are anatomic GI defects such as strictures, stenosis, and Hirschsprung disease; muscular diseases such as cerebral palsy and systemic lupus erythematosus (SLE); and endocrine disorders such as hypothyroidism.

A consequence of constipation may be encopresis, enuresis, and chronic urinary tract infections (UTIs). Stool-holding behaviors cause a dilated rectum to become less sensitive to rectal fullness and stool retention follows. The inability to pass stool does not stop the process of digestion, so softer, more-liquid stool leaks around the retained stool (encopresis) in children with chronic constipation.[37]

Epidemiology

As one of the most common pediatric complaints, constipation is noted to start in the toilet-training years (2–3 years old) and persists throughout childhood. Althoughthe prevalence of constipation peaks at 5 to 6 years old, visits to pediatricians for constipation constitute 3% of visits to office-based practices throughout the pediatric age spectrum. Males are more commonly afflicted with retentive constipation than females in childhood, but this reverses in adulthood.[38]

Clinical Presentation

Patients with constipation present with a 2-month history of fewer than three bowel movements per week, weekly episodes of involuntary soiling, passage of stool so large that it clogs the toilet, pain with defecation, active fecal withholding with retentive posturing, and/or stool impaction. They may also present with frequent urination. The exam typically notes no abdominal distension, normal bowel sounds, mild tenderness, or fullness in the lower left quadrant (LLQ), and a full rectum on digital rectal exam.

Diagnosis

Diagnosis is typically made after a thorough dietary and elimination history, but an abdominal x-ray can help identify a large stool load. If organic causes are suspected, referral to a pediatric gastroenterologist is warranted for further testing, such as biopsies, manometry, and contrast studies.

Management

Increasing ingestion of high-fiber foods and stool softeners are the mainstay of management once the stool has been disimpacted. Disimpaction can be achieved with enemas, stool softeners, and milk of magnesia. The primary stool softener used in pediatrics is polyethylene glycol at 0.8 to 1.0 g/kg/d. Formulated as a powder, the powder is mixed in water or juice and taken in divided doses twice a day or in a full dose once a day. Typically, treatment is needed until the child is having two to three soft stools daily for 1 to 2 months and then the dose can be tapered to a maintenance dose or stopped and used as needed for recurrences.

> **CLINICAL PEARL:** Mixing polyethylene glycol with pear juice or Gatorade can make it much more palatable.

GASTROENTERITIS: ACUTE

Etiology

Acute gastroenteritis (AGE) is most commonly caused by viral infections, including rotavirus, enteric adenovirus, enteroviruses, and norovirus. *Campylobacter, Clostridium difficile, Escherichia coli, Salmonella, Shigella, Cryp-*

tosporidium, and *Giardia* should also be considered in patients with foreign travel, untreated water ingestion, or animal exposures.

Epidemiology

AGE can occur during any time of the year, but is more common in the winter months and requires hospitalization more frequently in children younger than 5 years old and those with an underlying medical disease or immunocompromised state. Those children younger than 18 months old and those who are premature and not breastfed may suffer the most severe clinical course. Because AGE is spread by fecal–oral route, outbreaks can be seen in childcare centers and schools.

Clinical Presentation

In mild disease, patients usually present without fever, but may have anorexia, nausea, and vomiting, followed by diarrhea and abdominal cramps. In more serious disease, signs of systemic illness may be present, such as fever, headache, and rash. Most viral AGE is self-limited and mild, but those patients with severe disease may have complications related to dehydration. Gastroenteritis may mimic other abdominal disease, such as appendicitis and intussusception, so it is important that you differentiate a self-limited illness from a more serious abdominal pathology. Patients typically show signs of disease 1 to 3 days after infection and on average symptoms last 3 to 7 days. Distinguishing between viral, bacterial, and parasitic infections is not always easily done without stool studies, but you should have a higher suspicion for a bacterial infection if the patient has blood or mucus in the stool and parasitic infections with greasy, malodorous stools with increased bloating and flatulence. Exam is usually unremarkable, but diffuse abdominal pain without lateralization or localization is common, as are hyperactive bowel sounds.

Diagnosis

History and a relatively normal exam are typically enough to make the diagnosis clinically; however, if you are concerned about bacterial or parasitic infections, a stool culture, leukocytes, and ova and parasite studies are key.

Management

The first line of care for AGE is managing and/or preventing dehydration. As this is usually a mild self-limited infection, supportive care with oral rehydration therapy (ORT) with an electrolyte fluid is normally sufficient. Encouraging families to offer oral rehydration slowly and at regular intervals is the best approach. Many practitioners will offer the "prescription" of 5 mL of fluid every 5 minutes for the first hour. If tolerated, families can increase to 10 mL every 10 minutes for the second hour, 15 mL every 15 minutes for the third hour, and then ad lib on demand. If a child vomits during the first 3 hours of offering oral rehydration, you should recommend that the family wait 1 to 2 hours and then start the ORT protocol again. If disease is severe, IV rehydration may be needed to correct electrolyte disturbances and hydration.

Probiotics *Lactobacillus rhamnosus, Saccharomyces boulardii,* and *Lactobacillus reuteri* DSM 17938 have been shown to shorten the duration of diarrheal symptoms and can be recommended as an adjunct to ORT.[39] The use of antidiarrheal medications is not recommended, but a single dose of ondansetron may be useful in preventing dehydration and hospitalization.

> **CLINICAL PEARL:** Starting a BRAT (**b**ananas, **r**ice, **a**pplesauce, **t**oast) diet 24 hours after vomiting stops can help with diarrheal losses.

Antibiotics should be started if the infant is younger than 3 months old, the child is immunocompromised, or there is isolation of *Shigella*, enterotoxigenic *E. coli, Vibrio cholerae, Yersinia enterocolitica,* or *Entamoeba histolytica.* *Campylobacter* colitis can be treated with antibiotics, but treatment is effective only if administered within the first 2 days of symptoms.[39]

GASTROESOPHAGEAL REFLUX

Etiology
Secondary to the relaxation of the lower esophageal sphincter during swallowing, gastric contents that are under pressure, due to high-volume feeds in a small stomach, move up the esophagus in normal infants without much indication of discomfort, but older children may have comorbid conditions that increase the risk of persistent, bothersome reflux symptoms. GER disease (GERD) occurs when GER becomes symptomatic or causes pathologic changes in the esophagus.

Epidemiology
Although more common in adults, the prevalence of gastroesophageal reflux has been increasing in pediatric populations with up to 25% of children and teens complaining of symptoms. Obesity and family history are risk factors for GERD,[40] so the increasing prevalence of obesity may be related to the increasing prevalence of GERD. Access to increasingly spicy food additives may also contribute to the abdominal pain associated with GERD.

Clinical Presentation
With infants, parental reporting of spitting up or nonbilious vomiting after feeding is commonly the presenting history, but may also include associated crying, irritability with feedings or postprandial back arching, cough, or apnea.[40] Older children present with symptoms similar to adults, including regurgitation into the mouth, heartburn, abdominal pain, and occasionally painful swallowing or cough.[40] Younger children tend to present with complaints of epigastric pain, whereas tweens and teens describe heartburn and regurgitation.[41]

Diagnosis

GER and GERD are diagnosed clinically, but you may see providers order an upper GI series to rule out anatomic abnormalities as the cause of the vomiting. In older children, first-line diagnostics include dietary modifications and a trial of acid suppressants. If symptoms persist, you can order an upper GI series, endoscopy, pH probe, or refer to a specialist for more specialized studies.

Management

Treatment is often determined by how the infant responds to the reflux. If parents report significant crying, back arching, or significant fussiness, treatment may need to expand beyond the feeding modifications typically recommended. For infants with mild symptoms of reflux, reassuring parents that 85% of infants spontaneously improve by 1 year of age may be sufficient.[37] When discussing GER with families, you can suggest that parents feed/nurse the baby in a more upright position, offer smaller feedings at more frequent intervals, watch for cues that indicate the baby is satisfied and use a bottle designed to reduce air intake with feedings with a nipple with the appropriate flow rate for the baby's age and intake.

For older children and teens, weight loss and dietary modification, such as avoiding caffeine, chocolate, alcohol, and spicy foods as potential symptom triggers, are advised.[42] Postprandial sugarless gum chewing can also reduce reflux symptoms.[43]

If continuing to be symptomatic, infants and children can be given a trial of ranitidine (5 mg/kg/d divided BID) or omeprazole (0.5–1.0 mg/kg/d), which may reduce pain, but likely will not reduce the reflux itself. Surgical intervention with a fundoplication is indicated only for patients with severe symptoms unresponsive to medications.

INTUSSUSCEPTION

Etiology

Created when a proximal section of ileum telescopes into the colon, the swelling, vascular compromise and necrosis associated with the invagination of the ileum causes paroxysmal abdominal pain. In 85% of intussusceptions, an underlying cause is not identified, but Meckel diverticulum, intestinal duplication, celiac disease, Henoch–Schonlein purpura, lymphoma, parasites, and viral enteritis have all been associated with intussusception.[37]

Epidemiology

With a 3:1 male-to-female ratio, intussusception occurs more often in children under the age of 2.

Clinical Presentation

An infant typically presents appearing lethargic and febrile with recurring episodes of abdominal pain marked by screaming and drawing up the knees toward the chest. In 90% of cases, infants have vomiting and diarrhea and about 50% of cases have bloody stools with mucus or "currant jelly stools." On exam, the infant may have a distended and tender abdomen with a sausage-shaped mass palpable in the upper to middle abdomen.

Diagnosis

Historically, intussusception has been diagnosed and treated with enema, but more recently US has become a modality for diagnosis with a sensitivity of 97.9% and specificity of 97.8%, as well as its ability to assess for alternative diagnoses.[44] If you are using an enema for diagnosis and treatment, the enema is administered under standardized pressures to reduce the invagination. Radiologic findings are classically described as a target or pseudokidney sign.[44] Air insufflation is safer and has a success rate of 82.7%, compared to barium enema at 69.6%.[45]

Management

Given the child's typical ill or even toxic appearance, transfer to an emergency setting is warranted. Perforation, and subsequent peritonitis, can be a complication of strangulated bowel; and qualified specialists should be involved in determining whether the patient is a candidate for a diagnostic and therapeutic enema or if surgical correction is preferred. If perforation is suspected, surgery is required.

PINWORMS

Etiology

Pinworms, scientifically known as *Enterobius vermicularis*, are transmitted when embryonic eggs are ingested, hatch in the stomach, and then larval parasites migrate to the cecum to mature into adults. As humans are the only host for this obligate parasite, breaking the cycle of infection is critical. Adult females migrate at night to lay eggs on the perianal region. This migration and egg laying causes nocturnal pruritus, which then allows eggs to transfer from the anus to underneath the fingernails. Without proper hygiene, this allows for direct transmission into the GI tract. As there is no tissue invasion, the body's ability to mount a response is somewhat limited and the consequences of infection are more bothersome than medical.

Epidemiology

Children between the ages of 5 and 14 years have the highest prevalence, but pinworms can occur at any age and socioeconomic status. However, living in congested areas can predispose individuals and families to the infection.

Clinical Presentation

Children infected with pinworms will present with a history of rectal itching that is worse at night and impacts sleep. In young girls, this may manifest as vulvovaginal pruritus or vulvovaginitis.

Diagnosis

Definitive diagnosis is established with the "Scotch tape test" first thing in the morning. By pressing clear adhesive tape to the perianal region in the morning, you are able to lift parasites or their eggs onto the tape for investigation under the microscope. Identifying eggs or worms under the microscope is diagnostic.

Management

The infected individual and family members should be treated empirically with the following:

- Albendazole 400 mg by mouth once with a repeat dose in 2 weeks
- Mebendazole 100 mg orally with repeat dosing in 2 weeks
- Pyrantel pamoate 11 mg/kg orally up to a maximum dose of 1 g with repeat dose in 2 weeks

Treating family members, washing bedding in hot water, encouraging personal hygiene, and cutting the nails short may help decrease transmission and excoriations.

> **CLINICAL PEARL:** Having a child wear clean cotton mittens at night can minimize excoriations and the potential for superinfections.

PYLORIC STENOSIS

Etiology

The cause of pyloric stenosis is not clear, but a family history can be noted in about 10% of patients. Studies have shown conflicting data on the role of macrolides in pyloric stenosis.

Epidemiology

With a 4:1 male predominance and no significant racial or ethnic predilections, pyloric stenosis typically presents in 0.8% of neonates and infants.

Clinical Presentation

A patient is classically described as a very hungry neonate with nonbilious, projectile vomiting after feeding. Pyloric stenosis may present as a distended upper abdomen with left-to-right peristaltic waves seen immediately after feeding. Occasionally an "olive" or mass can be felt in the right upper abdomen after vomiting. If not identified early, these infants may present with weight loss, dehydration, electrolyte abnormalities, and lethargy.

> **CLINICAL PEARL:** An infant with bilious vomiting should be evaluated for malrotation or volvulus, as pyloric stenosis does not present with bilious vomiting.

Diagnosis

A classic history of projectile vomiting should raise suspicion for pyloric stenosis and emergent evaluation of the infant should be done, as IV access and immediate labs are often required. Definitive diagnosis is made with a US finding of hypoechoic pylorus greater than 4-mm thick and a pyloric channel greater than 15 mm in length. You may see providers order an upper GI series with barium contrast, but US is less invasive.

Management

Correction of the hypochloremic alkalosis and potassium deficits is the first order of management. After the child is stabilized, surgical intervention with a laparoscopic Ramstedt pyloromyotomy is curative.

GENITOURINARY SYSTEM

Although it may seem unusual to think about genitourinary issues in pediatrics, especially in reference to prepubescent children, issues affecting the genitalia or urinary systems are actually quite common in pediatrics. Being comfortable with the most common genitourinary diagnoses in pediatrics is important, as your comfort with these issues, how to assess them, and their treatment puts parents at ease during an often uncomfortable visit. The most common issues in primary care pediatrics are phimosis, paraphimosis, vulvovaginitis, and UTIs.

PHIMOSIS AND PARAPHIMOSIS

Etiology

Phimosis is a tight penile foreskin that cannot be retracted to expose the glans penis, whereas paraphimosis is retracted foreskin that becomes caught behind the coronal sulcus and cannot be returned to its normal position. Males are born with a naturally tight foreskin that loosens between the ages of 5 and 7 years with penile growth, so phimosis is a physiologically normal state, but paraphimosis can cause constriction, edema, and pain secondary to occlusion of blood flow. The paraphimosis can be caused by retracting the foreskin too far for cleaning, balanitis, sexual activity, or catheterization.

Epidemiology

Present in both prepubescent and pubescent uncircumcised males, it can be a concerning and urgent complaint in primary care pediatrics.

Clinical Presentation

Phimosis presents with a band-like tissue ring at the tip of the penis or as only partial movement of the foreskin with minimal pain with manipulation. Paraphimosis, on the other hand, presents with penile swelling/edema, erythema (or possibly cyanosis if there is ischemia), painful foreskin, painful urination, and possibly a weak urinary stream.

Diagnosis

Both phimosis and paraphimosis are clinical diagnoses.

Management

In the case of paraphimosis, urgent treatment is needed to prevent ischemic damage. Manually retracting the foreskin over the coronal sulcus is the main goal, but providing vasoconstriction and pain control are also critical. In severe cases, urologic interventions with a dorsal slit procedure may be required. As noted earlier, phimosis often resolves spontaneously without any treatment; however, if the phimosis is compromising hygiene or the urine stream or causes discomfort, daily gentle retraction with or without the use of corticosteroids may be initiated. In severe cases, circumcision may need to be considered.[46]

The mainstay of management should be prevention. Educating families about the role of the foreskin and how to clean the diaper area of an uncircumcised male, reminding young males not to forcefully retract the foreskin, and teaching teens to return the foreskin to its normal position after cleansing and intercourse are important preventative measures.[47]

UTI AND PYELONEPHRITIS

Etiology

UTIs are caused by a bacterial infection, with *E. coli, Klebsiella, Proteus, Enterococcus, Pseudomonas,* and *Staphylococcus* as the primary agents. Fungal infections are rarely a cause. Infections localized to the bladder (cystitis) are more common than those that ascend into the ureters and kidney (pyelonephritis); however, in neonates hematogenous spread can cause a group B *Streptococcus, Staphylococcus,* or *Candida* pyelonephritis.[50]

Epidemiology

As the most common bacterial infection in childhood, UTIs account for 7% to 10% of febrile illnesses in infancy and childhood.[50] When trying to determine whether to evaluate a pediatric patient's urine, understanding the factors that put patients at greater risk is important. Patients with abnormalities of the renal or urinary tract anatomy, females younger than 4 years of age, uncircumcised males younger than 12 months of age, dysfunctional elimination, and a family history of UTI and/or vesicoureteral reflux (VUR) increase the risk of UTIs in young children. Changes in periurethral flora and sexual activity increase the risk of UTI in adolescent females.[51] About 6% to 12% of females under 1 year of age will have a UTI, whereas males have a 2.5% to 20% risk depending on whether they are circumcised or uncircumcised, respectively.[50] This risk drops precipitously after age 1, with males, regardless of circumcision status, dropping to less than 1% and females to less than 2%.

Clinical Presentation

2–24 months old: Fever without an obvious source may be the only presenting symptom of UTI in children younger than 2 years old. Occasionally, fussiness, poor feeding, and/or foul-smelling urine can be identified. If a fever is present, it is assumed that patients younger than 24 months have pyelonephritis.

>24 months old: As children become verbal, they have the ability to localize their symptoms and may describe dysuria, frequency, urgency, and suprapubic pain. A patient with pyelonephritis may have systemic symptoms, such as fever and headache, while also complaining of flank pain and costovertebral angle tenderness.

Diagnosis

Determining the pretest probability of UTI can be done using point-of-care clinical decision support tools such as UTICalc.[52] Other similar diagnostic risk determiners, such as the Diagnosis of Urinary Tract infections in Young children (DUTY) protocol, use signs, symptoms, and dipstick findings to determine the risk of UTI.[53]

With various options for urine collection, it can be confusing as to which options to use, but the type of collection will greatly impact diagnosis and confirmation with urine culture. In nontoilet-trained children, urine should be collected via urethral catheterization or suprapubic aspiration, as these samples have less contamination than a bagged urine sample and can be used for urine culture. In older children, a clean-catch urine is acceptable for diagnosis and confirmation.

After the urine has been collected, UA is the first step in diagnostic process. Single components on the UA tend to be less sensitive and specific than a combination of leukocyte esterase, nitrites, and microscopy, with the exception of the 98% specificity of a positive nitrite test. Urine with both positive leukocyte esterase and nitrites should be sent for confirmation with bacterial identification. Urine culture is usually considered positive with bacterial growth greater than 10,000 to 50,000 colony-forming units (CFU) for a catheterized specimen and positive if more than 100,000 CFU for a clean-catch specimen.

Management

Determining when to treat empirically for a UTI or pyelonephritis involves the use of risk calculators and posttest probability. However, if UTI is suspected, especially for a child younger than 24 months, empiric treatment should be started, as the early treatment of UTI can prevent pyelonephritis and complications of upper UTI such as renal scarring. Older children can often defer treatment until the culture results return in 12 to 24 hours. The AAP has identified several acceptable empiric therapies (cephalexin 50–100 mg/kg divided into three or four doses daily × 7–10 days or ceftriaxone 50 mg/kg intramuscularly every 24 hours until they demonstrate clinical improvement and can tolerate oral therapy) for UTI treatment, but using local susceptibility patterns is best when choosing an empiric treatment. Antibiotic duration should be no less than 7 days and up to 14 days depending on clinical judgment. Parental antibiotics can be transitioned to oral dosing when a child is able to tolerate oral intake and is symptomatically improving.

Febrile infants should have a renal and bladder US (RBUS) to evaluate for anatomic abnormalities. Indications of hydronephrosis, scarring, high-grade VUR or obstructive uropathy should be followed up with a voiding cystourethrogram (VCUG). Recurrent UTIs with or without fever should be evaluated and underlying etiologies, such as bowel dysfunction, should be treated accordingly.

VULVOVAGINITIS

Etiology

Thin, sensitive skin that is located close to the rectum and is unprotected in the genital area of premenarchal females is easily irritated by rubbing, scratching, moisture; and contact with detergents, soaps, and bubble baths. Irritation in prepubertal girls typically starts at the vulva and extends to the vagina, whereas tweens and teens typically have vulvovaginitis that starts with a vaginal infection.[48] Most vulvovaginitis is nonspecific and results from poor hygiene. However, bacterial vulvovaginitis is usually a result of sexually transmitted infections (STIs) and anaerobic bacteria.

Epidemiology

Present in both prepubescent and pubescent females, vulvovaginitis is a common chief complaint in primary care pediatrics. It is also important to remember that up to 5% of girls with chronic symptoms are being sexually abused.[49]

Clinical Presentation

Typically presenting as a nonodorous, mucus discharge with genital itching and occasionally painful urination, irritant vulvovaginitis (usually from residual soap or bubble bath) appears as erythematous labia majora with evidence of excoriation. Bacterial vulvovaginitis presents with a malodorous, mucopurulent discharge that may or may not be associated with scant blood. The vulva is erythematous and painful. Candidal vulvovaginitis, more common in adolescent females, presents with a nonodorous, thick, white discharge with associated itching. On physical exam, you may see "beefy red" erythema of the vulva and surrounding area with satellite lesions. The discharge is typically adherent and is noted to have pseudohyphae when prepared for wet mount with 10% potassium hydroxide.[48]

Sexually transmitted organisms, such as *Trichomonas vaginalis,* herpes simplex virus, gonorrhea, and chlamydia, can also cause vulvar irritation, but are rare in prepubertal females and, if noted, should raise the suspicion of sexual abuse. These infections are covered in more detail in the gynecology section of this chapter.

Diagnosis

Most often diagnosed clinically, swabs of the discharge may help differentiate bacterial from fungal infections.

Management

Because the primary cause of vulvovaginitis is poor hygiene, the mainstay of treatment is education about proper hygiene after toileting, avoiding prolonged soaking in a bubble bath and soap to the vaginal area in prepubertal females, removing chemical irritants, and rectifying humid conditions in the vaginal area.

> **Clinical Pearl:** If vulvovaginitis does not improve with changes in hygiene, consider evaluating or treating for pinworms, as they may present as vulvovaginitis in girls.

Electronic Resources

UTI Risk Calculator (UTICalc):
https://uticalc.pitt.edu

Gynecologic System

With the average age of menarche at 12 ½ years old, gynecologic complaints are quite common in pediatrics, especially if you are in a setting that cares for tweens and teens on a regular basis. Although problems with menses are the most prevalent concerns, issues surrounding sexarche, family planning, and high-risk sexual behaviors also fall under the purview of the pediatric provider.

Dysmenorrhea

Etiology

Caused by high levels of prostaglandin $F_2\alpha$, uterine contractions, along with hypersensitive pain fibers, are the root of the dysmenorrhea (painful periods in the absence of pathology).[37]

Epidemiology

Some studies have reported up to 90% of adolescent girls complain of dysmenorrhea, with increasing prevalence up to the peak age in the mid-20s. Of 90% of females with dysmenorrhea, 15% consider their symptoms severe or disabling enough to miss school.[54]

Clinical Presentation

Starting days to hours prior to menstrual flow, dysmenorrhea is described as cramping or "labor-like" pain with pain in the lower abdomen that may radiate to the back or upper thighs. The pain may be associated with nausea or vomiting. The pelvic exam may reveal lower abdominal tenderness or uterine tenderness, but otherwise is normal. Dysmenorrhea secondary to other pathologic causes may be associated with metromenorrhagia, vaginal discharge, pain with intercourse, and abnormal findings on physical exam.[54]

Diagnosis

Diagnosis is typically made clinically after collecting a thorough history and performing a pelvic exam, if the patient is sexually active. If a secondary cause of dysmenorrhea is suspected, a pelvic exam is mandatory and will typically be followed by pelvic imaging.

Management

Primary dysmenorrhea can be managed in a stepwise fashion with increasingly more potent treatments that act at the myometrium and target suppression of ovulation and subsequent withdrawal bleeding/menstruation. Figure 2.6 shows a pragmatic approach to dysmenorrhea in adolescent patients.

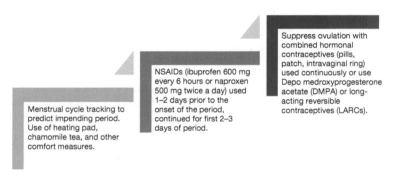

Suppress ovulation with combined hormonal contraceptives (pills, patch, intravaginal ring) used continuously or use Depo medroxyprogesterone acetate (DMPA) or long-acting reversible contraceptives (LARCs).

NSAIDs (ibuprofen 600 mg every 6 hours or naproxen 500 mg twice a day) used 1–2 days prior to the onset of the period, continued for first 2–3 days of period.

Menstrual cycle tracking to predict impending period. Use of heating pad, chamomile tea, and other comfort measures.

Figure 2.6. Stepwise approach to dysmenorrhea treatment.
NSAIDs, nonsteroidal antiinflammatory drugs.

Ectopic Pregnancy

Etiology

Implantation of a zygote with rapid cellular division and increasing size into any structure outside of the uterine cavity causes the symptoms of an ectopic pregnancy. It is well documented that a history of a previous ectopic pregnancy or tubal surgery, along with pelvic infections and smoking, increase the risk of ectopic pregnancy. Although effective in preventing pregnancy and ectopic pregnancy, if a contraceptive method fails, those women using intrauterine devices and progesterone-only contraception have a higher risk of an ectopic pregnancy than those using combined hormonal contraceptives.[55]

Epidemiology

It is estimated that ~2% of pregnancies are ectopic, with Black women affected almost twice that of White women and multigravida women affected significantly more often than nulliparous women.[56]

Clinical Presentation

You should suspect an ectopic pregnancy in any women of childbearing age who present with abdominal pain, vaginal bleeding, and a history of 6 to 8 weeks of amenorrhea. An ectopic pregnancy can be confused with appendicitis, ovarian torsion, pelvic inflammatory disease (PID), nephrolithiasis, and a ruptured ovarian cyst, as it may present with lower abdominal pain, guarding, rebound tenderness, cervical motion tenderness, and sometimes a palpable adnexal mass. However, nearly 40% of ectopic pregnancies present with only abdominal pain and vaginal bleeding without any other risk factors or physical exam findings.[57]

Diagnosis

A positive urine pregnancy test, beta-hCG levels and transvaginal US are used in combination to confirm diagnosis of an ectopic pregnancy. The algorithm shown in Figure 2.7 demonstrates how the diagnostic modalities are used synergistically.

Management

As with all conditions, patient stabilization is the number one priority. If the patient is unstable or presents with signs of shock, immediate critical care should be sought with an emergent surgical consultation awaiting the patient's arrival. If the patient is stable, medical management may include methotrexate, and surgical management may include a laparoscopic salpingostomy.[57]

PELVIC INFLAMMATORY DISEASE

Etiology

Infection of the upper reproductive tract occurs when organisms ascend into the uterus, fallopian tubes, and rarely, the peritoneum. Although pelvic inflammatory disease (PID) is classically considered a sexually transmitted disease associated with *Neisseria gonorrhoea* and *Chlamydia trachomatis*, normal genital flora, enteric bacteria, and respiratory organisms have been found to cause nearly 70% of PID cases.[58]

Epidemiology

Disproportionately higher rates of PID are seen in adolescents and minority women, with nearly 200,000 cases annually. Teens who initiate vaginal intercourse at younger than 15 years of age, have multiple sexual partners, and who do not use hormonal contraception are at higher risk of PID.[59] Hormonal contraception increases the cervical mucus barrier, thus reducing the ascension of bacteria into the endometrial cavity.

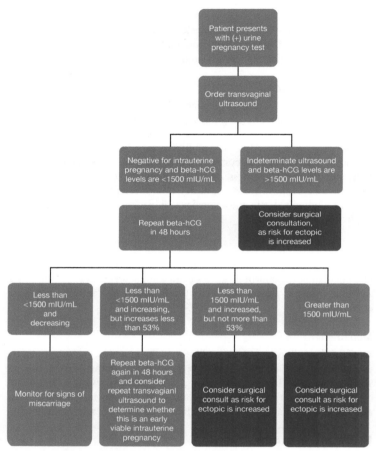

FIGURE 2.7. Ectopic pregnancy algorithm.
HCG, human chorionic gonadotropin.

Clinical Presentation

The classically described presentation for PID of acute onset of lower abdominal pain and a positive "chandelier sign" or cervical motion tenderness (CMT) on exam is actually fairly rare and most women with PID will present with mild nonspecific abdominal pain, vaginal discharge, bleeding, or dyspareunia.[58] Some may present with fever (>38.3°C) as well. Therefore, any patient at risk for an STI, with a positive STI screen for *N. gonorrhoea/C. trachomatis* or with wet-mount findings consistent with bacterial vaginosis, should have PID in the differential.

Diagnosis

As there is a large proportion of adolescents who will present with "silent" PID, the diagnosis is often made clinically and empirically based on the current Centers for Disease Control and Prevention (CDC) recommendations.[60] The CDC currently recommends women with lower abdominal or pelvic pain with uterine, adnexal, **or** CMT be diagnosed with PID. Mucopurulent discharge with WBCs on saline microscopy can also help solidify the diagnosis. If the patient is febrile, many practitioners will evaluate the patient with a CBC and acute phase reactants. An elevated ESR or CRP is also considered a supportive clinical finding for the diagnosis of PID.

Management

Treatment of PID should begin immediately upon clinical diagnosis. If cultures are not already available, genital swabs for *N. gonorrhoeae*/*C. trachomatis* nucleic acid amplification test (NAAT) should be taken prior to initiating antibiotic therapy. A presumptive diagnosis of PID should also warrant an HIV test.

The decision to hospitalize a patient for PID treatment should be made on an individual basis, taking into consideration the patient's appearance, severity of illness, ability to tolerate oral medications, patient adherence, and the possibility of comorbid conditions such as pregnancy, tubo-ovarian abscess, appendicitis, and so on. Inpatient treatment of PID consists of parenteral second-generation cephalosporins (cefoxitin 2 g IV every 6 hours or cefotetan 2 g IV every 12 hours) until clinical improvement for 24 to 48 hours. Oral doxycycline (100 mg twice a day for 14 days) can be added after improvement is noted.

Outpatient treatment of PID consists of a broad-spectrum antibiotic regimen that includes an injectable cephalosporin (ceftriaxone 250 mg IM once or cefoxitin 2 g IM once), oral doxycycline (100 mg twice daily for 14 days), and oral metronidazole (500 mg twice a day for 14 days).[60] Patients treated in the outpatient setting should be monitored closely with follow-up in 72 hours to assess for clinical improvement.

Educating teens with PID about disease transmission, abstaining from intercourse while completing treatment, and partner notification and treatment are essential. The CDC also recommends that any female diagnosed with chlamydial or gonococcal PID be retested 3 months after treatment or as soon as possible after the 3-month anniversary.[60] Because human papillomavirus (HPV) infection is also high during adolescence, you should consider providing the unvaccinated patient with HPV, hepatitis B, and hepatitis A vaccinations after she shows clinical improvement.

SEXUALLY TRANSMITTED INFECTIONS

Etiology

Generally speaking, STIs occur when bacteria, viruses, fungus, and/or parasites are transferred from one human to another via bodily fluids/secretions. As sexual intercourse is an intimate comingling of bodily fluids, some organisms thrive in this environment and are easily passed from one person to another. The bacterial diseases commonly associated with STIs include *Mycoplasma genitalium, C. trachomatis, N. gonorrhoeae, Treponema pallidum,* and bacterial vaginosis, whereas trichomoniasis, scabies and lice are the most common parasitic diseases. The viral STIs include HIV, genital herpes, and HPV. Fungi can also cause STIs, most notably *Candida albicans*, which is the cause of vulvovaginal candidiasis.

Epidemiology

The CDC estimates that 10 million new STIs occur every year in the United States, but only 12% of adolescents are tested for STIs each year.[61] Chlamydia is the most commonly reported STI at nearly 770,000 adolescent and young-adult cases in 2017.[62] Rising rates of syphilis and gonorrhea are occurring in gay adolescent males.

Clinical Presentation

The various STIs present a multitude of symptoms; Table 2.17 shows the most common presentations for each of the STIs.

TABLE 2.17. Common STIs and Their Clinical Presentations

Clinical Presentation	Common Causative STIs	Classic Signs and Symptoms
Urethritis	Gonorrhea	Symptoms start 4 days to 2 weeks after contact and men may be asymptomatic or may present with yellow, green, brown, or blood-tinged discharge; dysuria at the meatus and distal penis; urethral itching; orchalgia; fever and chills are usually absent, but if present may represent disseminated disease. Some patients may present with joint pain and a reactive arthritis.
	Chlamydia	May be asymptomatic or may present with subacute dysuria without discharge.
Epididymitis	GC/CT Enteric organisms	Gradual onset of unilateral scrotal pain accompanied by dysuria, frequency, and/or urgency. A large majority of younger patients with epididymitis present with fever and chills.
Cervicitis	Chlamydia Gonorrhea	Often asymptomatic and diagnosed on clinical exam by visualizing a purulent or mucopurulent endocervical exudate at/in the cervical os with an erythematous or friable endocervical canal. If symptoms are present, they are usually vague and include increased vaginal discharge, dysuria, urinary frequency, and breakthrough bleeding or postcoital bleeding.
PID	GC/CT Respiratory, enteric, vaginal flora	Rarely presents as acute abdominal pain with a (+) chandelier sign and instead is more likely to cause mild nonspecific abdominal pain, vaginal discharge, bleeding, or dyspareunia.

(continued)

TABLE 2.17. Common STIs and Their Clinical Presentations (*continued*)

Clinical Presentation	Common Causative STIs	Classic Signs and Symptoms
Recurrent or persistent urethritis, cervicitis, or PID	*Mycoplasma genitalium*	Will present similarly to urethritis, cervicitis, or PID as described previously, but symptoms will usually not abate after treatment.
Genital ulcers	Genital herpes	Genital herpes may present with a foreshadowing itch or tingle before the actual appearance of a blister. The vesicle ulcerates and may take 2–4 weeks for complete crusting and healing. The lesions may be associated with dysuria.
	Syphilis	Primary syphilis manifests as firm, round, and painless ulcers or chancre on/or around the anogenital area. Secondary syphilis presents with a nonpruritic, faint, rough, red or reddish-brown rash on the palms and soles. The rash may or may not be accompanied by a fever, lymphadenopathy, pharyngitis, and constitutional symptoms such as headaches, weight loss, myalgia, and fatigue. Tertiary syphilis is unlikely in pediatric rotation, so details are not included here.
Genital warts	HPV	Painless, clusters of irregularly shaped bumps that appear more commonly on the penile shaft or vulvovaginal and cervical areas. They may appear pearly, filiform, fungating, cauliflower, or plaquelike.[63]
Vaginal discharge	Bacterial vaginosis	Initial and most common symptom is a fishy vaginal odor after intercourse. It may present with moderately increased gray, thin, homogenous, and mildly adherent discharge. Small bubbles may be observed in the fluid,[64] but the external and internal mucosa appears normal without evidence of inflammation.
	Trichomoniasis	Classically described as a "frothy" greenish-gray vaginal discharge with vulvovaginal pruritus. Exam may reveal petechiae, or "strawberry cervix." If infecting the urethra or Skene's glands, it may be asymptomatic.
	Vulvovaginal candidiasis	Vulvar burning and pruritus that causes vulvar erythema and edema. Associated discharge is thick, white, adherent, and curd like.
Pruritus	Scabies	Classically presents as intractable nocturnal pruritus with papules and vesicles found on the scrotum and penile shaft for men and areola for women. Burrow lines are pathognomonic for scabies.

(*continued*)

TABLE **2.17.** Common STIs and Their Clinical Presentations (*continued*)

Clinical Presentation	Common Causative STIs	Classic Signs and Symptoms
	Lice	Migratory itching and burning in the genital, axillary, and intertriginous areas is the hallmark of lice infestation. Wheals may also be found as a reaction to the lice. As with scabies, itching is often worse at night.
Flu-like symptoms	HIV	It is important to have a high index of suspicion, as primary HIV infection may be confused with other illnesses that present with fever, fatigue, rash, headache, nausea, vomiting, diarrhea, and pharyngitis. Only a small proportion of patients present with painful ulcers on the mouth or genitalia.

GC/CT, gonorrhea and chlamydia; HPV, human papillomavirus; PID, pelvic inflammatory disease; STI, sexually transmitted infection.

Diagnosis

Diagnosis is typically made using viral or bacterial cultures, in-office microscopy with wet mount or KOH prep, NAAT, or skin scrapings. Table 2.18 notes diagnostic methods for the most common STIs.

Management

Treatment of STIs is complicated and requires specific treatment guidelines to ensure eradication of the infection. Table 2.18 gives a brief overview of the first-line treatment recommended by the CDC, but the CDC also provides more extensive treatment guidelines by organism and can be accessed at itunes.apple.com/us/app/std-tx-guide/id655206856?mt=8 (Apple platform) or play.google.com/store/apps/details?id=gov.cdc.stdtxguide&hl=en (Android platform).

TABLE **2.18.** Common Sexually Transmitted Infections and Their Diagnoses and Treatments

Clinical Presentation	Diagnosis	Treatment
Urethritis	NAAT	Azithromycin 1 g PO × 1 **OR** Doxycycline 100 mg PO BID × 7 days
	NAAT	Ceftriaxone 250 mg IM × 1 **AND** Azithromycin 1 g PO × 1
Persistent or recurrent urethritis, cervicitis, or PID	NAAT—clinical research setting only	No clinical trials have been done, but based on drug MOA, moxifloxacin 400 mg PO QD × 14 days can be considered for recurrent or persistent infections

(*continued*)

TABLE 2.18. Common Sexually Transmitted Infections and Their Diagnoses and Treatments (*continued*)

Clinical Presentation	Diagnosis	Treatment
Epididymitis	NAAT	See GC/CT treatments previously described
	Gram stain of urethral discharge, if present	Levofloxacin 500 mg PO QD × 10 days
Cervicitis	NAAT	See GC/CT treatments previously described
PID	NAAT	See treatment options under PID
	Wet mount and KOH microscopy that evaluates fluid for leukorrhea (>10 WBC/high-power field; >1 WBC/epithelial cell); leukorrhea is the most sensitive laboratory indicator of PID; the absence of leukorrhea is a negative predictor of PID	
Genital ulcers	Viral culture	Acyclovir 400 mg PO TID × 7–10 days
	Positive nontreponemal test, such as VDRL or RPR, must be confirmed by a treponemal test such as FTA-ABS or an EIA	Penicillin G 2.4 million units IM × 1
Genital warts	Clinical exam or Pap smear of lesions	Imiquimod 5% cream AAA prior to sleep and leave on skin for 8 hours; wash with mild soap; repeat three times a week until total clearance of warts or for a maximum of 16 weeks
Vaginal discharge	Saline wet-mount microscopy that demonstrates clue cells, a pH >4.5 and a (+) whiff test	Metronidazole 0.75% gel 5g intravaginally QD × 5 days
	Wet-mount microscopy with motile trichomonads and a pH >4.5 or *Trichomonas vaginalis* culture	Metronidazole 2 g PO × 1
	Microscopic identification of Candida via wet mount or KOH preparation	Clotrimazole 2% cream 5g intravaginally QD × 3 days
Pruritus	Visualization of live lice or nits; Wood's lamp will cause nits to fluoresce yellow-green	Permethrin 1% cream rinse AAA and wash off after 10 minutes

(*continued*)

TABLE 2.18. Common Sexually Transmitted Infections and Their Diagnoses and Treatments (*continued*)

Clinical Presentation	Diagnosis	Treatment
	Clinically if linear burrows are seen; confirm with skin scraping viewed under microscopy	Apply permethrin 5% cream from neck down; rnse off after 8–14 hours
Flu-like symptoms	Blood test for EIA	Treatment regimen is complex and outside the scope of this book

AAA, applied to affected area; BID, twice a day; EIA, enzyme immunoassay; FTA-ABS, fluorescent treponemal antibody absorbed; GC/CT, gonorrhea and chlamydia; HPV, human papillomavirus; HSV, herpes simplex virus; IM, intramuscular; KOH, potassium hydroxide; MOA, mechanism of action; NAAT, nucleic acid amplification test; PID, pelvic inflammatory disease; PO, per os; QD, quaque die; RPR, rapid plasma reagin; TID, ter in die; VDRL, Venereal Disease Research Laboratory; WBC, white blood cell.

Sources: Adapted from Workowski KA, Bolan GA. Sexually transmitted diseases treatment guidelines, 2015. *MMWR Recomm Rep.* 2015;64(3):78–82. https://www.cdc.gov/mmwr/preview/mmwrhtml/rr6403a1.htm; Tough DeSapri KA, Christmas MM. Pelvic inflammatory disease workup. In: Karjane NW, ed. Medscape. https://emedicine.medscape.com/article/256448-workup#c7. Updated May 3, 2019

HEAD, EYES, EARS, NOSE, AND THROAT (HEENT)

Otolaryngologic disorders comprise more than 25% of a pediatric primary care provider's daily practice. Families present with children complaining of ear pain, ear discharge, and hearing changes, as well as persistent or purulent runny noses, mouth sores, and sore throats. Once again, taking a good history and performing a good, focused, exam will usually lead you down the correct path to the appropriate diagnosis.

ACUTE OTITIS MEDIA

Etiology

Acute otitis media (AOM) is one of the most frequent reasons children visit their primary care providers. Infants, toddlers, and younger children tend to be more at risk for bacterial infections of the ear because of the angle of the eustachian tubes and their immature immune systems. Most patients will have a viral upper respiratory infection (URI) that instigates the AOM by causing increased pressure and inflammation in the upper respiratory tract. The microbiologic organisms attributed to AOM have changed over the past 20 years due to introduction of vaccines. The pneumococcal-7 vaccine helped to reduce some types of AOM but saw an increase in other serotypes. When the pneumococcal-13 vaccine was introduced in the early 2000s, the number of bacterial AOM cases attributed with *Streptococcus pneumoniae* decreased and even young infants appeared to have some protection due to herd immunity.

Streptococcus pneumoniae is still the most frequently obtained organism in AOM. Other microbes that cause AOM include *Haemophilus influenza* (Hi) and *Moraxella catarrhalis*. Vaccination with the *H.influenza* type B vaccine (HiB) did not help reduce the number of AOM cases as many of the infections caused by Hi are caused by nontypeable serotypes. A common AOM syndrome is otitis–conjunctivitis complex caused by a nontypeable *H.influenza* (NTHi), which is important to identify as NTHi is resistant to most first-line agents. Many children present to their primary care provider with symptoms consistent with viral AOM and these patients tend to have other symptoms of upper respiratory infection.[65]

CLINICAL PEARL: Acute otitis media is the second most frequent diagnosis made by pediatricians and is the most common indication for antibiotic use in children in North America.

Epidemiology

Despite advances in medicine and with vaccines, the number of visits to primary care providers for the diagnosis of otitis media (OM) has increased. OM can occur in all pediatric age groups but is most commonly seen in those between 3 and 36 months. Those who attend day care or spend their day surrounded by larger groups of children, those with a family history of OM, those with immunodeficiency, and children who live with a cigarette smoker have a higher risk of recurrent OM.

Clinical Presentation

Unilateral or bilateral otalgia is the most common symptom in children older than 2 years and is a great predictor of AOM. Infants and children with AOM may present with nonspecific symptoms and signs, including fever, irritability, headache, apathy, disturbed or restless sleep, poor feeding/anorexia, dizziness, and/or vomiting.

Diagnosis

The diagnosis of AOM must include signs of sudden onset (<48 hours) of inflammation and middle ear effusion. Acute inflammation may include bulging or erythema of the tympanic membrane (TM), fever, and otalgia. Middle ear effusion may be indicated by an air–fluid level or decreased mobility of the TM with pneumatic otoscopy. Children will often have a fever but a temperature higher than 40°C (104°F) is unusual.

Management

Pain is a common symptom of AOM and analgesics (acetaminophen or ibuprofen) should be utilized with or without concurrent antibiotics. Treatment of uncomplicated AOM can range from observation to oral antibiotics. The AAP recommends amoxicillin for most patients and their recommended dose is 90 mg/kg/d divided in two doses. They recommend treating children younger than 2 years for 10 days and those 2 years and older for 5 to 7 days. For children with severe otalgia, recurrent symptoms, or those refractive to amoxicillin, consider changing the antibiotic after 48 to 72 hours or refer to an ear, nose, and throat (ENT) specialist to consider tympanostomy tubes. Additional recommendations for specific antimicrobials can be found on the AAP's website.

> **CLINICAL PEARL:** Most children recover well from acute otitis media, even without antibiotic therapy. In most patients, the choice of treatment is empirical and should be based on the available local epidemiologic information on the most common pathogens and their susceptibility patterns.

GINGIVOSTOMATITIS AND HERPANGINA

Etiology
Gingivostomatitis is an enanthem caused by the herpes simplex virus, while herpangina is an enanthem caused by Group A coxsackievirus.

Epidemiology
All ages can be affected by both the herpes and coxsackieviruses, but both tend to be more devastating in infants and younger children.

Table 2.19 describes the differences in clinical presentation, diagnosis, and management of gingivostomatitis and herpangina.

MONONUCLEOSIS

Etiology
The Epstein–Barr virus (EBV) is responsible for infectious mononucleosis and is also known as "HHV-4".

Epidemiology
Approximately 90% of U.S. adults have antibodies to EBV but may not recall having symptoms of mononucleosis as most cases in infants and young children are mild. Mononucleosis's nickname of the "kissing disease" comes from the infection's increased risk for transmission through saliva and close personal contact.

Clinical Presentation
The typical patient with classic signs and symptoms is a teenager or young adult presenting with fever, sore throat, cervical lymphadenopathy, and significant malaise. The appearance of the anterior tonsils may be confused with streptococcal pharyngitis. Associated symptoms may include left upper quadrant abdominal pain or tenderness from splenomegaly.

TABLE **2.19.** Gingivostomatitis and Herpangina: Clinical Presentation, Diagnosis, and Management

Disease		Clinical Presentation/Diagnosis	Management
Gingivostomatitis	Herpes simplex virus (all ages affected but occurs more often in infants and children)	Ulcerative lesions of gingiva and mucous membranes usually begin 1 week after contact with source. The eruption on the oral mucosa begins with red, edematous marginal gingivae that bleed easily and clusters of small vesicles. The vesicles become yellow after rupture and are surrounded by a red halo. Vesicles coalesce to form large, painful ulcers of the oral mucosa. Associated symptoms include fatigue, fever, malaise, and cervical lymphadenopathy. Diagnosis is usually made clinically but viral culture and serology may be used PRN to identify HSV-1.	Fluid management is the most important aspect to prevent dehydration. Analgesics and antipyretics, such as acetaminophen and ibuprofen, are helpful for painful lesions. Most patients will not need oral antivirals but for immunocompromised patients and those with severe pain, a 7-day course of oral acyclovir is appropriate.
Herpangina	Group A Coxsackievirus	Onset of symptoms may be sudden and begins with high fever (40°C) and sore throat. Additional symptoms may include neck stiffness, cervical lymphadenopathy, headache, and malaise. Papules usually erupt on anterior tonsils and occasionally on hard palate and tongue. After 24 hours the papules become vesicles and these usually measure 1 to 2 mm in diameter and are surrounded by an areola of erythema. After approximately 24 hours, the vesicles rupture, leaving shallow, yellow/grayish ulcerations 3 to 4 mm in diameter, with a rim of intense erythema. Diagnosis is usually made clinically but viral cultures and serology may be used PRN to identify Coxsackievirus.	Supportive measures are the mainstay of treatment for herpangina as there are no antiviral medications available. Analgesics are helpful and hydration will help manage this generally mild illness. If patients are not able to manage oral hydration due to painful oral lesions, hospitalization should be considered to start IVF and analgesia.

HSV, herpes simplex virus; IVF, in vitro fertilization; PRN, pro re nata.

> **CLINICAL PEARL:** Patients with Epstein–Barr virus (EBV) who are treated with ampicillin or amoxicillin after a misdiagnosis of streptococcal pharyngitis may return a few days later complaining of a generalized rash covering the face, neck, trunk, and extremities. This rash usually resolves within a week of discontinuing the antibiotic and is not due to an allergic reaction to the medication.

Diagnosis

The heterophile antibody response primarily is IgM, which spikes during the first 2 weeks of illness and gradually disappears over a 6-month period. Heterophile antibody tests (including the rapid monospot) identify approximately 85% of cases of classic infectious mononucleosis in older children and adults during the second week of illness but there may be an increase in false negative results when the test is performed earlier. An absolute increase in atypical lymphocytes during the second week of illness with infectious mononucleosis is a characteristic but nonspecific finding.

Serology for EBV is available in a variety of antibody tests or can be ordered as a panel. The most commonly performed test is for antibody against the viral capsid antigen (VCA). Because IgG antibodies against VCA occur in high titer early in infection and persist for life, testing of acute and convalescent serum specimens for anti-VCA may not be useful for establishing the presence of active infection. Testing for presence of IgM anti-VCA antibody and the absence of antibodies to Epstein–Barr nuclear antigen (EBNA) is useful for identifying active and recent infections. Because serum antibody against EBNA is not present until several weeks to months after onset of infection, a positive anti-EBNA antibody test excludes an active primary infection.[66]

Management

Patients are advised to increase fluid intake and may take analgesics for sore throat and fever. Prescribe rest, reduced activity, and reassure patients that symptoms usually improve in 3 to 6 weeks. Occasionally, oral steroids are required for severe tonsillar hypertrophy, hepatosplenomegaly, hemolytic anemia, and myocarditis. Athletes should be restricted from contact sports until symptoms have improved and the spleen is no longer palpable. Splenomegaly can be determined by palpation of an enlarged spleen, but clinical studies have shown historically that palpation has poor sensitivity. Imaging modalities, such as ultrasonography or CT, offer greater sensitivity and accuracy and may be useful in determining whether an athlete safely can be returned to competition in a contact sport.[66]

SINUSITIS

Etiology

Sinusitis, also known as "rhinosinusitis," may be caused by myriad viruses and bacteria. The most common bacterial causes are *H.influenzae* (nontypeable), *S. pneumoniae*, and *M.catarrhalis*.

It is essential that the primary care clinician understand the differences between the signs and symptoms of a viral sinusitis and a bacterial sinusitis as to avoid antibiotic overprescribing. Table 2.20 differentiates these signs and symptoms of various types of sinusitis. Most viral sinusitis begins with 2 to 3 days of fever; sore throat; cough; clear nasal drainage; intermittent, alternating nasal congestion; and headache. Most viral sinusitis infections resolve within 7 to 10 days. The risk for bacterial infection of the paranasal sinuses begins with a viral URI, especially if the patient has increased chronic risk factors such as concomitant allergic rhinitis, nasal polyps, first- or secondhand cigarette smoke exposure, abnormal anatomy of the nose or sinus openings, and has recurrent symptoms. Children do not have preformed frontal bone sinuses as these tend to develop by around 6 years of age.

> **CLINICAL PEARL:** The paranasal sinuses consist of four paired cavities or collections of air cells—maxillary, ethmoid, frontal, and sphenoid sinuses—that ultimately drain into the nasal cavity via channels called ostia. The paranasal sinuses are in close proximity to the orbits and intracranial cavity.

TABLE 2.20. Signs and Symptoms of Bacterial and Viral Sinusitis

Symptoms and Signs	Viral Sinusitis	Bacterial Sinusitis
Fever	Early in course for 1–2 days	Fever worsens after day 7 as infection worsens
Headache and/or facial pain	Early: First 3–5 days; diffuse facial tenderness	Worsens after day 7 regionally over infected sinus
Cough	Yes	No
Purulent nasal drainage	No	Yes
Appearance of nasal mucous membranes	Pale to mildly erythematous, boggy, and mild anterior/inferior turbinate hypertrophy	Moderate to severe erythema and anterior/inferior turbinate hypertrophy; purulent drainage may be visible

Diagnosis

A diagnosis of acute bacterial rhinosinusitis (ABRS) may be reached clinically as nasal cultures are rarely obtained to determine the cause of infection.

Antimicrobial therapy should be initiated at the time of presentation for children with ABRS who also have:

- A clinical presentation of severe symptoms or worsening symptoms
- Complications or suspected complications
- Recent use of antibiotics in the previous 4 weeks
- Concurrent bacterial infection (e.g., pneumonia, group A streptococcal pharyngitis, AOM)
- Certain underlying conditions, including asthma, cystic fibrosis, immunodeficiency, previous sinus surgery, or anatomic abnormalities of the upper respiratory tract

Management

When initiating antibiotics, the primary care clinician should consider antimicrobial coverage, including *S.pneumoniae, H.influenzae,* and *M.catarrhalis.* The proportion of isolates of *S.pneumoniae* that are not susceptible to penicillin varies from community to community. Isolates obtained from surveillance centers nationwide indicate that 10% to 15% of upper respiratory tract isolates of *S.pneumoniae* are nonsusceptible to penicillin. However, values as high as 50% to 60% have been reported in some areas. First-line therapy for mild/moderate ABRS without complication is amoxicillin–clavulanate 45 mg/kg/d orally divided into two doses for 10 days. For those with penicillin allergy the following are recommended:

- For children with uncomplicated ABRS who have a severe type I allergy to penicillin, levofloxacin 10 to 20 mg/kg/d orally divided every 12 or 24 hours
- For children with uncomplicated ABRS who have a nontype I allergy to penicillin, start with a third-generation cephalosporin, such as cefdinir 14 mg/kg/d orally divided every 12 or 24 hours

Streptococcal Pharyngitis

Etiology

Pharyngitis is more commonly caused by a wide variety of viruses. Streptococcal pharyngitis is caused by Group A beta-hemolytic *Streptococcus* (GABHS).[65] Most pharyngeal infections by GABHS are benign, self-limited, and uncomplicated processes. In fact, most patients improve without any prescribed treatment. However, a small number of children will go on to develop renal and cardiac complications following GABHS infection, it is important to diagnose and treat these infections appropriately.

Epidemiology

Streptococcal pharyngitis, also known as "strep throat," is a common disease among children and adolescents, especially during the winter and spring. Close, interpersonal contact in schools and families with several children appear to be risk factors for the infection.

Clinical Presentation

Signs and symptoms of strep throat include acute onset of sore throat, fever, cervical lymphadenopathy, enlarged tonsil with exudate, headache, and occasionally stomach pain or nausea. Absence of cough, rhinorrhea, conjunctivitis, and hoarseness are important because if they are present, they help point to a viral cause.

Diagnosis

The evidence-based, validated Centor Score helps to estimate probability that a patient's pharyngitis is streptococcal and suggests a management course. Although its use in children aged 3 to 14 with symptoms for 3 days or fewer is best, the Centor criteria can help providers determine how likely it is that GABHS is the cause of their patients' symptoms in older children and adults. Using the patient's age, presence or absence of tonsillar exudate, tender or swollen anterior cervical lymph nodes, temperature higher than 38°C (100.4°F), and presence or absence of a cough, the provider can estimate the patient's likelihood of having a Group A *Streptococcus*-positive culture.

Most primary care offices will have a rapid strep test that can be completed quickly, but care should be taken to obtain the culture from the tonsils and not the hard or soft palate, buccal mucosa, or tongue. Many pediatric clinicians will swab the patient to obtain samples for a rapid strep test and swab again for a "send-out" throat culture. If the rapid test is negative but your clinical judgment, based on a Centor score of 4 or more, suspects the diagnosis of GABHS, treating the patient empirically for bacterial infection is a reasonable course. In pediatrics, backup cultures should be collected and analyzed, as 14% of GABHS infections can be missed with rapid testing alone.

Management

To date no strains of GABHS have developed penicillin resistance or increased minimum inhibitory concentrations so the drug of choice remains penicillin. The standard length of dosing for penicillin or amoxicillin is 10 days. For those who are penicillin-allergic, an azithromycin dose once daily for 5 days is a reasonable alternative. Patients should be monitored for fluid intake, analgesia, and impending suppurative complications such as peritonsillar abscess.[65]

UPPER RESPIRATORY INFECTION

Etiology

Among young children, nasopharyngitis is caused by viruses, typically in the colder months. Adenoviruses, influenza viruses, rhinoviruses, respiratory syncytial viruses, parainfluenza viruses, and enteroviruses are the most common causes of viral URIs.

Epidemiology

Children who attend day care or elementary school are exposed to viral infections throughout the year but the risk for transmission increases in the winter when they go outside less and environmental humidity drops. Rhinoviruses, parainfluenza viruses, and respiratory syncytial viruses tend to occur more often in infants and preschool children, whereas adenovirus is more common in older children and adolescents. Influenza viruses frequently affect all age groups.

Clinical Presentation

Children will present with typical common-cold symptoms such as sudden onset of fever, chills, headache, sore throat, nasal drainage, rhinitis, nasal congestion, cough, myalgias, arthralgias, malaise, and GI upset.

Diagnosis

Diagnosis is usually made on clinical judgment, although there are rapid tests available for influenza and respiratory syncytial virus. There are further serological and polymerase chain reaction (PCR) tests available if an exact diagnosis is required.

Management

Supportive measures, such as control of fever, hydration, and analgesia, are the mainstay for most viral URIs. Parents must be given reassurance and specific instructions for return to clinic if symptoms worsen.

MUSCULOSKELETAL/RHEUMATOLOGIC SYSTEM

Unlike adults, musculoskeletal disorders seen in pediatrics are often related to the unique anatomy associated with powerful ligamentous structures, open growth plates, and growth spurts. Although trauma is a leading cause of musculoskeletal pain in both adults and children, the majority of musculoskeletal problems in pediatrics are adeptly managed in the primary care setting. The musculoskeletal problems reviewed in this section represent only a small sample of possible diagnoses in the pediatric years.

CHONDROMALACIA PATELLAE: SECONDARY TO PATELLOFEMORAL SYNDROME

Etiology

Caused by tightness or weakness of the muscles associated with the knee, abnormal patellar positioning (patellofemoral syndrome) creates uneven wear on the femur and underside of the patella as it rubs against the patellar groove of the femur. This misalignment, combined with continued flexing and extending at the knee, leads to loss of protective cartilage and subsequent femur and patellar contact with inflammation and pain (chondromalacia patellae). Pes planus can contribute to chondromalacia patellae as well, as the anatomic posture turns medially, placing uneven stress at the patella.

Epidemiology

With a female predominance, chondromalacia patellae is also more common in those who are exercising regularly and, ironically, in those who are overweight. Frequency of chondromalacia patellae increases in adolescence; however, it can be seen in children as young as 6 or 7 years old.

Clinical Presentation

Patients typically report knee pain on the front or sides of the knee that is worsened with walking up and down stairs, squatting, or when getting up from sitting for prolonged periods of time. Patients may also describe crepitus at the knee, a fullness or tightness at the knee, and rarely swelling. On exam, compression of the patella while tightening of the quadriceps produces pain.

Diagnosis

Clinically diagnosed in most cases, especially with classic history and physical exam findings in a female teenage athlete, imaging is rarely needed unless symptoms do not improve with conservative management or if you suspect trauma.[67]

Management

For most patients, RICE (**r**est, **i**ce, **c**ompression, and **e**levation) therapy, nonsteroidal anti-inflammatory drugs (NSAIDs) and strengthening of quadriceps, hip adductor, and hamstring are able to halt the patellofemoral pain and control the symptoms. Physical therapy, bracing, and orthotic supports can help correct mechanical forces to relieve the underlying pathology.

DEVELOPMENTAL DYSPLASIA OF THE HIP

Etiology

Developmental dysplasia of the hip (DDH) is thought to occur secondary to abnormal development of the hip and/or its associated structures. This may include abnormal ossification of the acetabulum or femoral head, abnormal formation of the labrum, hip capsule, or other ligamentous structures of the hip. Thus, DDH ranges from instability to dislocation with or without a malformed acetabula. A shallow acetabulum at birth, along with ligamentous laxity, may allow for flattening of the femoral head and subsequent instability.

Epidemiology

Noted in about one in 1,000 births, DDH is more prevalent in females born in a breech position. A total of 75% of all DDH diagnoses are made in females. Breech position late in pregnancy is correlated with DDH in up to 25% of DDH diagnoses. Family history of a parent with DDH increases the risk for DDH 12 times. According to Shaw and Segal, the left hip is more commonly affected than the right hip.[68] White infants are diagnosed more than Black infants.[69]

> **CLINICAL PEARL:** The four Fs can help you remember the risk factors for developmental dysplasia of the hip (DDH). A **f**irstborn **f**emale, who was born **f**eet first with a **f**amily history of DDH.

Clinical Presentation

Because newborns are asymptomatic as they are not yet weight bearing and walking, physical exam techniques currently serve as a screening exam for hip dysplasia.[68] Detecting limb length discrepancies, asymmetric thigh or gluteal creases, instability on Ortolani test, and limitation in abduction should be done periodically during well-child exams.

> **CLINICAL PEARL:** To remember which test does which component of the hip exam, remember Ortolani pushes the hip out and Barlow pushes it back in.

Diagnosis

If a screening exam technique is positive or an infant is in a higher risk group, hip ultrasonography can be considered between the ages of 6 weeks and 6 months; anteroposterior and frog pelvis x-rays can be considered after 4 months of age.

> **CLINICAL PEARL:** You need to order ultrasound to confirm exam findings until the infant is 4 months old, as the hip is not sufficiently ossified until after this time.

Management

Referral to an orthopedist for evaluation and management of unstable or dislocated hip on clinical examination is appropriate. However, any child with limited hip abduction or asymmetric hip abduction after 1 month of age, an infant with risk factors, and any questionable examination should also be referred to a pediatric orthopedist. The orthopedist will likely manage confirmed hip dysplasia with the use of a Pavlik harness, but may manage US abnormalities without clinical findings with close monitoring.[68]

DISLOCATION

Etiology

Trauma is the leading cause of dislocations in children and many are associated with fracture. The main exceptions are a nursemaid's elbow and DDH. In children younger than 5, a dislocation can occur without fracture due to the strength of ligaments in young children. Dislocation from trauma may occur in any joint, but are most common in the hip, knee, or finger.

Epidemiology

Joint dislocations are rare in children, with the exception of subluxation of the radial head and DDH.

Clinical Presentation

The child will be in significant pain regardless of the joint affected and will present with some level of deformity. Dislocations at the hip typically present after a high-velocity injury with groin or buttock pain and a shortened limb that is adducted, internally rotated, and flexed. Although most spontaneously reduce, patellar dislocations present with a history of feeling the "knee give out" while performing a rapid change in direction, a knee effusion, apprehension secondary to increased patellar mobility, and tenderness at the medial patella. Interphalangeal joint dislocations usually present with a history of hyperflexion or hyperextension during a sporting activity, pain, edema, and ecchymosis. If not treated quickly and correctly, these can result in lasting deformity.

Diagnosis

Dislocations themselves are relatively obvious on clinical exam, but radiographs are often obtained to rule out associated fractures. These should be done prior to reduction attempts.

Management

Hip dislocation: Surgical reduction under general anesthesia, immobilization, and months of physical therapy are required for a good outcome. Avascular necrosis is an unfortunate complication, particularly when treatment is delayed for longer than 6 hours.

Patellar dislocation: Treatment includes ice, rest, and knee immobilization before return to play.

Shoulder dislocation: Associated fractures of the humerus must be ruled out. Performed under sedation, reduction requires manual traction, or the use of counterweights. Recurrent shoulder dislocations usually are due to a Bankart lesion and should be managed accordingly by orthopedics.

Finger dislocation: Using local anesthesia, most finger dislocations can be reduced in the office, but when tendons have avulsed bony fragments, open reduction under general anesthesia may be necessary. The finger should remain immobilized for 14 to 21 days before buddy taping and range-of-motion (ROM) exercises can be started. Early follow-up and the involvement of an occupational therapist (OT) or physical therapist (PT) is important to prevent a proximal interphalangeal joint deformity (boutonniere injury) or a distal interphalangeal deformity (mallet finger).

JUVENILE IDIOPATHIC ARTHRITIS

Etiology

The cause of juvenile idiopathic arthritis (JIA) is unknown, but the synovium becomes inflamed and proliferates, which increases secretion of synovial fluid in the joint space. The inflammation associated with JIA results in increased blood flow to the joint and resultant swelling. Inflammation of the synovium can cause damage to cartilage, ligaments, and tendons. Eventually, the long-standing inflammation can cause bone destruction as well.[70] There are four types of JIA that are classified by the number and types of joints affected. Oligoarticular JIA affects less than five medium to large joints. Polyarticular JIA is seen in small and large joints with five or more joints affected. Enthesitis-associated JIA can affect any number of joints, but affects primarily the large joints of the lower extremities, including the sacroiliac joints. Finally, systemic JIA affects any number of small and large joints and has systemic features.

Epidemiology

As the most common rheumatologic condition, it is no surprise that there is a family history of autoimmune disease. Like many other autoimmune diseases, females are more affected than males (3–5:1 for poly- and oligoarticular JIA). Systemic JIA, however, is equally distributed between males and females.

Clinical Presentation

To meet the diagnostic criteria, a patient must have pain, swelling, decreased ROM, and stiffness in one or more joints for 6 weeks. JIA must present prior to 16 years of age or the diagnosis of rheumatoid arthritis is made. These patients may present with a limp or complaints of morning stiffness, joint swelling, or loss of ROM and function. Systemic findings, such as the salmon-pink rash, lymphadenopathy, and high fevers, can be confused with other diagnoses, such as infectious and malignant conditions.[70]

Diagnosis

There is no one particular diagnostic test for JIA, but meeting the criteria for JIA in the setting of elevated inflammatory markers and a positive antinuclear antibody (ANA) is sufficient. Only about 5% of children with JIA have a positive rheumatoid factor, so this is useful only in categorizing polyarticular JIA. Enthesitis-associated arthritis, like ankylosing spondylitis, may be associated with a positive HLA-B27 antigen.

Management

The primary goal of JIA management is to reduce inflammation and its long-term sequelae, as well as to improve function and relieve pain. NSAIDs and disease-modifying rheumatoid arthritis medications (DMARDs) are the mainstay of treatment in children, but involving a pediatric rheumatologist will help to ensure that the patient is followed appropriately for the JIA subtype and that routine screenings are appropriate for the child's condition.

LEGG–CALVE–PERTHES DISEASE

Etiology

The exact etiology of the avascular necrosis of the femoral head, also known as Legg-Calve-Perthes disease (LCP), is unclear, but it has been hypothesized that there is a congenital malformation of the vascular supply near the femoral neck. A disruption in the blood supply to the intricate neurovascular structures around the femoral neck leads to necrosis with bone fragmentation. The subsequent reossification and remodeling of the femoral head can lead to gait disturbances and potentially leg-length discrepancies, if not followed closely.

Epidemiology

Patients affected by LCP are typically skeletally immature (ranging from 4 to 10 years old) males, who are shorter than their peers. In many patients, there is a family history of LCP in a first-degree relative and there may also be a history of transient synovitis (TS).

Clinical Presentation

There is an insidious onset of a Trendelenburg gait with a persistent, dull, achy pain that refers to the anterolateral thigh and/or knee. The pain tends to worsen with activity and improves with rest, so symptoms may wax and wane for several weeks before a parent considers a visit to the pediatrician. If severe, pain may lead to disuse and subsequent atrophy of the thigh and buttocks, but the classic physical exam finding is limited internal rotation and abduction.

Diagnosis

You should have a high index of suspicion for this diagnosis in a limping child with a Trendelenburg gait, as initial plain films may be normal. Serial radiographs are needed to differentiate LCP from TS, as both can present with a widening of the medial joint space. Later radiographs may show fragmentation and then healing of the femoral head.[71] Because of the location of the avascular necrosis, it is not uncommon to see a widened and flattened femoral head that remains as a residual deformity. MRI may show marrow changes and a bone scan would show decreased perfusion of the femoral head.

Management

Long-term management of LCP is aimed at preventing hip irritation, preventing epiphyseal collapse, and attaining a spherical shape to the femoral head with reossification. For children younger than 6 years old with mild symptoms, often LCP can be managed with observation, serial x-rays, anti-inflammatories, physical therapy exercises, and avoiding high-impact activities. If the symptoms are progressive, with limited ROM or radiographic evidence of a deformity, casting or bracing may be needed to keep the femoral head in the acetabulum. For older patients or more severe initial presentation, surgical osteotomy may be necessary.[71]

LITTLE LEAGUER'S SHOULDER (OVERUSE SYNDROME)

Etiology

Little Leaguer's shoulder, or proximal humeral epiphysitis, is a shoulder injury common in skeletally immature baseball pitchers, tennis players, swimmers, and gymnasts that is thought to occur secondary to the opposing rotational and rotator cuff forces at work in overhead motions. It is unclear whether the proximal humeral pain associated with repetitive over-the-shoulder movements causes a stress fracture at the proximal humeral physis or if there is underlying proximal epiphyseal inflammation secondary to overuse.[72] Either way, the injury causes the physis of the proximal humerus to widen with demineralization, sclerosis, and/or fragmentation of the metaphysis possible.

Epidemiology

Patients between 11 and 16 years old are most commonly diagnosed with Little Leaguer's shoulder, with boys affected more often than girls. As this is a growth plate injury, patients have not yet completed puberty and may be at the height of their growth spurt.

Clinical Presentation

An athletic child or early adolescent will usually present with diffuse, proximal arm pain that has gotten progressively worse over the preceding 2 to 3 months, especially with overhead movements. Pitchers will note a decrease in their pitching velocity, along with a decreased accuracy, and the need for progressively longer recovery periods to be pain free. If examined while acutely inflamed, you may elicit pain with palpation over the lateral proximal humerus or when the shoulder is abducted and internally or externally rotated against resistance. However, there are rarely external signs suggesting effusion, atrophy, or loss of ROM.

Diagnosis

Anteroposterior in external rotation, axillary, and scapular Y x-ray views should be ordered. These will show a widening of the physis.[72]

Management

Little Leaguer's shoulder is managed with anti-inflammatories in the acutely painful phase, rest, and then physical therapy. Most athletes must stop exacerbating activities for a minimum of 3 months and use a graduated return-to-use protocol. Physical therapy is essential to strengthen the rotator cuff, stretch the posterior shoulder capsule, and build core strength. Educating the patient and the family on the risks of returning to throwing or overhead activities too soon, improper overhead shoulder mechanics, exceeding recommended pitch counts, and the importance of rest days cannot be overemphasized.

NONACCIDENTAL TRAUMA

Etiology

The cause of nonaccidental trauma (NAT) is multifactorial, with a personal history of abuse, high-stress situations with few coping skills, poverty, and care of nonbiologic children as factors that can lead to abuse. There are four recognized types of abuse: neglect, physical, sexual, and psychological. There are often several forms of abuse coexisting in an abused child's life. NAT refers primarily to the 18% of abuse categorized as physical abuse.[73]

Epidemiology

Children at risk for physical abuse are typically younger than 5 years old, the product of an unplanned pregnancy, or the firstborn. They may also have a history of being born prematurely or having a physical disability, like cerebral palsy. From a parental perspective, there may be a history of abuse for the abusing parent. Other social factors that contribute to family stress in cases of NAT include the following:

- A single-parent house
- Drug abuse
- Financial instability
- Frequent moves
- Lower socioeconomic status
- Minimal social supports

Clinical Presentation

Although there is no "classic" presentation for child abuse, there are some red flags that should make you keep child abuse/neglect high on the differential. These red flags include the following:

- A parent who delays seeking care for the child
- No history of witnessed injury or an inconsistent/changing story
- Multiple bruises or burns, as skin lesions are the number one finding in abused children
- Long-bone fractures (especially the femur) in a nonambulatory child; a total of 50% of fractures in infants younger than 1 are caused by abuse, whereas 30% of fractures in children younger than 3 years of age are attributable to abuse[73]
- Fractures that are highly correlated with physical abuse such as a corner fracture (avulsion of the metaphysis) and bucket handle fractures (horizontal avulsion fracture); both occur when there is a violent twisting or pulling of the extremity; posteromedial rib fractures indicate a grabbing mechanism, whereas scapular fractures indicate a high-velocity injury
- Fractures in various stages of healing
- Skull fractures indicate a violent and potentially life-threatening injury

Diagnosis

Suspicions of NAT are often confirmed with x-rays and a skeletal survey to evaluate for fractures in various stages of healing and the highly correlated NAT fractures noted earlier. Head injuries may need to be evaluated by CT scan to determine the severity of the injury and assess for intracranial bleeding.

Management

The first item of care for the child is to report the abuse to the appropriate agency and involve child protective services. With a diagnosis of NAT, a child should be admitted to the hospital for evaluation by medical and social services. Medical treatment of the injury should not differ from the standards used for nonabuse cases. Fractures should be reduced and/or casted; burns should be debrided, if necessary, and medicated bandages applied; and head injuries should involve neurology or neurosurgery, if these services are available.

Osgood–Schlatter Syndrome

Etiology

Repetitive contraction of the quadriceps applies a traction force to the patellar ligament, which in turn creates traction at the apophysis of the tibial tubercle. The repetitive traction creates irritation of the tibial growth plate, inflammation, and microfracturing at the apophysis.

Epidemiology

Children ages 10 to 15 years old who participate in running and jumping activities are frequently diagnosed with Osgood–Schlatter syndrome.

Clinical Presentation

There is typically a history of knee pain that is worse when starting a physical activity, after play, and when sitting with the knee flexed for prolonged periods of time. There may be a palpable prominence at the anterior tibial tubercle that is nearly always tender when pressure is applied to the area.

Diagnosis

Diagnosis is typically made clinically based on a convincing history and physical exam findings.

Management

Osgood–Schlatter is typically managed with supportive care, anti-inflammatories, ice, and elevation. If symptoms are significant, activity modification and physical therapy may need to be implemented until the patient is able to participate in activities without pain. Stretching the quadriceps and hamstrings are often a core part of the rehabilitation with Osgood–Schlatter. Educating patients and families on the course of the syndrome is important, as the symptoms may continue until the child completes his or her growth spurt. The tibial prominence typically persists despite resolution of the pain.

OSTEOMYELITIS

Etiology

Direct inoculation, spread from adjacent tissues, or hematogenous spread of an occult bacteremia underlies the infection of the femur, tibia, and fibula. As all of these bones have highly vascular metaphyses, hematogenous spread is the most common mechanism in children. Bacterial virulence factors, such as bacterial adherence, resistance to host defense mechanism, and proteolytic activity, contribute to the ability of bacteria to invade and replicate within the bone.[74] *Staphylococcus aureus* is the most common organism cultured from osteomyelitis in children.

Epidemiology

More commonly seen in children younger than 5 years old, boys are affected twice as often as girls. Typically, the incidence of osteomyelitis decreases with increasing age in pediatric patients, with the exception of patients with sickle cell disease, indwelling catheters, and immunocompromised states.

Clinical Presentation

Patients with osteomyelitis typically present with a history of vague malaise and body aches for several days prior to the onset of high fevers and a toxic appearance; severe, local tenderness over the metaphysis; and pain on palpation of the bone. These patients may tolerate passive ROM, but typically resist active ROM and weight bearing secondary to pain.

Diagnosis

Laboratory data, x-rays, and bone scan are used to confirm the diagnosis of osteomyelitis. The CBC with differential usually reveals very elevated WBC counts, whereas the ESR is usually between 50 and 100 and blood cultures confirm the occult bacteremia etiology. Alkaline phosphate, calcium, and phosphate are typically normal in osteomyelitis.[74]

Radiographs are usually negative early in the course of the disease and may not show any periosteal changes for 10 to 14 days. A bone scan will show an increased uptake of the radioactive material, but MRI has become the mainstay in most facilities, as it can evaluate for abscess and can guide surgical irrigation and drainage.

Management

As these children are toxic appearing, immediate hospitalization with orthopedic and infectious disease consultations would be appropriate. Orthopedics will debride, irrigate, and collect culture samples in the operating room. Empiric antibiotic therapy varies by age with neonates receiving vancomycin and cefotaxime and older children receiving clindamycin. Antibiotics are usually continued for 1 to 2 months and ESR and CRP levels are followed throughout the antibiotic treatment course.[75]

Septic Arthritis

Etiology

A hematogenous spread of bacteria into the highly vascular synovium and joint space or local invasion from a nearby osteomyelitis cause inflammation and infection. The most common pathogen for all age groups is *S.aureus*. Neonates may also be susceptible to Group B *Streptococcus* and some Gram-negative bacilli and toddlers to school-aged children may have septic arthritis secondary to a GABHS and *S. pneumonia* infection. Teenagers with septic arthritis should be questioned about high-risk behaviors, such as IV drug use and risky sexual behaviors, as these factors may predispose them to *Pseudomonas* and *Neisseria* infections.

Epidemiology

Primarily a disease of the very young, 50% of septic arthritis occurs in children younger than 3 years old and typically affects one joint in the lower extremity.

Clinical Presentation

Septic arthritis presents with acute onset of unilateral joint pain without a history of trauma, with the hip and knee being the most commonly affected joints. The child is typically febrile and ill-appearing and refuses to bear weight on the affected limb. If they do bear weight, an antalgic gait often accompanies the movement. If the hip is affected, when the child is at rest he or she holds the hip in flexion, abduction, and external rotation. If the knee is affected, the joint is most comfortable when partially flexed. Periarticular warmth and swelling is more notable at the knee than the hip secondary to the deep-seated structure of the hip.

Diagnosis

As this can be confused with TS, reactive arthritis, SLE, cellulitis, and osteomyelitis, laboratory data can help narrow the differential for a limping child. A CBC will reveal an elevated WBC count and the ESR and CRP will be elevated. Using Kocher's criteria of fever >38.3°C, nonweight bearing, an ESR >40, and a WBC count >12,000, a child who presents with two of the four criteria has a 40% probability of having septic arthritis. This increases to 93% with three of the criteria and 99% with all four of the criteria.[76] Definitive diagnosis is made with arthrocentesis and a positive blood culture.

Plain films are not very useful for diagnosing septic arthritis, as they may show an effusion, but they may also be normal. US and MRI with contrast are most useful for identifying joint fluid and identifying surrounding structure involvement.

Management

Collaboration with orthopedic specialists is essential in the case of septic arthritis, because the patient will likely need emergent joint aspiration to decompress the joint capsule and decrease permanent risk of cartilage and bone damage. An operative irrigation and drainage of the joint is often used in the hip or shoulder, but may be needed at other joints if a co-occurring osteomyelitis is suspected. Empiric IV antibiotics should be based on the most likely organisms, with special attention on Gram-negative coverage in neonates and adolescents. After the synovial fluid Gram stain and culture results return, directed antibiotic therapy can be determined. Antibiotics are typically continued for 4 to 6 weeks with a transition to oral antibiotics with clinical improvement and a 50% reduction in the CRP.[75]

SLIPPED CAPITAL FEMORAL EPIPHYSIS (SCFE)

Etiology

The etiology of an SCFE is not completely understood, but during periods of rapid growth there is increased mechanical force at the epiphysis[77] and the femoral head begins to slip backward at the growth plate.[78]

CLINICAL PEARL: Slipped capital femoral epiphysis (SCFE) is essentially a Salter–Harris type 1 fracture that is commonly described as a "scoop of ice cream slipping off the cone."

Epidemiology

SCFE is most commonly associated with overweight and obese tweens, with more than 75% of patients with SCFE above the 90th percentile for BMI.[75] SCFE is more common in Blacks, Hispanics, and Pacific Islanders in a 4:1 male-to-female predominance. The disease occurs shortly after the onset of puberty, with the most common age ranges between 12 and 16 in boys and 10 and 14 in girls.[78] There is some association with underlying endocrine and metabolic disorders, as well as an increased risk if there is a parent with a history of SCFE.

Clinical Presentation

The classic SCFE presentation is an early adolescent with a protracted course of nonradiating, dull, achy hip, groin, thigh or knee pain in an otherwise healthy adolescent. The pain is typically chronic or intermittent, is worse with activity, and causes a waddling, antalgic gait. There may be a history of a fall or direct trauma to the hip, but often this is not readily available in the history. The physical exam reveals stiffness, hip pain on palpation and limited internal rotation and flexion. In unstable SCFE cases, the patient may present with a leg-length discrepancy and the leg may be held in external rotation.

Diagnosis

Lateral (not frog-leg lateral) and AP hip films are usually sufficient to make the diagnosis, as they usually reveal a displacement of the capital femoral epiphysis from the femoral neck at the physeal plate.

Management

Because slippage of the capital femoral epiphysis can compromise blood supply to the femoral head, the diagnosis of an SCFE is considered an orthopedic emergency. Intervention by a pediatric orthopedist will provide the child with the best outcome and decrease the risk for arthritis as an adult. Surgical fixation is the treatment of choice for SCFE.[78]

SPRAIN/STRAIN

Etiology

Sprains (injury to a ligament) and strains (injury to a tendon or muscle) are both the result of sudden oppositional forces, such as a stretch, twist, or tear, that changes the anatomic placement of a ligament or tendon in relation to the joint or bone, respectively. In younger children, tendons are stronger than the growth plates of the bones, so when there is a stretch of the tendon or muscle, the strength of the tendon may actually create such pull on the bone that a fracture occurs.

Epidemiology

Sprains and strains are found primarily in teens and young adults, as their physes are closed and the bone strength now overpowers the ligaments, muscles, and tendons.

Clinical Presentation

A child or teen will present with a history of trauma that was followed by pain, swelling, bruising, redness, weakness and limited function. There may be point tenderness over the injured area and many of the special exam techniques for the various joints are designed to assess for muscle strain, ligamentous laxity, and tendon irritation. With a strain or a sprain, these special maneuvers may be positive and painful.

> **CLINICAL PEARL:** A young patient with a history of sudden deceleration of the leg with a simultaneous twisting motion should be evaluated for a tibial spine fracture, while an adolescent with a similar mechanism is more likely to have an anterior cruciate ligament tear.

Diagnosis

Often the diagnosis can be made on history and physical exam alone; however, if there is a question of underlying bony pathology, special testing of the affected area may be needed. X-rays are useful to ensure that there is not a concomitant fracture, whereas CT and MRI can provide detailed images of the soft tissues. This is helpful in determining the severity of the sprain/strain and may direct therapies.

> **CLINICAL PEARL:** To determine whether your patient with knee pain needs an x-ray, you can use the Ottawa Knee Rules, as it has 100% sensitivity for clinically significant fractures. The rules suggest that if a patient has isolated patellar tenderness or tenderness at the head of fibula, an inability to flex knee to 90°, or an inability to bear weight immediately after injury, *and* is unable to take four steps in the ED, you should order radiographs.

Management

For the majority of sprains and strains, the RICE protocol is sufficient for adequate recovery. Activity restrictions, splinting, remaining nonweight bearing, and anti-inflammatories are used in the early stages of injury treatment, while physical therapy can be a useful adjuvant for more serious or long-standing injuries.

SYSTEMIC LUPUS ERYTHEMATOSUS (SLE)

Etiology

SLE is an autoimmune inflammatory condition that is thought to be multifactorial in etiology. Antibody–antigen complexes are deposited in the joints, skin, kidneys, central nervous system (CNS), and serosa. These complexes elicit an inflammatory response that signals leukocytes, neutrophils, and complement to the sites. These inflammatory cells then wreak havoc at the tissue sites and cause tissue damage that can manifest as cutaneous reactions; cardiovascular inflammation; renal damage with resultant proteinuria, hematuria, and hypertension; musculoskeletal arthropathies; and CNS aberrations.

Epidemiology

Girls at the peak ages of 9 to 15 years old are more affected than boys. Genetic links to SLE have been found.

Clinical Presentation

Patients may present with any of the manifestations of localized inflammation or may present with more systemic symptoms noted earlier. The classic photosensitivity rash in a malar distribution on the cheeks and nose is the most pathognomonic symptom, but not all patients have this presentation. Some may present with a discoid rash or just a photosensitivity reaction with painless oral and nasal ulcers.

Diagnosis

The American College of Rheumatology has set criteria to establish a diagnosis of SLE. Patients must meet four of the criteria, which include the following:
- Malar rash, discoid rash, photosensitivity, and/or oral/nasal ulcerations (cutaneous)

- Arthritis (musculoskeletal)
- Proteinuria >3+ and/or cellular casts (renal abnormalities)
- Seizures or psychosis (neurologic abnormalities)
- Pericarditis (serosal involvement)
- Pleuritis (serosal involvement)
- Positive ANA with titer >1:320, anti-double stranded DNA, anti-Smith, and/or antiphospholipid antibodies (autoimmune evidence)
- Hematologic abnormalities such as anemia, leukopenia, lymphopenia, or thrombocytopenia

  If a patient meets the criteria for diagnosis and has a positive ANA (95% of children have a positive ANA), you should consider ordering an antiphospholipid antibody, as a positive antiphospholipid antibody places the child at higher risk of venous thrombosis.[79]

Management

Treatment and subspecialty involvement depend on the organ system affected and may include NSAIDs, oral steroids, DMARDs, and antimalarial medications. Patients with SLE should be referred to a pediatric rheumatologist for long-term management of the disease and help in slowing disease progression.

TORTICOLLIS

Etiology

The cause is not 100% known, but torticollis is thought to occur due to positioning in the uterus or crowding in the uterus. The sternocleidomastoid muscle (SCM) becomes tense and shortened and this causes the chin to move down and away from the side of the shortening. Prolonged positioning and tightness of the SCM leads to scarring of the musculature.

Epidemiology

Typically noted at the 1- to 2-month well-child exam, as most infants are 6 to 8 weeks old when diagnosed. Torticollis tends to occur in firstborn children and can coincide with DDH.

Clinical Presentation

Parents' biggest concern regarding torticollis is that the infant preferentially tilts his or her head to one side (75% of the time it is the right side of the neck). As the infant typically does not have full head/neck control at the time of diagnosis, passive ROM may indicate some limitations on ROM or you may feel a palpable prominence in the affected neck musculature. You may also notice some plagiocephaly secondary to preferential head position. Head position can also make breastfeeding difficult, so you should always consider torticollis on the differential for poor breastfeeding or latch difficulties.

Diagnosis

Typically this is diagnosed clinically based on history and physical exam.

Management

The standard treatment for torticollis is a referral to a physical therapist and/or a home exercise program to stretch the SCM. Parents are asked to gently turn the baby's neck side to side several times a day. Tummy time and playtime can help babies with torticollis as well. Parents can position toys and cribs so that the baby has to turn his or her head. No medications are used in primary care pediatrics for torticollis, but sometimes in specialty service, BOTOX injections can be used.

Toxic Synovitis/Transient Synovitis

Etiology

"Toxic synovitis" is quite the misnomer, as there is no toxicity or toxic appearance associated with this disease. The underlying etiology is thought to be a reactive arthritis secondary to a viral illness, as nonspecific inflammation and hypertrophy of the synovial membrane are seen and synovial fluid has increased proteoglycans.[80]

Epidemiology

TS is the most common cause of limping and hip pain in the United States. Males between the ages of 3 and 10 years old are twice as likely as females to be diagnosed with TS.

Clinical Presentation

Patients with TS may present with a protracted course of hip pain without a clear precipitant, but there may be a history of preceding viral URI or diarrheal infection. These patients are typically well-appearing, afebrile with an antalgic gait. As with septic arthritis, these patients prefer to hold the hip flexed, abducted, and externally rotated. ROM is limited, particularly on internal ROM, but the patient will tolerate passive ROM with the most pain noted at the extremes of ROM and less pain during the ROM arc.

> **Clinical Pearl:** Transient synovitis (TS) typically improves within 24 to 48 hours within nonsteroidal anti-inflammatory drugs (NSAIDs) alone.

Diagnosis

This is primarily a clinical diagnosis to which you could apply the Kocher criteria in an effort to sort out those patients with septic arthritis from those with TS. From a laboratory data standpoint, the CBC, CRP, and ESR are in normal ranges and arthrocentesis reveals clear fluid with WBC levels between 5,000 and 15,000 with neutrophils at <25%.

If radiographs are obtained, they show nonspecific changes with soft-tissue swelling around the joint. US will usually show an effusion.

Management

Conservative therapy with activity limitation and NSAIDs over a 1- to 2-month period are typically sufficient. Educating the family about the recurrence rate is important, as 4% to 15% of patients will have similar symptoms in the future.

NEUROLOGIC SYSTEM

Unlike adults, most pediatric neurologic disorders are not manifested as discrete nerve deficits, paralysis, or paresthesias. Instead, neurologic disorders in pediatrics are quite broad and can include developmental delays, seizures, headaches, dizziness, learning disorders, and behavioral problems.

AUTISM SPECTRUM DISORDER

Etiology

The etiology and pathophysiology of autism spectrum disorder (ASD) is not fully understood, but genetic, neural, and metabolic anomalies have been found in ASD patients. Functional MRIs have shown neuroanatomic differences between ASD and neurotypical peers, including abnormal cellular configurations in the frontal, temporal, and cerebellar regions; enlargements of the amygdala and hippocampus; thinning of the corpus callosum; and evidence of poor pruning of neurons in the prefrontal cortex.[81] The abnormalities in the frontal and temporal brain regions correspond to the deficits in social and communication skills, whereas the cerebellar differences may explain the clumsiness and repetitive behaviors seen in ASD.

Epidemiology

Previously separate diagnoses, such as autism, Asperger's disorder, childhood disintegrative disorder, and pervasive developmental disorder not otherwise specified, are now all classified under the umbrella term "ASD." Grouping these disorders together has now made ASD one of the most common childhood developmental disabilities. It is estimated that 400,000 Americans have the condition.[81] Male-to-female ratio varies from 3.5 to 5:1.[81]

Clinical Presentation

As the name implies, ASD has a variable presentation along a spectrum that includes qualitative abnormalities or deficits in interaction, aberrant communication skills and restricted repetitive behaviors, interests, and activities. Typically presenting prior to 30 months of age, symptoms of ASD limit or impair daily function. The patient with ASD is often identified via a screening or surveillance tool, but parental or provider concerns for developmental regression; absence of protodeclarative pointing; abnormal reactions to environmental stimuli; abnormal social interactions, including failing to make eye contact, absence of symbolic play, and repetitive and stereotyped behaviors can be indicative of the diagnosis.[81]

> **CLINICAL PEARL:** Developmental "red flags" for possible autism spectrum disorder (ASD) include not babbling by 12 months; not pointing, showing, or reaching by 12 months; not speaking any words by 16 months; not speaking two-word meaningful phrases (without imitating or repeating) by 24 months; or loss of speech or social skills at any age.

Diagnosis

A screening questionnaire, such as the Modified Checklist for Autism in Toddlers (M-CHAT), is the first step in identifying children with suspicious behaviors. After the child is identified as being at risk for ASD, a level-two screening tool, such as the Screening Tool for Autism in Two-Year-Olds (STAT), can be administered, along with referrals to early intervention, audiology, and a developmental pediatrician or pediatric neurologist, as the diagnostic tools are very specialized and require significant training to administer.

Management

Multimodal therapies are implemented with ASD, with a goal to integrate these therapies as soon after diagnosis as possible. Early interventions greatly improve the outcomes. Patients are typically followed by a speech–language pathologist, behavioral therapist, special education teacher, and possibly an OT or PT to help with motor development and repetitive behaviors.

DIZZINESS

Etiology

"Dizziness" can be described as lightheadedness or feeling woozy or disoriented, whereas "vertigo" has a spinning component. Children and adolescents who present with complaints of dizziness or vertigo will usually have an inner ear disorder with a viral cause or, more common, benign paroxysmal positional vertigo (BPPV). Both are noted to have inner ear inflammation and/or otoliths that disrupt the normal vestibular functions of the ear, causing dizziness.

Epidemiology

Several studies have shown between 5% and 20% of children experience dizziness or vertigo at some point in childhood.

Clinical Presentation

Table 2.21 describes the most common disorders underlying dizziness and provides comparative presentations, as many vestibular disorders present very similarly. Management is outlined here as well.

Diagnosis

A well-documented history, including the frequency and duration of symptoms, is vital to determine what diagnostic testing is appropriate. Many vestibular disorders may be diagnosed clinically, but it is not unusual to see primary care clinicians refer patients to neurology, otolaryngology, or neuro-otology specialists for further assessment. Testing methods vary from in-office maneuvers to assess for nystagmus, caloric irrigation of the ears, head impulse testing, rotational testing, vestibular-evoked myogenic potentials (VEMP), and MRI of the brain.

FEBRILE SEIZURE

Etiology

The pathophysiology of febrile seizures is not well understood, but it is hypothesized that children have a lower seizure threshold and that fevers themselves may result in a seizure. A fever triggers the release of interleukin 1 beta (IL-1), which is an endogenous pyrogen thought to increase neuronal excitability.[82] The higher the fever, the more IL-1 produced, leading to increased neuronal excitability.[83] Children with a family history of febrile seizures, high temperature, developmental delay, perinatal illness requiring hospitalization, and day-care attendance are at increased risk for a febrile seizure. A child with two of these risk factors has a 30% probability of having a febrile seizure, whereas those exposed to alcohol or cigarette smoking in utero have a twofold increased risk.[82]

TABLE 2.21. Vestibular Disorders in Pediatric Populations

	Etiology/Epidemiology	Clinical Signs/Symptoms	Management
Central			
VM	Most common reason for dizziness in children VM can affect all age groups >50% of children who suffer from vertigo or dizziness also have headaches	All patients with episodic vertigo that occurs together with headache, autonomic signs, and increased sensitivity to light and sound should be diagnosed as having VM	Acute therapy for migraine (NSAIDs or triptans) does not work well for the vestibular symptoms Prophylactic treatment may be indicated for >3 episodes per month or severe, prolonged attacks (>72 hours)
BPV	Most common reason for episodic vertigo in children 2–8 years old Considered a precursor to migraine but those with BPV do not get migraines Typically attacks begin in children <4 years and disappear by 8–10 years of age Often a family history of migraine	BPV is characterized by recurrent brief attacks of vertigo (seconds to minutes), occurring without warning, and resolving spontaneously in otherwise healthy children Normal exam and testing	Attacks are usually brief and randomly occur so acute therapy is not necessary
Motion sickness	A sensory mismatch between otolith and semicircular canal signals is likely to be at least as relevant as a vestibular–visual mismatch Children between the ages of 4 and 10 years are more susceptible than most Prevalence of motion sickness in ages 7–12 years is >40% when traveling by car or bus	Exposure to otolith stimulation (e.g., road bumps) in combination with semicircular canal stimulation (e.g., head turns) is a typical trigger of motion sickness and is difficult to recreate clinically Physical exam is usually normal and diagnosis is usually made clinically and without further testing	Motion sickness can be prevented by controlling visual stimuli, such as looking out of the car window and avoiding head movements Drug prophylaxis is indicated in severe cases using dimenhydrinate (1–2 mg/kg) 1 hour before exposure to such situations. Dosing can be repeated every 6 hours

(continued)

TABLE 2.21. Vestibular Disorders in Pediatric Populations (*continued*)

	Etiology/Epidemiology	Clinical Signs/Symptoms	Management
Neurogenic tumors	Central vestibular disturbances are due to lesions in the brainstem Tumors of the brainstem and the cerebellum can cause vertigo in children Supratentorial lesions rarely cause rotatory vertigo, but affected patients can present with dizziness	Children and adolescents present with complaints of headache, nausea, and vomiting May have a variety of other symptoms based on the location of the tumor Infants usually present with enlarging macrocephaly Gait disturbances and impaired vision may lead to increased dizziness	MRI should be performed if the clinical examination reveals central ocular motor signs Sometimes symptomatic treatment is useful but generally treatment revolves around the underlying etiology
Peripheral			
BPPV	BPPV is a common cause of vertigo in adults, but only accounts for about 5% of childhood vertigo The pathophysiologic basis of the disorder is the presence of particles of calcium carbonate crystals within the semicircular canals (canalolithiasis) The posterior canal is affected in about 90% of cases	Patients present with complaints of attacks of rotatory vertigo when changing the position of the head relative to gravity (e.g., lying down, turning over in bed, looking up); The physical exam is usually normal, but the Dix–Hallpike maneuver will reveal a rotary nystagmus in the case of BPPV, essentially solidifying the diagnosis	The Epley maneuver is the most successful therapy for BPPV; this can be taught to the patient or family to do at home
Labyrinthitis/ vestibular neuritis	Vestibular neuritis is understood to be a viral or postviral inflammatory disorder affecting the vestibular portion of the eighth cranial nerve	Patients are brought to their PCP or ED with symptoms of vertigo, nausea, vomiting, and gait impairment; Patients present with spontaneous nystagmus beating to the unaffected side, pathologic head impulses to the affected side, and reduced responsiveness to caloric irrigation of the affected ear	Treatment depends on the etiology; in the acute stage, dimenhydrinate 1mg/kg–2 mg/kg is helpful; however, it should not be given for >3 days Mobilization should start as soon as possible in order to support recalibration of the vestibular system by mechanisms of central compensation

			Labyrinthitis in acute otitis media is treated by antibiotics, if bacterial infection is present; in vestibular neuritis, unrelated to an acute infection, steroids can improve vestibular recovery
Somatoform dizziness	Functional (somatoform) dizziness is common in adolescence The terms *"phobic postural vertigo"* and *"psychiatric/psychogenic dizziness" "phobic postural vertigo and psychiatric/psychogenic dizziness* are used interchangeably Patients with somatoform syndromes often present with chronic dizziness that worsens in certain situations (e.g., at school, in stores) Most often affects female adolescents	Comprehensive history and physical exam point to a psychogenic etiology	Therapy begins by providing information on the illness to both patients and parents; desensitization to visual and self-motion by vestibular rehabilitation, regular walks, and/or sports; behavioral therapy
OD	OD accounts for 5% of dizziness in patients who attend specialty clinics OD is by far the most frequent complaint in older children and adolescents and it is more common in girls than boys	The key to the diagnosis is the history of dizziness after getting up from a supine or sitting position or during prolonged standing; An important diagnostic test is the assessment of blood pressure in supine and upright positions (orthostatic testing)	Where there is concomitant syncope and relevant impairment, a cardiac workup is recommended For most patients, counseling on behavioral measures, including sufficient fluid intake, activation of muscle pump (leg movements) before getting up, avoidance of fast rises, and avoidance of prolonged standing without leg activity is the treatment of choice

BPV, benign paroxysmal vertigo; BPPV, benign paroxysmal positional vertigo; NSAIDs, nonsteroidal anti-inflammatory drugs; OD, orthostatic dizziness; PCP, primary care provider; VM, vestibular migraine.
Sources: Jahn K. Vertigo and dizziness in children. In: Furman JM, Lempert T, eds. *Handbook of Clinical Neurology 137: Neuro-otology.* Cambridge, MA: Elsevier; 2016:353–363. doi:10.1016/B978-0-444-63437 -5.00025-X; van Esch A, Steyerberg EW, Berger MY, et al. Family history and recurrence of febrile seizures. *Arch Dis Child.* 1994;70(5):395-399. doi:10.1136/adc.70.5.395

Epidemiology

Febrile seizures occur in children between 3 months and 5 years with a temperature higher than 100.4°F. To qualify for the diagnosis, children may not have an underlying seizure disorder or developmental problem. There is a slight male predominance, but no racial predominance. Children with a first-degree relative with history of febrile seizures are at increased risk for repeat febrile seizures.[84]

Clinical Presentation

Children will often present after a febrile seizure has occurred and may have a mild postictal state or appear to be back to baseline. There is typically a history of a preceding respiratory or GI illness or first dose of measles, mumps, rubella and varicella (MMRV) vaccine, with most seizures occurring in the first 24 hours of fever onset. Parents or caregivers may describe generalized tonic–clonic seizure activity that lasts less than 15 minutes. Many times the underlying cause of the fever is found on physical exam, but if not elicited, meningitis and other serious bacterial infections (SBIs) must be considered on the differential and management plan. Complex seizures, seizures that last longer than 20 minutes, should be evaluated further for underlying neurologic abnormalities.

Diagnosis

Diagnosis is clinical after exclusion of other causes.

Management

Patients with active seizures should be treated with airway management, high-flow oxygen, supportive care, and anticonvulsants as necessary. Most children with febrile seizures should be given antipyretics and the underlying cause of the fever should be treated with antibiotics, if treatment is warranted. Reassure worried parents and discuss the slightly increased risk of recurrent febrile seizures (upward of 35%) and the risk for epilepsy (slightly increased over the general population, but still very small at 1%).

HEADACHES: MIGRAINE, TENSION, AND CLUSTER HEADACHES

Etiology

Headache is one of the most common complaints in all age groups, including children, and usually increases in incidence with increasing age. Headaches caused by acute viral illness, sinusitis, or migraine are the most common causes.[85] Discussion of emergent headaches is covered in Chapter 5, Urgent Management in Pediatrics.

The three broad primary headache syndromes—migraine, tension, and cluster—have been grouped in terms of symptoms and attack patterns. These occur through all ages though with some variations in the transition from child to adulthood.[85]

Epidemiology

Headaches are common in children and adolescents. In a systematic review of 50 population-based studies, nearly 60% of children reported having had headaches (ranging from 1 month to "lifetime"). By age 18 years, more than 90% of adolescents report having had a headache. Before 12 years of age the prevalence of headache between boys and girls is equal but after 12 years of age girls report more headaches than boys.

Clinical Presentation

Migraines: Migraine headache in children is typically episodic, bifrontal, or bitemporal and lasts hours to several days. Nausea and/or vomiting and abdominal pain may be abrupt and greatly distressing.

Tension-type headaches: Tension-type headaches are characterized by headaches that are diffuse in location, have a squeezing character, are mild to moderately severe, and do not worsen with activity (although the child may not wish to participate in activity). These can last from 30 minutes to 7 days. Tension-type headaches may be associated with nausea, photophobia, or phonophobia, but usually are not accompanied by vomiting and virtually never have an aura.

Cluster headaches: Cluster headaches are typically unilateral and located in the frontal–periorbital area. The pain of cluster headaches is severe, but lasts less than 3 hours. Cluster headaches are characterized by multiple headaches that occur in a very short period of time. Cluster headaches usually are associated with ipsilateral autonomic findings, including lacrimation, rhinorrhea, ophthalmic injection, and occasionally Horner syndrome (ipsilateral miosis, ptosis, and facial anhidrosis).

Diagnosis

The patient or parents should be encouraged to keep a headache diary before arriving for the appointment. Significant information can be retrieved from a diary that lists specifics about headaches, details about the pain, associated symptoms, possible triggers, and resolution patterns. All of this information can assist with diagnosis. Although CT and MRI are easy and efficient diagnostic tools, you must determine whether they are truly necessary. Exposing a child to radiation for a CT or using sedation to get a quality MRI does not always pay off with pertinent information.

If a child has experienced a crescendo headache pattern; recent onset of headaches; an abnormal exam, in particular, evidence of increased intracranial pressure; alteration of consciousness; or clinical profile suggestive of seizure, imaging should be undertaken urgently.[85]

The challenge for most primary care clinicians from the outset is to distinguish headache syndromes that are primary from those that are secondary headache disorders.

Management

Behavior modifications (based on information received from a headache diary, review of systems, and history gathering) may help to drastically reduce the severity and recurrence of headaches. When occurrences do happen, ibuprofen or acetaminophen are first-line agents. If behavior modification and analgesics are not sufficiently effective, the 5-hydroxytryptamine (5-HT) agonists (triptans) may be useful in children.

If acute tension-type headache has to be treated by a prescription medication other than ibuprofen or acetaminophen, butalbital/acetaminophen may be tried in those patients older than 12 years. To avoid analgesic-induced headache, analgesic headache medication should be used no more than 10 days a month.

Cluster headaches are treated with oxygen as a first-line agent and if this does not help, subcutaneous sumatriptan 6 mg may abort the headache.

Prophylactic medication is also indicated in juvenile migraine, especially if acute attack therapy is not effective; if attack frequency, headache intensity, or attack duration are high; or if aura symptoms are extreme. Medication should be started slowly, and patients and their families should be educated that during the first few weeks, side effects may predominate. As a rule, after 8 weeks it is possible to judge the effect. After 6 months, a patient may try to taper the medication.

LEARNING DIFFICULTIES

Etiology

"Learning difficulties" is a broad term that encompasses brain-based differences that can affect processing of information and attention. Not all learning difficulties qualify as learning disabilities, but they may impact the ability to learn. Issues with vision, hearing, and motor skills may impact learning, but have a distinctly different underlying etiology from learning difficulties/disorders.

There does appear to be a genetic component to learning difficulties, but the etiology has not been clearly established. What is known is that the temporal and parietal lobes of the brain are underactive. In reading disorders, they have poor information exchange and in math disorders the parietal lobe is underactive. Learning difficulties can manifest as mild to severe and affect reading, writing, math, organization, concentration, listening comprehension, social skills, motor skills, or a combination of these.[86]

Epidemiology

One in five children have a learning or attention issue, with upward of 50% of children with learning disorders having concomitant attention deficits.[86] Seventy to 80% of people with a learning disorder have a reading disorder, with dyslexia being the most common. Familial history of learning disability or attention deficit hyperactivity disorder (ADHD) is common, with boys identified more often than girls. There are no racial or ethnic disparities noted for learning difficulties.

Clinical Presentation

A child with a learning disorder may present for evaluation after the school has identified him or her as performing below what is expected for his or her academic skills.[87] Children with learning disorders can be diagnosed only after formal education starts.[87] The learning difficulties are seen by the early school years in most children, manifesting as difficulties recognizing and writing letters, recognizing rhyming words, and breaking down spoken words into syllables in kindergarten. However, for some the learning difficulties may not be apparent until later, when academic demands are greater. By third grade, students may struggle to connect sounds, read slower, and have difficulty with spelling and math, and by adolescence and adulthood the difficulties affect academic achievement, comprehension, and computation.

> **CLINICAL PEARL:** Signs of a possible learning disorder may appear as early as preschool years, with children experiencing delays in attention, language, or motor skills.

Diagnosis

A learning disorder is diagnosed based on a combination of medical and family history, observation, interviews, history of the learning difficulty, school reports, educational and psychological assessments, and standardized tests. To be diagnosed with specific learning disorder, a child must have at least 6 months of difficulty in at least one of the following areas, despite targeted interventions:

1. Reading (e.g., inaccurate, slow, and only with much effort)
2. Reading comprehension
3. Spelling
4. Writing (e.g., problems with grammar, punctuation, or organization)
5. Understanding number concepts, number facts, or calculation
6. Mathematical reasoning (e.g., applying math concepts or solving math problems)[87]

In addition, the difficulties cannot be comorbid with limited English proficiency, intellectual disabilities, economic disadvantage, vision or hearing diagnoses, or neurologic conditions.[87] The most common learning disorders include the following:

- *Dyslexia*: Learning difficulties related to word recognition, decoding, and spelling
- *Dysgraphia*: Difficulties with writing (e.g., organization, handwriting, grammar)
- *Dyscalculia*: Difficulties learning math facts and performing math calculations

- *Dyspraxia:* Difficulties planning and completing motor tasks
- *Processing disorders in auditory, visual, sensory, and social realms:* Challenges in receiving, processing, retrieving, and communicating information[86]

Management

The first step typically involves an individual educational plan (IEP) that outlines the specific short- and long-term educational objectives, special education services, and timelines for reevaluation.[88] Treatment will vary depending on the specific diagnosis, but in general those children with mild severity (some difficulties in one or two academic areas) may benefit from behavioral and educational intervention that help the child compensate for the disorder. Moderate to severe learning disorders (those that affect several academic areas) usually require specialized teaching, accommodations, and support services. Those children with comorbid attention issues may find that stimulant medications help address this piece of the puzzle. Instructional interventions, assistive technology, and accommodations are also reasonable management options for specific learning disorders.[88]

ELECTRONIC RESOURCES

M-CHAT:
https://mchatscreen.com/m-chat/
STAT training:
http://stat.vueinnovations.com/about

PSYCHIATRIC ISSUES

Psychiatric issues in the pediatric population are quite similar to those found in adult populations. They are often diagnosed in childhood and carry forward into adulthood. Anxiety and depression are common conditions diagnosed in pediatrics, especially in teenagers. Although there are a few subtle pharmacologic issues to consider in pediatric populations, for the most part, both anxiety and depression are treated as in adult patients. In an effort to present information specific to pediatrics, anxiety and depression have not been covered in a breakout section.

ATTENTION DEFICIT HYPERACTIVITY DISORDER

Etiology

The pathophysiology of ADHD has not yet been clearly elucidated by researchers, but what is known is that ADHD is likely a multifactorial disorder with a brain-based, neurobiological component that includes neurotransmitter levels and response, functional anatomic differences of the brain, and environmental triggers.

Epidemiology

ADHD is one of the most common psychiatric diagnoses in children and is more common in boys than girls. Approximately 8% of school-aged children have ADHD difficulties, but these appear to improve as they mature into adulthood, with only 4% of adults having ADHD.[89] There appears to be a genetic influence, as ADHD tends to run in families and 75% of children with ADHD have a relative with the disorder.[89]

Clinical Presentation

Children with ADHD may present with a range of symptoms or difficulties. These difficulties are typically arranged in three categories: inattention, hyper-activity/impulsivity, or a combination. Children with inattention-type ADHD may have a history of struggling to pay attention to details or pay attention to the wrong details, have difficulty sustaining attention, are easily distracted, are disorganized, and have trouble following through and/or completing tasks. Children with hyperactive/impulsive-type ADHD appear to have a low-level motor drive at all times. They are squirmy and fidgety, need tactile stimulation and therefore touch, grab, and hold things, and have difficulty waiting for their turn and may blurt out frequently. They also tend to get frustrated easily and have a difficult time recuperating from this frustration.

Most commonly, children have features of each ADHD type and these manifest as problems in executive function. According to The National Center for Learning Disabilities, they tend to have difficulty with the following:

- Working memory
- Getting started on work consistently
- Sustaining and completing tasks
- Listening and waiting
- Emotional control
- Reading social cues
- Mood swings
- Transitioning from one task to another
- Problem-solving
- Organization
- Time management[90]

Diagnosis

The diagnosis of ADHD is made based on meeting the *Diagnostic and Statistical Manual of Mental Disorders* (*DSM-5*) criteria, many of which are listed earlier, in more than one setting with impairments in school performance and function. The Vanderbilt ADHD Diagnostic Rating Scale (VADRS) is a psychological assessment tool that can be completed by parents/caregivers and teachers of 6- to 12-year-olds. The assessment tool is designed to measure the severity of ADHD symptoms, but also assesses for other comorbid psychiatric disorders like mood disorders, conduct disorder, and oppositional defiant disorder.[91] There is no single assessment instrument for the diagnosis, but a combination of patient and parent interview, assessment tools like the VADRS, and ruling out other psychiatric and behavioral disorders are necessary for the diagnosis.

Management

Management of ADHD is typically handled in several different ways. Behavioral therapy, in combination with medications, has been shown to be the most effective management for moderate to severe ADHD. There are two classes of medications used for ADHD—stimulant and nonstimulant. Stimulant medications include methylphenidate and amphetamines and the nonstimulant medications are atomoxetine and guanfacine. Dosing of these medications is often based on age and weight with a slow titration until symptom improvement or bothersome side effects occur.

SCHOOL AVOIDANCE/SCHOOL REFUSAL

Etiology

Often manifesting as vague abdominal discomfort, nausea, dizziness, or headache, underlying all school avoidance are anxiety and fear. These children may have separation anxiety (especially in younger school-aged children), a fear of something at school (a bully or an intimidating teacher), or a social phobia (fear of being exposed or embarrassed, especially in specific subject matter areas).

Epidemiology

Found equally in males and females, three peaks of school avoidance occur—around first or second grade, fourth to fifth grade, and again in eighth to tenth grade.[92] Often tied to family stress, parents may be noted to have anxiety or mood disorders.

Clinical Presentation

Starting after a vacation or weekend, children with anxiety-related school avoidance often report vague abdominal discomfort, nausea, headaches, and/or dizziness that increases as the time to leave for school draws closer. Often symptoms will improve once the child is allowed to stay home.[92] Adolescents may present with more depressive symptoms and should be screened for a mood disorder.

Diagnosis

Organic causes for the somatic symptoms should be ruled out prior to making the diagnosis of school nonattendance, but school avoidance is diagnosed based on history and interview.

Management

Educating the patient and family on the somatic symptoms associated with anxiety and depression, treating mood disorders with medications, if necessary, and creating a plan with the patient and the family around returning to school are key elements of management. Collaborating with the school administrators, counselors, and the school nursing staff can offer secondary support when the child returns to school and reassures anxious parents that any situations that arise in school will be managed in a multidisciplinary fashion.[93]

RESPIRATORY SYSTEM

Although there are many reasons children present to their primary care provider for respiratory illness, these are the most common reasons why children cough. The parents' description of the cough, time of day or night that it may flare, noticeable triggers, and associated symptoms play a large part in developing your diagnosis. As there is considerable overlap among respiratory diseases and they can often look very similar, Table 2.22 outlines the most common respiratory diseases, their etiology and epidemiology, how they might present, and the diagnosis and management for the disease.

TABLE 2.22. Common Pediatric Respiratory Disease: Etiology, Epidemiology, Clinical Presentation, and Diagnosis and Management

	Etiology/Epidemiology	Clinical Presentation	Diagnosis/Management
AR	AR is an inflammatory disorder of the nasal mucosa marked by nasal congestion, rhinorrhea, and itching, often accompanied by sneezing and itchy, watery eyes The symptoms may appear in infancy, with the diagnosis generally established by the time the child reaches 6 years old The highest prevalence peaks late in childhood A critical period exists early in infancy when the genetically susceptible individual is at greatest risk of sensitization; new research shows a decreased risk of asthma, AR, and atopic sensitization with early introduction to wheat, rye, oats, barley, fish, and eggs	On initial presentation, symptoms may include Clear rhinorrhea Rhinitis Sneezing Conjunctival irritation Nonproductive cough Headaches Reduced taste and smell Dry mouth (mouth breathing) Sleep difficulty On exam, patients may give the "allergic salute," as well as present with Conjunctival edema "Allergic shiners" Edematous, boggy, bluish mucus membranes Swollen turbinates Wheezing	*Diagnosis* Initial diagnosis may be made clinically but to determine specific allergens, skin testing is the gold standard Patients should be >2 years and antihistamines should be held for 2–7 days before testing *Management* Allergen trigger avoidance Sedating antihistamines Nonsedating antihistamines Leukotriene antagonists Antihistamine nasal sprays Intranasal corticosteroid sprays Allergy immunotherapy (subcutaneous injection or sublingual drops) is very effective, although sublingual drops are not yet licensed by the FDA

| Asthma | Asthma is a chronic inflammatory condition of the pulmonary airways resulting in hyperresponsiveness to provocative exposures leading to episodic airflow obstruction

The cause of childhood asthma has not been determined, but environmental exposures and inherent biologic and genetic susceptibilities have been implicated

Ongoing inflammatory exposures appear to worsen asthma, driving disease persistence, and increasing the risk of severe exacerbations (2)

Approximately 80% of all asthmatic patients report disease onset prior to 6 years of age but most outgrow symptoms by adolescence

Approximately 14% of U.S. children have asthma, with male gender, poverty, and African American race increasing risk | Presenting symptoms may include
Intermittent, nonproductive cough
Shortness of breath
Chest congestion
Chest tightness
Respiratory symptoms that are worse at night, especially with viral infections or allergy season
Activity-induced daytime symptoms
Risk factors, such as a history of other allergic conditions and parental asthma, help support the diagnosis of asthma

On exam, patients may have
Expiratory wheezing
Prolonged expiratory phase
Decreased breath sounds on auscultation
Increased respiratory rate
Accessory muscle use | *Diagnosis*
Clinical signs and symptoms, as well as obstructive patterns on PFTs, can help to confirm the diagnosis of asthma; however, PFTs may be difficult for children younger than 6 years old, so clinical judgment is key in these cases
Bronchodilator response to an inhaled beta-agonist (e.g., albuterol) shows reversibility of the airway constriction and is a hallmark feature of asthma

Management
Treatment options for urgent or emergent asthma exacerbations are found in Chapter 5, Urgent Management in Pediatrics. Asthma management outside of exacerbations can include
Avoiding triggers
Inhaled beta-agonists as needed
Daily preventative medications, such as leukotriene inhibitors, corticosteroid inhalers, and long-acting bronchodilators
Regardless of treatment regimen, families and patients should be educated about regular peak flow measurements, how to step up or step down therapy based on symptomology and regular clinic visits to reassess and maintain good control |

(continued)

TABLE 2.22. Common Pediatric Respiratory Disease: Etiology, Epidemiology, Clinical Presentation, and Diagnosis and Management *(continued)*

	Etiology/Epidemiology	Clinical Presentation	Diagnosis/Management
Bronchitis	Acute bronchitis is a syndrome, usually following a viral infection, with cough as a prominent feature; bronchitis is more common in the winter when more viral pathogens circulate Exposure to environmental irritants, such as tobacco smoke and air pollution, can incite or aggravate the cough There is a well-established association between tobacco exposure and pulmonary disease, including bronchitis and wheezing	Presenting symptoms may include Nonspecific URI symptoms Frequent, dry, hacking cough Purulent sputum, indicating leukocyte migration but not necessarily bacterial infection Many children swallow their sputum, which can produce emesis, nausea, and pharyngitis On exam, patients may have No findings Low-grade fever URI symptoms Raspy sounds on chest auscultation Coarse and fine crackles Scattered high-pitched, wheezes	*Diagnosis* Chest x-rays are usually normal or can have increased bronchial markings Absence of abnormal vital signs (tachycardia, tachypnea, fever) and a normal exam of the chest reduce the likelihood of pneumonia and increase the likelihood of bronchitis *Management* Bronchitis is typically managed with supportive measures such as Analgesia Antipyretics Mucolytics Increased hydration Rarely, a patient may require a short burst of corticosteroid to reduce severe bronchial inflammation

| CAP | Pneumonia is the leading cause of death worldwide for children <5 years of age

In the U.S., childhood mortality has dropped significantly due to vaccines and antibiotic use

Streptococcus pneumoniae is the most common causative organism in children under 4, whereas Mycoplasma pneumoniae and Chlamydophila pneumoniae are the most common bacterial agents for patients >4 years of age | Presenting symptoms may include

Symptoms similar to other viral URIs

Rhinitis

Fever (usually more severe with bacterial forms)

Cough

On exam, patients may present with

Tachypnea

Increased work of breathing

Crackles and wheezing on auscultation, although it can be difficult to localize sounds in the young | *Diagnosis*
Definitive diagnosis requires isolation of organism from the blood, pleural fluid, or lung, but chest x-ray and a CBC can help discern a clinical diagnosis

Viral CAP is characterized by hyperinflation and bilateral interstitial infiltrates, although there is a predominance of lymphocytes on the CBC

Lobar consolidation is often seen in bacterial CAP, although alone is not diagnostic

Management
Recommendations for empiric treatment for bacterial pneumonia include high-dose amoxicillin, amoxicillin-clavulanate or azithromycin

Supportive therapy for those with bacterial infection and for those with viral pneumonia include antipyretics, analgesics, and hydration |

(continued)

TABLE 2.22. Common Pediatric Respiratory Disease: Etiology, Epidemiology, Clinical Presentation, and Diagnosis and Management (*continued*)

	Etiology/Epidemiology	Clinical Presentation	Diagnosis/Management
Croup	PIV types 1 and 2 are the major cause of laryngotracheobronchitis (croup) Different serotypes have distinct epidemiologic patterns Type 1 tends to produce outbreaks of croup in the autumn of every other year Type 2 outbreaks, although less common, also occur in the fall in conjunction with type 1 outbreaks, but tend to be less severe and more irregular PIV infections do not confer complete protective immunity; therefore, reinfections can occur with all serotypes and at any age; reinfections usually are mild and limited to the upper respiratory tract Primary infection with all types usually occurs by 5 years of age.[94]	Presenting symptoms may include Symptoms of viral URI Combination of rhinorrhea, pharyngitis, mild cough for 1–3 days before upper airway obstruction become apparent Fever that ranges from low grade to as high as 40°C (104°F) Characteristic "barking" cough Hoarseness Inspiratory stridor Symptoms worse at night On exam, patients may present with Hoarse voice Coryza Normal to moderately inflamed pharynx Slightly increased respiratory rate	*Diagnosis* Croup is a clinical diagnosis and does not require a radiograph of the neck, although it can show the typical subglottic narrowing, or steeple sign, of croup on the posteroanterior view[94] *Management* Croup is managed differently depending on the severity of the illness, which can be determined using the Westley Croup Score. A Westley Croup Score takes into account level of consciousness, cyanosis, stridor, air entry, and retractions. A score of ≤2 is mild, 3–7 is moderate, 8–11 is severe, and ≥12 indicates impending respiratory failure;[95] Primary management is to reduce agitation, place the child in a comfortable position, and administer oxygen if hypoxemic or severe respiratory distress. Once stable, patients should be treated with Dexamethasone (0.15–0.6 mg/kg once) Budesonide Methylprednisolone Nebulized racemic epinephrine, if moderate to severe croup

Influenza	Epidemic disease is caused by influenza virus types A and B, with antigenic drift in the circulating strain(s) associated with seasonal epidemics	Presenting symptoms typically include	*Diagnosis*

Epidemic disease is caused by influenza virus types A and B, with antigenic drift in the circulating strain(s) associated with seasonal epidemics

During community outbreaks, the highest incidence occurs among school-aged children, with secondary spread to adults and other children within a family

Peak influenza activity in the U.S. most commonly occurs in January and February (ranging from November to May)

Influenza is spread by respiratory droplets created by coughing or sneezing

Patients may become infectious during the 24 hours before onset of symptoms, but viral shedding in nasal secretions peaks during the first 3 days of illness

Although all children younger than 5 years of age are considered at higher risk for complications from influenza, the highest risk is for those younger than 2 years of age; the highest hospitalization and mortality are in children <6 months old

Presenting symptoms typically include
Sudden onset of fever
Chills or rigors
Headache
Malaise
Diffuse myalgia
Nonproductive cough
Sore throat
Nasal congestion
Conjunctival injection
Abdominal pain, nausea, and vomiting and diarrhea can occur, but are less common

On exam, patients may present with URI symptoms that are indistinguishable from other URIs
Fever
Tachycardia
Crackles

Diagnosis

Although confirmation of influenza virus infection by diagnostic testing is not required to prescribe antiviral medications, prompt suspicion, or diagnosis of influenza may allow for antiviral therapy to be initiated and reduce inappropriate use of antibiotics

Management

The most frequently prescribed antiviral for influenza A or B is oseltamivir (Tamiflu)

Infants younger than 1 year old are dosed at 3 mg/kg/dose twice daily for 5 days

In those older than 1 year, the dose varies by weight

Supportive measures should also be initiated and include
Analgesics
Antipyretics
Increased hydration
Rest

School-aged children should not be cleared to return to school or activities until the fever has been <99°F for >24 hours; *prevention* influenza vaccination is the best means of preventing severe disease caused by influenza

(*continued*)

TABLE 2.22. Common Pediatric Respiratory Disease: Etiology, Epidemiology, Clinical Presentation, and Diagnosis and Management (*continued*)

	Etiology/Epidemiology	Clinical Presentation	Diagnosis/Management
Pertussis	Caused by *Bordetella pertussis*, which is vaccine preventable (DtaP; Tdap) Increasing prevalence in adults as immunity wanes over a 3–10 year period Cases occur year-round with increased numbers in late summer and fall Pertussis is most severe in first 6 months of life, with >60% of infants hospitalized for pertussis[94]	Pertussis has three phases with the initial-phase (catarrhal stage) symptoms including Mild fever Chills Rhinorrhea Mild cough Phase 2 occurs 2–3 weeks after initial presentation and is characterized by worsening, paroxysmal cough; severe, choking, hacking cough; and/or "whooping" secondary to inhalation after coughing spasm. Last phase is the convalescent or recovery phase with overall improvement in symptoms; on exam, patients may present with Mild URI symptoms Low-grade fever Cough Minimal or no adventitious lung sounds	*Diagnosis* Gold standard is nasopharyngeal culture, although a PCR assay is being used more frequently *Management* Antimicrobial agents administered during the catarrhal stage may ameliorate the disease. After the cough is established, antimicrobial agents have no discernible effect on the course of illness, but are recommended to limit spread of organisms to others. The first-line antibiotics of choice are Azithromycin Erythromycin Clarithromycin Infants <6 months of age may need to be managed in the hospital

AR, allergic rhinitis; CAP, community-aquired pneumonia; CBC, complete blood count; FDA, Food and Drug Administration; PCR, polymerase chain reaction; PFTs, pulmonary function tests; PIV, parainfluenza virus; Tdap, tetanus, diphtheria, acellular pertussis; URI, upper respiratory infection.

REFERENCES

1. Centers for Disease Control and Prevention. Congenital heart defects: data and statistics on congenital heart defects. CDC website. https://www.cdc.gov/ncbddd/heartdefects/data.html

2. Lary JM, Paulozzi LJ. Sex differences in the prevalence of human birth defects: a population-based study. *Teratology.* 2001;64(5):237–251. doi:10.1002/tera.1070

3. Frank JE, Jacobe KM. Evaluation and management of heart murmurs in children. *Am Fam Physician.* 2011;84(7):793–800. https://www.aafp.org/afp/2011/1001/p793.html

4. Naik RJ, Shah NC. Teenage heart murmurs. *Pediatr Clin North Am.* 2014;61(1):1–16. doi:10.1016/j.pcl.2013.09.014

5. Newburger JW, Alexander ME, Fulton DR. Innocent murmurs, syncope, and chest pain. In: Keane J, ed. *Nadas' Pediatric Cardiology.* 2nd ed. Philadelphia, PA: Saunders; 2006:357–371. https://www.macpeds.com/documents/InnocentmurmursSyncopeChestpain.pdf.

6. Flynn JT, Kaelber DC, Baker-Smith CM, et al. Clinical practice guideline for screening and management of high blood pressure in children and adolescents. *Pediatrics.* September 2017;140(3):e20171904. doi:10.1542/peds.2017-1904

7. Dalton T, Wang NE. Pediatric syncope: current status of diagnostic evaluation and management. *Pediatric Emergency Medicine Reports.* Published May 1, 2017. https://www.reliasmedia.com/articles/140535-pediatric-syncope-current-status-of-diagnostic-evaluation-and-management

8. Paris Y, Toro-Salazar OH, Gauthier NS, et al. Regional implementation of a pediatric cardiology syncope algorithm using standardized clinical assessment and management plans (SCAMPS) methodology. *J Am Heart Assoc.* 2016;5(2):8. doi:10.1161/JAHA.115.002931

9. Gahagan S. Overweight and obesity. In: Kleigman RM, ed. *Nelson Textbook of Pediatrics.* 20th ed. Philadelphia, PA: Elsevier; 2016:307–316.

10. Galbraith SS. Acne. In: Kleigman RM, ed. *Nelson Textbook of Pediatrics.* 20th ed. Philadelphia, PA: Elsevier; 2016:3228–3235.

11. Bussel JB. Immune thrombocytopenia (ITP) in children: initial management. In: Mahoney, DH, Jr., ed. *UpToDate.* https://www.uptodate.com/contents/immune-thrombocytopenia-itp-in-children-initial-management. Updated September 10, 2018.

12. Wolff K, Johnson RA, Suurmond D. *Fitzpatrick's Color Atlas & Synopsis of Clinical Dermatology.* 5th ed. New York, NY: McGraw-Hill; 2005:844–860.

13. Sperling MA, Tamborlane WV, Battelino T, et al. Diabetes mellitus. In: Sperling MA, ed . *Pediatric Endocrinology.* 4th ed. Philadelphia, PA: Saunders; 2014:846–900.

14. Elsevier Point of Care. Clinical overview: diabetes mellitus type 2 in children. *Clinical Key.* https://www-clinicalkey-com.proxy.hsl.ucdenver.edu/#!/content/clinical_overview/67-s2.0-079280b1-585e-4533-955d-f801116edd43?scrollTo=%23toc-7.

15. Sirotnak AP, Chiesa A. Failure to thrive. In: Pataki C, ed. *Medscape.* https://emedicine.medscape.com/article/915575-overview. Updated November 05, 2018.

16. Homan GJ. Failure to thrive: a practical guide. *Am Fam Physician.* 2016;94(4):295–299. https://www.aafp.org/afp/2016/0815/p295.html

17. Jensen MD. Obesity. In: Goldman L, Schafer AI, eds. *Goldman-Cecil Medicine*. 25th ed. Philadelphia, PA: Elsevier-Saunders; 2016:1458–1466.e3.

18. Graydanus DE, Agana M, Kamboj MK, et al. Pediatric obesity: current concepts. *Dis Mon*. 2018;64:98–156. doi:10.1016/j.disamonth.2017.12.001

19. Cunningham SA, Kramer MR, Venkat Narayan KM. Incidence of childhood obesity in the United States. *N Engl J Med*. 2014;370:403–411. doi:10.1056/NEJMoa1309753

20. Basman CL. Obesity. In: Ferri, FF, ed. *Ferri's Clinical Advisor 2019*. New York, NY: Elsevier; 2019:969–972.

21. Barlow SE, Walter H, Rao G, et al. Expert Committee recommendations regarding prevention, assessment, and treatment of child and adolescent overweight and obesity: summary report. *Pediatrics*. 2007;120(suppl 4):S164–S192. doi:10.1542/peds.2007-2329C

22. MaineHealth. Let's go!'s response to latest national childhood obesity data. https://mainehealth.org/news/2018/03/lets-gos-response-to-latest-national-childhood-obesity-data. Published March 9, 2018.

23. Vine J, Rodgers VW. Let's go! Evaluation report 2015-16 program year 10. 2017. https://mainehealth.org/lets-go/impact.

24. Czernichow S, Lee CM, Barzi F, et al. Efficacy of weight loss drugs on obesity and cardiovascular risk factors in obese adolescents: a meta-analysis of randomized controlled trials. *Obes Rev*. 2010;11(2):150–158. doi:10.1111/j.1467-789X.2009.00620.x

25. Rogol AD. Diagnostic approach to children and adolescents with short stature. In: Geffner ME, ed. *UpToDate*. https://www.uptodate.com/contents/diagnostic-approach-to-children-and-adolescents-with-short-stature Updated March 2, 2018.

26. Shah SS, Ronan JC, Alverson B. *Step-Up to Pediatrics*. Baltimore, MD: Lippincott Williams & Wilkins; 2014:93–94.

27. Hanley P, Lord K, Bauer AJ. Thyroid disorders in children and adolescents: a review. *JAMA Pediatr*. 2016;170(10):1008–1019. doi:10.1001/jamapediatrics.2016.0486

28. Shah SS, Ronan JC, Alverson B. *Step-Up to Pediatrics*. Baltimore, MD: Lippincott Williams & Wilkins; 2014:107–112.

29. Sinha SK. Pediatric hypothyroidism medication. In: Bowden SA, ed. *Medscape*. https://reference.medscape.com/article/922777-medication#2. Updated December 20, 2016.

30. Kravets I. Hyperthyroidism: diagnosis and treatment. *Am Fam Physician*. March 1, 2016;93(5):363–370. https://www.aafp.org/afp/2016/0301/p363.html

31. Sicherer SH, Allen K, Lack G, et al. Critical issues in food allergy: a National Academies consensus report. *Pediatrics*. 2017;140(2):e20170194. doi:10.1542/peds.2017-0194

32. Heyman MB. Lactose intolerance in infants, children, and adolescents. *Pediatrics*. 2006;118(6):1279–1286. doi:10.1542/peds.2006-1721

33. Baker RD. Acute abdominal pain. *Pediatr Rev*. 2018;39(3):130–139. doi:10.1542/pir.2017-0089

34. Fitzmaurice GJ, McWilliams B, Hurreiz H, Epanomeritakis E. Antibiotics versus appendectomy in the management of acute appendicitis: a review of current evidence. *Can J Surg*. 2011;54(5):307–314. doi:10.1503/cjs.006610

35. Barr M. What is the period of PURPLE crying? *The Period of PURPLE Crying*. http://purplecrying.info/what-is-the-period-of-purple-crying.php

36. Shah SS, Ronan JC, Alverson B. *Step-Up to Pediatrics*. Baltimore, MD: Lippincott Williams & Wilkins; 2014:445.

37. Hay WW, Jr., Levin MR, Deterding RR, Abzug MA, eds. *Current Diagnosis and Treatment Pediatrics*. 24th ed. New York, NY: McGraw-Hill; 2018.

38. van Ginkel R, Reitsma JB, Büller HA, et al. Childhood constipation: longitudinal follow-up beyond puberty. *Gastroenterology*. 2003;125(2):357–363. doi:10.1016/S0016-5085(03)00888-6

39. Guarino A, Lo Vecchio A, Dias JA, et al. Universal recommendations for the management of acute diarrhea in nonmalnourished children. *J Pediatr Gastroenterol Nutr*. 2018;67(5):586–593. doi:10.1097/MPG.0000000000002053

40. Rybak A, Pesce M, Thapar N, Borrelli O. Gastro-esophageal reflux in children. *Int J Mol Sci*. 2017;18(8):1671. doi:10.3390/ijms18081671

41. Nelson SP, Chen EH, Syniar GM, Christoffel KK. Prevalence of symptoms of gastroesophageal reflux during childhood: a pediatric practice-based survey. *Arch Pediatr Adolesc Med*. 2000;154:150–154. doi:10.1001/archpedi.154.2.150

42. Lightdale JR, Gremse DA. Gastroesophageal reflux: management guidance for the pediatrician. *Pediatrics*. 2013;131(5):e1684–e1695. doi:10.1542/peds.2013-0421

43. Moazzez R, Bartlett D, Anggiansah A. The effect of chewing sugar-free gum on gastro-esophageal reflux. *J Dent Res*. 2005;84(11):1062–1065. doi:10.1177/154405910508401118

44. Al-Mubarak L, Alghamdi E, Alharbi S, Almasoud H. Air enema versus barium enema in intussusception: an overview. *Int J Community Med Public Health*. 2018;5(5):1679–1683. doi:10.18203/2394-6040.ijcmph20181487

45. Sadigh G, Zou KH, Razavi SA, et al. Meta-analysis of air versus liquid enema for intussusception reduction in children. *Am J Roentgenol*. 2015;205(5):W542–W549. doi:10.2214/AJR.14.14060

46. University of California, San Francisco Department of Urology. Phimosis. https://urology.ucsf.edu/patient-care/children/phimosis

47. Shah SS, Ronan JC, Alverson B. *Step-Up to Pediatrics*. Baltimore, MD: Lippincott Williams & Wilkins; 2014:209.

48. Kokotos F, Adam HM. Vulvovaginitis. *Pediatr Rev*. 2006;27(3):116–117. doi:10.1542/pir.27-3-116

49. McGreal S, Wood P. Recurrent vaginal discharge in children. *J Pediatr Adolesc Gynecol*. 2013;26:205–208. doi:10.1016/j.jpag.2011.12.065

50. Balighian E, Burke M. Urinary tract infections in children. *Pediatr Rev*. January 2018;39(1):3–12. doi:10.1542/pir.2017-0007

51. Shah SS, Ronan JC, Alverson B. *Step-Up to Pediatrics*. Baltimore, MD: Lippincott Williams & Wilkins; 2014:296–297.

52. Shaikh N, Hoberman A, Hum SW, et al. Development and validation of a calculator for estimating the probability of urinary tract infection in young febrile children. *JAMA Pediatr*. 2018;172(6):550–556. doi:10.1001/jamapediatrics.2018.0217

53. Hay AD, Sterne JA, Hood K. Improving the diagnosis and treatment of urinary tract infection in young children in primary care: results from the DUTY Prospective Diagnostic Cohort Study. *Ann Fam Med*. 2016;14:325–336. doi:10.1370/afm.1954

54. Anton Calis K, Popat V, Dang DK, et al. Dysmenorrhea. In: Rivlin ME, ed. *Medscape*. https://emedicine.medscape.com/article/253812-overview#a6. Updated October 22, 2018

55. McCann M, Potter L. Progestin-only oral contraception: a comprehensive review. *Contraception.* 1994;50(6)(suppl 1):S9–S13. doi:10.1016/0010-7824(94)90113-9

56. Sepilian VP, Wood E. Ectopic pregnancy. In: Rivlin ME, ed. *Medscape.* https://emedicine.medscape.com/article/2041923-overview#a5. Updated September 28, 2017.

57. Lozeau A-M, Potter B. Diagnosis and management of ectopic pregnancy. *Am Fam Physician.* 2005;72(9):1707–1714. https://www.aafp.org/afp/2005/1101/p1707.html

58. Trent M. Pelvic inflammatory disease. *Pediatr Rev.* 2013;34(4):163–172. doi:10.1542/pir.34-4-163

59. Trent M. Status of adolescent pelvic inflammatory disease management in the United States. *Curr Opin Obstet Gynecol.* 2013;25(5):350–356. doi:10.1097/GCO .0b013e328364ea79

60. Workowski KA, Bolan GA. Sexually transmitted diseases treatment guidelines, 2015. *MMWR Recomm Rep.* 2015;64(RR3):1–137. https://www.cdc.gov/mmwr/preview/mmwrhtml/rr6403a1.htm

61. American Sexual Health Association. Statistics. http://www.ashasexualhealth.org/stdsstis/statistics

62. Centers for Disease Control and Prevention. Reported STDs in the United States, 2016. *CDC Fact Sheet.* https://www.cdc.gov/std/healthcomm/fact_sheets.htm.

63. Ghadishah D. Genital warts clinical presentation. In: James WD, ed. *Medscape.* https://emedicine.medscape.com/article/763014-clinical#b2. Updated October 16, 2018.

64. Girerd PH. Bacterial vaginosis clinical presentation. In: Rivlin ME, ed. *Medscape.* https://emedicine.medscape.com/article/254342-clinical#b4. Updated October 25, 2018.

65. Schoem S, Darrow D, eds. *Pediatric Otolaryngology.* Elk Grove, IL: American Academy of Pediatrics; 2012.

66. Pickering LK, Baker CJ, Kimberlin DW, eds. *Red Book.* 29th ed. Elk Grove, IL: American Academy of Pediatrics; 2012.

67. Dixit S, Difiori JP, Burton M, Mines B. Management of patellofemoral pain syndrome. *Am Fam Physician.* 2007;75(2):194–202. https://www.aafp.org/afp/2007/0115/p194.html

68. Shaw BA, Segal LS. Evaluation and referral for developmental dysplasia of the hip in infants. *Pediatrics.* 2016;138(6):e20163107. doi:10.1542/peds.2016-3107

69. Tamai J. Developmental dysplasia of the hip. In Jaffe WL, ed. *Medscape.* https://emedicine.medscape.com/article/1248135-overview#a8. Updated February 26, 2018.

70. Shah SS, Ronan JC, Alverson B. *Step-Up to Pediatrics.* Philadelphia, PA: Lippincott Williams & Wilkins; 2014:158–160.

71. American Academy of Orthopaedic Surgeons. Perthes disease. https://orthoinfo.aaos.org/en/diseases-conditions/perthes-disease

72. Kocher MS, MacDonald J, Ogunwole O. Little Leaguer's shoulder. In: Miller MD, Hart JA, MacKnight JM, eds. *Essential Orthopaedics.* Philadelphia, PA: Saunders Elsevier; 2010:864–867.

73. Basset A. Pediatric abuse. OrthoBullets website. https://www.orthobullets.com/pediatrics/4001/pediatric-abuse?expandLeftMenu=true

74. Kishner S. Osteomyelitis. In: Poduval M, ed. *Medscape*. https://emedicine.medscape.com/article/1348767-overview#a7. Updated March 1, 2018

75. Shah SS, Ronan JC, Alverson B. *Step-Up to Pediatrics*. Philadelphia, PA: Lippincott Williams & Wilkins; 2014:300–302.

76. Kocher MS, Zurakowski D, Kasser JR. Differentiating between septic arthritis and transient synovitis of the hip in children: an evidence-based clinical prediction algorithm. *J Bone Joint Surg Am*. December 1999;81(12):1662–1670. doi:10.2106/00004623-199912000-00002

77. Novais EN, Millis MB. Slipped capital femoral epiphysis: prevalence, pathogenesis, and natural history. *Clin Orthop Relat Res*. 2012;12(2):3432–3438. doi:10.1007/s11999-012-2452-y

78. American Academy of Orthopaedic Surgeons. Slipped capital femoral epiphysis. https://orthoinfo.aaos.org/en/diseases–conditions/slipped-capital-femoral-epiphysis-scfe

79. Shah SS, Ronan JC, Alverson B. *Step-Up to Pediatrics*. Philadelphia, PA: Lippincott Williams & Wilkins; 2014:162–163.

80. Whitelaw CC. Transient synovitis. In: Jung LK, ed. *Medscape*. https://emedicine.medscape.com/article/1007186-overview#a5. Updated December 20, 2018

81. Brasic JR. Autism spectrum disorder treatment and management. In: Pataki C, ed. *Medscape*. https://emedicine.medscape.com/article/912781-treatment. Updated November 27, 2018.

82. Tejani NR. Febrile seizures. In: Bechtel KA, ed. *Medscape*. https://emedicine.medscape.com/article/801500-overview#a5. Updated December 11, 2018.

83. Netea MG, Kullberg BJ, Van der Meer JWM. Circulating cytokines as mediators of fever. *Clin Infect Dis*. 2000;31(suppl 5):S178-S184. doi:10.1086/317513

84. van Esch A, Steyerberg EW, Berger MY, et al. Family history and recurrence of febrile seizures. *Arch Dis Child*. 1994;70(5):395-399. doi:10.1136/adc.70.5.395

85. Caviness V, Ebinger F. Headache in pediatric practice. In: Dulac O, Lassonde M, Sarnat HB, eds. *Handbook of Clinical Neurology 112: Pediatric Neurology Part II*. Cambridge, MA: Elsevier; 2013:827–838. doi:10.1016/B978-0-444-52910-7.00002-7

86. Understood Team. An overview of different kinds of learning disabilities [Video]. Understood.org. https://www.understood.org/en/learning-attention-issues/getting-started/what-you-need-to-know/video-an-overview-of-different-kinds-of-learning-disabilities

87. American Psychiatric Association. What is specific learning disorder? APA website. https://www.psychiatry.org/patients-families/specific-learning-disorder/what-is-specific-learning-disorder. APA website.

88. Navigator LD. Educational placement decisions: The IEP process. *LD.org*. http://ldnavigator.ncld.org/#/education-related/educational-placement-decisions

89. American Psychiatric Association. What is ADHD? APA website. https://www.psychiatry.org/patients-families/adhd/what-is-adhd

90. National Center for Learning Disabilities. What is ADHD? [Video]. https://www.youtube.com/watch?v=0Wz7LdLFJVM. Published February 20, 2013.

91. National Institute for Children's Health Quality. NICHQ Vanderbilt assessment scales. NICHQ website. https://www.nichq.org/resource/nichq-vanderbilt-assessment-scales

92. American Academy of Child & Adolescent Psychiatry. School refusal. https://www.aacap.org/AACAP/Families_and_Youth/Facts_for_Families/FFF-Guide/School-Refusal-007.aspx. Updated June 2018.

93. Fremont WP. School refusal in children and adolescents. *Am Fam Physician.* 2003;68(8):1555–1561. https://www.aafp.org/afp/2003/1015/p1555.html

94. Roosevelt GE. Acute inflammatory upper airway obstruction (croup, epiglottitis, laryngitis, and bacterial tracheitis). In: Kliegman RM, ed. *Nelson Textbook of Pediatrics.* 20th ed. Philadelphia, PA: Elsevier; 2016:2031–2036.

95. Smith DK, McDermott AJ, Sullivan JF. Croup: diagnosis and management. *Am Fam Physician.* 2018;97(9):575–580. https://www.aafp.org/afp/2018/0501/p575.html

Electronic Resources

AAP Asthma guidelines:
https://www.aap.org/en-us/Documents/medicalhome_resources_keypoints forasthma.pdf
Westley Croup Score:
https://www.mdcalc.com/westley-croup-score

3

Common Diagnostic Tests in Pediatrics

LABS

The most common diagnostic labs used in pediatric settings are ordered for a wide range of indications. Many of these labs are used to diagnose acute infections and guide treatment, whereas others are used to manage complex chronic conditions. Table 3.1 shows the most common labs used in pediatrics, their indications, and factors to consider when interpreting the labs. It is important to note that many labs have normal reference ranges that vary due to patient age and gender. Point-of-care (POC) options for some of the more frequently ordered laboratory tests are becoming more and more common in outpatient settings as well as in EDs. Most POC tests are rapid versions of long-standing laboratory tests and are usually less expensive and just as reliable. Check with the manufacturer's user manual to establish reference ranges. For tests sent to outside labs, always check with the laboratory to determine standard reference ranges when interpreting results.

TABLE **3.1** Common Pediatric Laboratory Tests

Test Name and Normal Reference Range	Indication	Notes
Acute phase reactants		
CRP: <1 mg/dL	To differentiate between viral and bacterial infection	Elevated results can occur in obese patients and in patients with diabetes, chronic infections, or

(*continued*)

TABLE 3.1 Common Pediatric Laboratory Tests (*continued*)

Test Name and Normal Reference Range	Indication	Notes
ESR: 0–10 mm/hr[a]	Assess and monitor inflammation	long-standing inflammation
Bilirubin		
Bilirubin, total: 1.0–12 mg/dL Indirect bilirubin: 0.2–0.8 mg/dL Direct bilirubin: 0.1–0.3 mg/dL	Neonatal jaundice	Treatment will depend on risk factors and the nomogram used Newborn levels >15 mg/dL require immediate treatment to prevent kernicterus
Blood culture		
No growth in two culture specimens	Bacteremia, sepsis	Obtain two culture specimens from two different sites to confirm bacteremia Perform cultures before giving antibiotics Preliminary reports may be available at 24 hours, but 48–72 hours are required to identify organism and/or confirm no growth
CBC with differential[a] (+/− peripheral smear)		
WBC: $5–17 \times 10^9$ /L RBC: $3.5–6 \times 10^{12}$ /L Hgb: 9.5–20 g/dL Hct: 29%–64% MCV: 80–95 fL MCH: 27–31 pg MCHC: 32–36 g/dL RDW:11%–14.5% Platelets: $150–475 \times 10^9$/L Neutrophils: 55%–70% Lymphocytes: 20%–40% Monocytes: 2%–8% Eosinophils: 1%–4% Basophils: 0.5%–1.0%	Varies; may be useful if you suspect: Infections/sepsis Anemias Nutritional deficiency Concerning weight loss Marrow failure Trauma/hemorrhage Hemolysis Renal failure Chronic illness	Increased WBC count usually indicates infection, inflammation, tissue necrosis, or leukemic neoplasia A persistent increase in WBC counts may indicate a worsening infection A decrease in WBC counts may indicate marrow failure The Hct is usually 3× the Hgb Hgb values are slightly increased in patients living at higher altitudes Hgb, Hct and MCV values are an integral part of the evaluation of anemic patients
CMP[a]		
Glucose (fasting): 30–110 mg/dL Sodium: 134–150 mEq/L Chloride: 90–110 mEq/L Potassium: 3.4–5.3 mEq/L	Varies; may be useful if you suspect: Diabetes Electrolyte imbalance Muscle injury	CMP is ordered frequently in pediatric settings, but if liver function tests are not needed for clinical decision-making, you could order a BMP

(*continued*)

TABLE 3.1 Common Pediatric Laboratory Tests (*continued*)

Test Name and Normal Reference Range	Indication	Notes
Calcium: 8.8–10.8 mg/dL Bicarbonate: 13–28 mEq/L BUN: 3–18 mg/dL Creatinine: 0.2–1.0 mg/dL ALT: 4–36 IU/L AST: 15–40 units/L Alk Phos: 30–235 units/L Bilirubin: 0.3–1.0 mg/dL Protein (total): 4.2–8 g/dL Albumin: 3–5.9 g/dL	Renal disease Liver disease Heart disease Malnutrition Dehydration Parathyroid disease Cancer	
Fecal fat		
0–6 g/24 hr	Failure to thrive Cystic fibrosis Celiac disease	A fat-retention coefficient determines the difference between ingested and fecal fat Increased levels represent steatorrhea, which may indicate malabsorption or maldigestion
Hemoccult stool test		
Negative	Blood in stool	Common POC test that can be done quickly in an office or ED Refer patients with positive test to gastroenterology
Hemoglobin A1C		
Nondiabetic: 4%–5.9% Good diabetic control: <7%	Obesity Types 1 and 2 diabetes	Used to monitor diabetic glucose control, but can now also be used to establish a diagnosis of type 2 DM
Influenza A and B		
Negative	Febrile with rapid onset of URI symptoms	Most POC Influenza swab values are highly specific but have low sensitivity
Lipid panel[b]		
Total cholesterol: 70–200 mg/dL LDL: <110 mg/dL HDL: >45–55 mg/dL Triglycerides: 0–160 mg/dL	Screening for CVD risk Obesity Familial hypercholesterolemia	The appropriate age to begin statin use in children is subject to debate

(*continued*)

TABLE **3.1** Common Pediatric Laboratory Tests (*continued*)

Test Name and Normal Reference Range	Indication	Notes
Monospot		
Negative	Cervical lymphadenopathy +/− fatigue, fever, sore throat, dysphagia	False-negative results may be reported if testing is done too early, as antibodies have not formed in sufficient numbers
Pregnancy test		
Negative	Secondary amenorrhea	Urine testing is a common POC test available in most office settings
Rapid strep test		
Negative	Bacterial (Group A *Streptococcus*) tonsillitis, pharyngitis	A common POC test Follow-up throat cultures can be done if rapid test is negative Obtain POC and culture swabs from oropharynx at the same time
RSV swab		
Negative	Child younger than 3 with cough, wheezing, and crackles during respiratory season	Bronchiolitis is often diagnosed using clinical judgment, physical exam, and CXR Many clinicians use rapid diagnostic assays to guide treatment
Skin scrapings prepared with KOH and saline		
Normal cells, no hyphae, or budding seen	Candida, tinea variants	Confirmation of infection can guide treatment for both candida and tinea Fungal cultures grow slowly, usually requiring 4 weeks for identification
Stool culture		
No growth	Suspect bacterial enteritis Acute to chronic diarrhea	A positive bacterial culture report will list the pathogen found as well as the sensitivities of various antibiotic therapies

(*continued*)

TABLE 3.1 Common Pediatric Laboratory Tests (*continued*)

Test Name and Normal Reference Range	Indication	Notes
Tissue culture with Gram stain		
No growth	Wound or soft tissue infection	Obtain culture before starting antibiotics Most labs will provide a culture and sensitivity report to guide antibiotic selection
TSH		
0.3–18 μU/mL[a]	Growth concerns Thyroid dysfunction	Additional labs can be ordered to help confirm a thyroid dysfunction and assist in monitoring the disease
Urinalysis (+/− culture)		
Appearance: Clear Color: amber yellow pH: 4.6–8.0 Protein: 0–8 mg/dL Specific gravity: 1.005–1.030 Leukocyte esterase: negative Nitrites: none Ketones: none Bilirubin: none Urobilinogen: 0.01–1 unit/mL Crystals: none Casts: none	Suspected UTI Dysuria Hematuria Type I diabetes Type II diabetes Renal disease	Obtain urine culture if leukocyte esterase and/or nitrites are positive, as that is suspicious for infection Suspect renal stones if crystals noted Protein is a sensitive indicator of kidney function, so consider ordering a 24-hour urine specimen, if significant protein found on UA
Glucose: none WBC: 0–4/LPF RBC: <2 Culture: No growth		If the urine has a red-to-orange color, ask the parent or patient whether they have taken a urinary tract analgesic, such as pyridium

Note: Laboratories may use different reference ranges than the ones listed to report values. You should always check with the laboratory at your institution to determine standard reference ranges when interpreting results.

[a] Values in children are age specific with normal values varying throughout the first 18 years.

[b] Values vary by age and gender.

AST, aspartate aminotransferase; Alk phos, alkaline phosphatase; ALT, alanine aminotransferase; BMP, basic metabolic panel; BUN, blood urea nitrogen; CBC, complete blood count; CMP, comprehensive metabolic panel; CRP, C-reactive protein; CVD, cardiovascular disease; CXR, chest x-ray; DM, diabetes mellitus; ESR, erythrocyte sedimentation rate; HDL, high-density lipoprotein; Hgb, hemoglobin; Hct, hematocrit; LDL, low-density lipoprotein; LPF, low-power field; MCV, mean corpuscular volume; MCH, mean corpuscular hemoglobin; MCHC, mean corpuscular hemoglobin concentration; POC, point of care; RBC, red blood cell; RDW, red blood cell distribution width; RSV, respiratory syncytial virus; TSH, thyroid-stimulating hormone; URI, upper respiratory infection; WBC, white blood cell.

Source: Adapted from Pagana KD, Pagana TJ. *Mosby's Manual of Diagnostic and Laboratory Tests.* 4th ed. Saint Louis, MO: Elsevier; 2010.

DIAGNOSTIC IMAGING STUDIES

Diagnostic imaging studies for pediatric patients range from simple to sophisticated, with most of the same technology that is available for adult patients. The most common diagnostic study in pediatrics is the x-ray. X-rays can help in the diagnosis of many conditions, are inexpensive, and can often be done in an outpatient provider's office or at an outpatient diagnostic imaging center. When ordering any diagnostic imaging, you should provide the radiology technician and the radiologist with as much clinical information as possible. This helps them provide a more comfortable setting for the patient, as well as allows the radiologist to prepare the most appropriate report and interpretation.

CT/ MRI

In ambulatory pediatric settings, CT and MRI are not typically first-line choices; however, for hospitalized patients, those seeing a specialist, or those needing surgery, a CT or MRI may be required to provide a more complete evaluation of a patient or before a surgical procedure to learn more about the patient's pathology and anatomical structures. CT and MRI are commonly used to visualize disease and injury to the brain and spinal cord as well as cardiovascular and vascular issues. Tumor diagnosis and disease of the bones and joints are other indications for these scans.

The use of CT imaging has declined during the last decade as providers have shifted to alternate modalities.[1] With advances in technology, many clinicians now order ultrasound for abdominal, chest, and musculoskeletal complaints. This is beneficial in the pediatric setting as the patients do not need sedation and the procedure is less costly.[2] CT is more specific and sensitive in many of the situations previously mentioned, but ultrasound is often technically easier for patients and families, which often outweighs the slight decrease in specificity and sensitivity. Choosing Wisely® (www.choosingwisely.org) and American College of Radiology (ACR) Appropriateness Criteria (www.acr.org/Clinical-Resources/ACR-Appropriateness -Criteria) are two resources useful for guiding your choice of diagnostic imaging based on pertinent clinical findings.

RADIOGRAPHS/X-RAYS

Head

- Indications: Injury, infection
  - Pertinent findings: Skull fracture, nasal fracture, and sinusitis. *Note:* Most ED clinicians will order a CT of the head for a head injury; however, with increased concern about exposing children to high levels of radiation, some clinicians are returning to skull x-rays. If a pediatric patient is found to have a skull fracture on x-ray, a CT of the head

should be highly considered. X-rays of the sinuses are done infrequently but may be helpful for determining fluid levels in the sinuses as well as polyps and cysts

Neck

- Indications: Injury, infection, stridor, cough, shortness of breath
  - Pertinent findings: Cervical spine fracture (best seen in lateral view), cervical misalignment, and soft-tissue swelling. If anterior soft tissue swelling is noted, consider anterior neck, while prevertebral swelling should make you think of a retropharyngeal abscess, a foreign body, or soft-tissue hypertrophy from stridor and/or snoring. Epidglottitis has a classic thumb-print sign, while croup has a classic steeple sign on neck x-rays a foreign body or soft-tissue hypertrophy from stridor and/or snoring; epiglottitis (thumb-print sign); and croup (steeple sign)

Chest

- Indications: Injury (e.g., sports injury, blunt-force trauma with shortness of breath), external catheter placement, infection, shortness of breath, and cough
  - Pertinent findings: Pneumothorax, rib fracture, pneumonia, bronchiolitis, bronchitis, foreign body, tuberculosis, and pleural effusion

Abdomen

- Indications: External catheter placement, ingested foreign body, injury (e.g., blunt-force trauma), infection, hematuria, abdominal pain, air enema, abdominal mass
  - Pertinent findings: Renal lithiasis, hydronephrosis, mass, umbilical vein catheter placement, intestinal obstruction, intussusception, and constipation

Pelvis (Often Ordered With Abdomen X-rays)

- Indications: Injury, infection
  - Pertinent findings: Pelvis fracture, lumbosacral vertebral fracture, pyelonephritis, and pelvic pain

Musculoskeletal

- Indications: Injury (e.g., sports injuries, trauma, soft-tissue injury), infection, mass
  - Pertinent findings: Anatomical fractures, osteomyelitis, dislocations, and benign and oncologic bony lesions

ULTRASOUND

Point-of-care ultrasound (POCUS) is now used frequently in medical offices and EDs, as well diagnostic imaging departments. Many providers now order ultrasound before more expensive modalities, such as CT.

Head

- Indications: Injury, mass, hydrocephalus, birth trauma
  - ○ Pertinent findings: Orbital fracture, craniosynostosis, cephalohematoma, subdural hemorrhage, and retinal tear

Neck

- Indications: Mass, infection, thyroid enlargement
  - ○ Pertinent findings: Thyroid neoplasm, thyroglossal duct cyst, lymphangitis, and sialadenitis

Cardiac (Echocardiogram)

- Indications: Injury, infection, congestive heart failure
  - ○ Pertinent findings: Coarctation of the aorta, pericardial effusion, congenital malformations, valvular anomalies, and murmurs

Chest

- Indications: Injury (e.g., blunt-force trauma), mass
  - ○ Pertinent findings: Pleural space fluid and breast mass

Abdomen

- Indications: Injury (e.g., blunt-force trauma), infection, obstruction, mass
  - ○ Pertinent findings: Splenomegaly, cholelithiasis, appendicitis, bowel obstruction, pyloric stenosis, and pancreatitis

Renal

- Indications: Injury, infection, mass, hematuria
  - ○ Pertinent findings: Congenital anomalies, renal calculi, hydronephrosis, and pyelonephritis

Pelvis

- Indications: Injury, infection, mass
  - ○ Pertinent findings: Ovarian mass, pregnancy, ectopic pregnancy, and intrauterine device (IUD) placement

Musculoskeletal

- Indications: Injury, infection, mass
  - ○ Pertinent findings: Compartment syndrome, deep vein thrombosis, Baker's cyst, hematoma, and osteomyelitis

OTHER DIAGNOSTIC TESTING

Some of the other tools used for diagnosis in pediatrics require specialized training, contrast materials, or specialized equipment. Even though they are ordered infrequently compared to the laboratory tests and imaging modalities noted earlier in the chapter, these diagnostic tests can be the gold standard for some diagnoses.

JOINT ASPIRATION (ARTHROCENTESIS) WITH SYNOVIAL FLUID ANALYSIS

- Indications: Injury, infection
  - ○ Interpretation/Pertinent findings: Hemarthrosis, pseudogout, large effusion, and septic joint

LUMBAR PUNCTURE WITH CEREBROSPINAL FLUID ANALYSIS

- Indications: Infection, subarachnoid hemorrhage, central nervous system (CNS) disease
  - ○ Interpretation/Pertinent findings: Meningitis, encephalitis, and subarachnoid hemorrhage

PULMONARY FUNCTION TEST

- Indications: Shortness of breath, cough with exercise
  - ○ Interpretation/Pertinent findings: Asthma, bronchospasm, restrictive lung disease, and vocal cord dysfunction
  - ○ The most common spirometry results show the following:
    - Forced vital capacity (FVC): Amount of air forcibly exhaled
    - Forced expiratory volume over 1 second (FEV1): Amount of air forcibly exhaled over 1 second
    - FEV1/FVC: This is the percentage of the FVC that person exhaled in the first second
    - Peak expiratory flow (PEF): An indication of effort as this is the flowrate the patient attains during exhalation and usually occurs at the beginning of exhalation
    - Normal for FVC, FEV_1, and PEF is between 80% and 120% of what has been predicted for the patient
  - ○ To adequately gauge the patient's effort, you have to include the patient's age, gender, and height; the patient has to be able to adequately perform the test, which involves holding the spirometry mouthpiece and tubing, taking a deep breath, placing teeth and lips securely around the mouthpiece, and blowing out as fast and hard as possible for as long as possible; the spirometer will trace the patient's effort throughout the attempt; patient should get a minimum of three attempts and a maximum of eight; the technician should monitor and encourage the patient during the test

VOIDING CYSTOURETHROGRAM

- Indication: Complicated/recurrent urinary tract infection (UTI)
  - ○ Interpretation/Pertinent fndings: Vesicourethral reflux by grade I to V, duplicated collecting ducts, and pyelonephritis

REFERENCES

1. Parker MW, Shah SS, Hall M, et al. Computed tomography and shifts to alternate imaging modalities in hospitalized children. *Pediatrics*. 2015;136(3):e573–e581. doi:10.1542/peds.2015-0995
2. Hiscock H, Neely RJ, Warren H, et al. Reducing unnecessary imaging and pathology tests: a systematic review. *Pediatrics*. 2018;141(2):e20172862. doi:10.1542/peds.2017-2862

4

The Well-Child Check and Preventative Care Guidelines

Well-child checks (WCCs) are regularly scheduled visits designed to evaluate a child's growth, physical health, and development, as well as to offer an open forum for patients or caregivers to ask questions about growth and/or development. Pediatric well visits tend to coincide with specific, well-established developmental milestones and immunization needs. Although there are general guidelines for what should be discussed during the WCC visit, it is important that you understand that these checks are dynamic and should be somewhat flexible, as pediatric patients are not always as cooperative as their adult counterparts.

HISTORY

A thorough and focused well-child history provides most of the information needed to differentiate between a child with normal, age-appropriate growth and development and the child who would benefit from further evaluation or interventions. As the age-adjusted normals for nutrition, elimination, sleep, developmental milestones, family interaction, and growth expectations change dramatically over time, you should develop a system for organizing this information or have a handy reference available to use until you begin to feel more comfortable with all the ages and stages of pediatrics.

When a healthy child presents for a routine well-child care visit, a systematic way of capturing information that will help determine your final assessment is very helpful. Starting with the fuel that helps kids grow is a logical first step.

DIET

Determining the appropriate nutritional status of a pediatric patient allows you to assess potential deficiencies and abundances, as well as offer patients and parents information on changing demands/needs. However, nutrition is more than feeding frequency and portion sizes. It is important to ask families and patients about fruit, vegetable, and protein sources, while recognizing that deficiencies in these areas may require supplementation. As iron-deficiency anemia is a common problem in pediatrics, inquiring about iron sources (natural or fortified), in addition to milk consumption, is key. Milk binds iron in the gut and makes it less bioavailable for absorption, so high dairy intake could put a child at risk for iron-deficiency anemia.

Encouraging whole grains and limiting added sugar and salt are key nutritional concepts that can help curb childhood obesity. The general recommendations for various age groups around fruit, vegetable, protein, carbohydrate, dairy, and vitamin intake will change with differing growth patterns and ages, so you should always tailor your information to the child's individual situation, and a family's cultural foods, keeping in mind that poverty contributes greatly to a child's nutritional status. For patients who struggle with food insecurity, asking about government assistance use, encouraging school breakfast and lunch program participation, and having resources for food banks, summer lunch programs, backpack programs, and how to apply for assistance are essential.

ELIMINATION

Elimination is a top parental observation during the early years, as parents are immersed in diaper changes and toilet training. Therefore, understanding normal elimination patterns and being able to provide reassurance and anticipatory guidance to families around elimination will serve you well in your pediatrics rotation. Elimination, both urination and defecation, are also helpful indicators of health. Baseline queries should include the type of elimination, how frequently that occurs, color, and consistency.

SLEEP

As we now know, sleep is hugely important in the homeostasis of the human body, so discussing sleep with families at all ages of well visits should be a priority. Sleep position, quality and quantity of sleep, routines around sleep, and sleep safety/sleep hygiene are important components to consider for a screening interview around sleep. Sleep apnea and sleep disorders have become more prominent in the pediatric field, so having a working knowledge of the indicators for further testing will impress your pediatric preceptors.

> **CLINICAL PEARL:** Sleep routines and sleep sites can vary from night to night or even throughout the night, so asking specifically about sleep will allow you to gain insight into the changes that can occur from night to night or even during the night.

FAMILY

Although not a common component of adult well care, understanding the family and the living environment of the pediatric patient can help add to the growth and developmental picture. Understanding the family structure (e.g., single-parent households, teen mother, divorced parents with shared custody, grandparents as caregivers) and outside resources for the family can give you clues as to the roles that each person in the house may have in regard to the child and provide you with clues about routines or daily stressors (e.g., a family with a parent on military deployment, mother who works nights or a single-parent family). Other questions you should ask include number of siblings and ages, plans for more children, childcare, and outside support such as friends, family, day-care providers, afterschool care, and support groups like religious organizations or parent groups. The family situation would not be complete without asking about financial resources, use of government supplement programs (if applicable), insurance, and housing.

> **CLINICAL PEARL:** Just asking about money may not reveal true issues of poverty. Poverty is multifactorial and includes the environment in which a child is raised. A family may have sufficient funds to buy food, but this may be at the expense of interactions with the child.

Once families are established and much of this information is known, the family situation may address only how the family is adjusting or handling a new age or stage. As children age, you may start asking patients these questions in an attempt to "break the ice" and move from low-stakes questions to more personal issues.

DEVELOPMENTAL MILESTONES

The vast majority of pediatric well care is focused on the physical, emotional, social, and cognitive development of infants, children, and adolescents. Early in the child's life, motor developments are the most overt developmental changes, and thus are the focus for much of the infant and early childhood years. These are slowly supplanted by the development of language, cognitive, and social–emotional skills. A renewed interest in physical development occurs during puberty, along with significant social–emotional transformations.

As one of the most important aspects of well-child care, assessing appropriate development at each and every visit is of key importance. Development builds on foundational skills, which if weak, may delay the progression of a developmental domain. Early identification and intervention for specific areas of delay or struggle is the single, most influential factor in future outcomes. In addition, providing caregivers with anticipatory guidance around the upcoming age or stage can help them prepare and provide the most appropriate supports to try to ensure the greatest success.

Development occurs in a predictable manner, starting centrally and moving peripherally. For example, brain development and myelination start in the core of the brain and move peripherally. Infant vision begins quite myopic and slowly improves to include peripheral and distance vision. The foundation of motor skills is gross motor truncal control with a slow march peripherally to fine motor control at the distal extremities. Social–emotional skills commence with a focus on understanding self and then move "peripherally" to relationships with others, whereas cognitive development begins with basic intelligence and then progresses to application and problem-solving. Finally, communication in infants is primarily nonverbal and slowly expands to repetitive sounds, single words, two-word phrases, and short sentences by early childhood, from which the full sentences and ideas of adolescence emerge.

CLINICAL PEARL: Children in bilingual families or those with older siblings should still reach developmental milestones at the appropriate age. If they do not, early referral is key for increasing the catch-up that might be required.

GROWTH CHARTS

Prior to seeing the patient, the first step in the evaluation is to review the child's growth chart, paying attention to the trajectory of previous points compared to today's point. In children younger than 2 years of age, length, weight, and head circumference should be plotted on a World Health Organization (WHO) growth chart. Beginning at 2 years old, height is measured using a stadiometer and can be combined with weight and age to plot body mass index (BMI). Evaluating the growth velocity and growth trends over time are more valuable than a single point on the graph, but a weight-to-length ratio can provide you with information on the proportionality of the child. Much of the tracking related to physical health comes via measuring vital signs. Blood pressure measurements should begin at 3 years old and hearing and vision exams should start at 4 years old. Beginning at 2 weeks of age, development can be tracked using serial surveillance (i.e., regular well-child exams that ask about development and monitor for "red flags" around development) and screening tools (standardized tools designed to identify delays by developmental domain) can be implemented as early as 2 months. Although much of the tracking done at well-child visits uses objective measures, the wise PA student will never fail to incorporate the anecdotal observations of the family. Even without formal medical or developmental training, parents are keen observers of their children and are often the first to note a change. Box 4.1 notes the components of a thorough well-child visit.

Box 4.1 COMPONENTS OF A THOROUGH WELL-CHILD VISIT

Diet
Natural foods
Vitamins
Iron sources
Grains
Added sugar

Elimination
What and when?
Color
Consistency

Sleep
Position
Quality
Routines
Sleep safety/sleep site

Family
Family structure, including siblings
Outside support
Adjustments
Money/finances

Developmental Milestones
Physical development (gross and
    fine motor skills)
Intelligence/cognition
Communication (verbal and
    nonverbal)
Social–emotional

Growth Chart

An important interview instrument that is commonly used in adolescent well visits is the HEADSS (**h**ome, **e**ducation, **a**ctivities/employment, **d**rugs, **s**exuality, **s**uicide/depression). The late Dr. Eric Cohen, a clinical professor and medical educator at the University of Southern California, developed this tool. It suggests asking about HEADSS.[1] The components of the HEADSS instrument are noted in Table 4.1.

TABLE 4.1 HEADSS Adolescent Interview Instrument and Sample Questions

Home	Who lives with the young person? Where? Does he or she have his or her own room? What are relationships like at home? What do parents/relatives do for a living?	Has he or she ever been institutionalized? Incarcerated? Recent moves? Running away? New people in home environment?
Education and employment	School/grade performance (any recent changes, any dramatic past changes)? Favorite subjects and worst subjects (including grades)? Any years repeated/classes failed?	Suspension, termination, dropping out? Future education/employment plans? Any current or past employment? Relations with teachers, employers, including school, work attendance?

(continued)

TABLE 4.1 HEADSS Adolescent Interview Instrument and Sample Questions (*continued*)

Activities	On own, with peers, with family (What do you do for fun? Where? When?) Sports (regular exercise)? Church attendance, clubs, projects? Hobbies/other activities? Reading for fun?	Favorite TV show? How much TV does he or she watch weekly? Favorite music? Does he or she have a car? Use seatbelts? History of arrests (acting out), crime?
Drugs	Use by peers? Use by young person? Use by family members (include tobacco, alcohol)?	Amounts, frequency, patterns of use/abuse, and car use while intoxicated? Source and how paid for?
Sexuality	Sexual orientation? Degree and types of sexual experience and acts? Number of partners? Masturbation? (normalize) History of sexual/physical abuse?	History of pregnancy/abortion? STI—knowledge and prevention? Contraception? Frequency of use? Comfort with sexual activity, enjoyment/pleasure obtained?
Suicide and depression	Sleep disorders (usually induction problems, also early/frequent waking or greatly increased fatigue, despite sleep)? Appetite/eating behavior changes? Feelings of "boredom"? Emotional outbursts and highly impulsive behavior? History of withdrawal/isolation? Hopeless/helpless feelings? Psychosomatic symptomology?	History of past suicide attempts, depression, psychological counseling? History of suicide attempts in family or peers? History of recurrent serious "accidents"? Suicidal ideation (including significant current and past losses)? Decreased affect on interview, avoidance of eye contact—depression posturing? Preoccupation with death (clothing, media, music, art)?

HEADSS, home, education and employment, activities, drugs, sexuality, and suicide/depression; STI, sexually transmitted infection.
Source: Goldenring JM, Cohen E. Getting into adolescent heads. *Contemporary Pediatrics.* July 1, 1988. http://www.contemporarypediatrics.com/pediatrics/getting-adolescent-heads/page/0/3. Accessed June 17, 2018.

PHYSICAL EXAMINATION

A well-child exam typically involves a thorough head-to-toe physical exam that pays particular attention to age-appropriate techniques. Table 4.2 lists some of the most common exam components, the age range at which it should be performed, and the findings, while Table 4.3 lists normal vital sign ranges by age. The physical exam may also include assessing physical milestones, cognitive and social abilities, confirming parental observations, and observing parent–child interactions.

TABLE 4.2 Physical Exam Findings Unique to the Pediatric Exam by Age

Body System	Specific Physical Exam Component	Age Range for Exam	What Are You Looking for?
Vital signs		See Table 4.3 for vital signs by age	Abnormal vitals
Head	Fontanelle size	Birth until anterior fontanelle is closed (usually by 12 months)	Premature closure of the fontanelle (craniosynostosis)
	Head shape	All age ranges, but critical from birth until 1 year	Evaluate for flat occiput or asymmetry growth (plagiocephaly)
Eyes	Red reflex	Birth until 5–6 years old, but most critical in infancy	Retinoblastoma
	Cover–uncover	Typically unable to perform reliably until 15–18 months and continues until 5–6 years old	Strabismus, which left uncorrected will lead to amblyopia
	Extraocular movements	Typically unable to perform reliably until 6–9 months	Intact cranial nerves III, IV, VI
	Pupillary light reflex	All ages	Esotropia, exotropia, convergence disorders, pupillary dilation/constriction disorder
Ears	Shape, position, presence of pits or tags, deformity	All ages	Presence of pits or tags should signal an evaluation for kidney disease Deformities may be related to hearing loss, syndromes, or trauma
Nose	Nasal patency	Birth	Choanal atresia can be further screened for by trying to pass a catheter through the nostril; if atretic, catheter will not pass
Mouth	Frenulum	Birth until speech becomes well defined	"Tongue-tied" (ankyloglossia) occurs when the frenulum prohibits upward tongue movement, which may affect latch, nursing, and speech
	Teeth	All ages	Natal teeth (should be referred to a dentist), malocclusion, caries, gingivitis

(continued)

TABLE **4.2** Physical Exam Findings Unique to the Pediatric Exam by Age (*continued*)

Body System	Specific Physical Exam Component	Age Range for Exam	What Are You Looking for?
Neck	ROM	All ages	Torticollis in the infant can indicate birth trauma or SCM paralysis
	Head lag	Birth to 6–9 months	Head lag should disappear by 6 months; retained head lag could indicate a neuromuscular deficit
	Strength	All ages	Weakness or asymmetry in forward and lateral flexion, extension, and lateral turning
Heart	Auscultation	All ages	Murmurs, tachycardia, bradycardia
Lungs	Auscultation	All ages	Adventitious sounds
Abdomen	Palpation	All ages	To detect umbilical hernia and diastasis rectus, organomegaly
MSK	Ortolani and Barlow maneuvers	Birth until 1 year or walking	Dislocation and/or relocation of the hip, also referred to as a click or a clunk, which indicates DDH
	Leg length discrepancy	Birth until 1 year or walking; anytime there is asymmetry	A shortened leg might indicate DDH
	Gait	Once the child is walking unassisted	To detect limp, asymmetry, neuromuscular disease
Pulses	Femoral pulses	All ages	Decreased femoral pulses could indicate a coarctation of the aorta
Extremity	Thigh skin-fold symmetry	Birth until 1 year	Asymmetry might indicate DDH
Genital	Labia	Until puberty	Labial adhesions
	Testicles	1 year	Retractile and cryptorchid testicle
	Sexual maturity rating (Tanner staging)	(8–15 females; 10–16 males)	Tanner stage out of proportion to chronologic age

DDH, developmental dysplasia of the hip; MSK, musculoskeletal; ROM, range of motion; SCM, sternocleidomastoid muscle.

Tᴀʙʟᴇ **4.3** Vital Signs by Age

Age	Heart Rate (bpm)	Respiratory Rate (bpm)	Blood Pressure (mmHg)
Premature	120–170	40–70	55–75/35–45
0–3 months	100–150	35–55	65–85/45–55
3–6 months	90–120	30–45	70–90/50–65
6–12 months	80–120	25–40	80–100/55–65
12–36 months	70–110	20–30	90–105/55–70
3–6 years	65–110	20–25	95–110/60–75
6–12 years	60–95	14–22	100–120/60–75
>12 years	55–85	12–18	110–120/65–80

Aɢᴇ-Aᴘᴘʀᴏᴘʀɪᴀᴛᴇ Sᴄʀᴇᴇɴɪɴɢs

The American Academy of Pediatrics (AAP) recommends that all children have screening exams periodically throughout the years, many of which are either questionnaires or laboratory tests. These are a means of detecting medical conditions that, if not detected and treated early, will adversely influence growth or development. These include congenital diseases, micronutrient deficiency, heavy-metal poisoning, developmental delays, autism, high-risk behaviors, and depression. Table 4.4 indicates recommended screenings by age.

Vᴀᴄᴄɪɴᴇs

Always remember to evaluate a child's immunization status at each visit, but this is most important at the well-child exam. The most recent immunization recommendations can be found on the Centers for Disease Control and Prevention (CDC) website, as well as downloaded as an app for your smartphone. Catch-up vaccinations should also be offered at any time vaccine doses have been missed. Table 4.5 shows the most commonly administered vaccines by WCC ages.

TABLE 4.4 Recommended Screenings by Age

	Example of Screening Exam	What It Is Screening for ...	Age(s)	Treat/Refer if ...
Laboratory data	Newborn blood screening	Hemoglobinopathies and congenital disease	Before hospital discharge Repeated within the first month of life	Abnormalities reported
	Hgb or Hct with confirmatory CBC, including MCV	Iron-deficiency anemia	12 months[a]	6 months to <5 years: Hgb <11g/dL and low MCV 5 to <12 years: Hgb <11.5 g/dL and low MCV
	Lead level	Lead exposure	12 months[a] 24 months	≥5 mcg/dL
	Lipid panel	Dyslipidemia	10 years old 20 years old	Abnormal results
	Oral mucosal HIV antibody testing; rapid HIV-1; EIA	HIV	Once between 16 and 18 years old, but more often as dictated by sexual activity risk level	Positive on confirmatory Western blot
	STI testing	Chlamydia, gonorrhea, syphilis, trichomoniasis	At sexual debut or as dictated by sexual activity risk level	Positive results need treatment
	Pap smear	Cervical dysplasia	Starting at 21 years old	LGSIL or higher
Vitals	Length/height and weight	Growth	Starting at birth	Crosses 2 percentile lines
	Head circumference	Micro- or macrocephaly	Starting at birth until 24 months	<5th or >95th percentile
	BMI	Nutritional status	Starting at 2 years old	<5th or >95th percentile
	BP	Essential hypertension	Starting at 3 years old	>90th percentile
	Snellen chart	Visual acuity	Starting at 3 years old and continue annually until 6, then at 8, 10, 12, and 15 years old	4 years old: worse than 20/40 >5 years old Worse than 20/30

(continued)

TABLE 4.4 Recommended Screenings by Age (*continued*)

	Example of Screening Exam	What It Is Screening for . . .	Age(s)	Treat/Refer if . . .
	Acoustic	Hearing	Prior to hospital discharge, annually between 4 and 6 years of age, 8, 10, 11–14, and 15–18 years of age	Failed
	Oral health assessment	Caries risk stratification	6 months 9 months	All patients should receive a referral to a dental home
	ASQ; CDI; PEDS, Denver-II Developmental Screening Test	Developmental progress	9 months 18 months 30 months[b]	Results warrant watchful waiting or referral
Questionnaires	M-CHAT	Autism	18 months 24 months	Failed
	CRAFFT	Alcohol and drug use	Annually starting at 11 years old	Positive results
	PHQ-2, PHQ-9	Depression	Annually starting at 12 years old	PHQ-2 positive → PHQ-9 PHQ-9 positive
	EPDS	Maternal postpartum depression	At every well visit from 2–6 months of age	>10

[a] May start earlier for high-risk infants, such as preterm infants.

[b] Not a standard WCC time interval, so some practices may do at 24 months WCC.

ASQ, Ages and Stages Questionnaire; BMI, Body mass index; BP, Blood pressure; CBC, complete blood count; CDI, Child Development Inventory; CRAFFT, car, relax, alone, forget, friends, trouble; EIA, enzyme immunoassay; EPDS, Edinburgh Postnatal Depression Scale; Hgb, hemoglobin; Hct, hematocrit; LGSIL, low-grade squamous intraepithelial lesion; M-CHAT, Modified Checklist for Autism in Toddlers; MCV, mean corpuscular volume; PEDS, Parents' Evaluation of Developmental Status; PHQ, Patient Health Questionnaire; STI, Sexually transmitted infection; WCC, well-child check.

Source: Adapted from information from American Academy of Pediatrics. Engaging patients and family: periodicity schedule. AAP website. https://www.aap.org/en-us/professional-resources/practice-transformation/managing-patients/Pages/Periodicity-Schedule.aspx; Hagan JF, Jr, Shaw JS, Duncan PM, eds. *Bright Futures: Guidelines for Health Supervision of Infants, Children, and Adolescents.* 4th ed. Elk Grove, IL: American Academy of Pediatrics; 2017; Powers JM, Mahoney DH, Jr. Iron deficiency in infants and children <12 years: screening, prevention, clinical manifestations, and diagnosis. In: Motil KJ, Drutz JE, eds. UpToDate. https://www.uptodate.com/contents/irondeficiency-in-infants-and-children-less-than12-years-screening-preventionclinical-manifestations-and-diagnosis. Updated January 21, 2019.

TABLE **4.5** Vaccine Schedule by Most Commonly Administered WCC Ages

Vaccine	Birth	2 mo.	4 mo.	6 mo.	12–15 mo.	15–18 mo.	24 mo.	4–5 yr	11–12 yr	15–16 yr
DTaP		#1	#2	#3		#4		#5		
HepA					#1	#2[a]				
HepB	#1	#2		#3						
Hib		#1	#2	#3[b]	#4					
HPV									#1 and #2	
IPV		#1	#2	#3				#4		
MenACWY									#1	#2
MenB										#1, #2, #3[b]
MMR					#1			#2		
PCV13		#1	#2	#3	#4					
RV		#1	#2	#3[b]						
Tdap									#1	
Var					#1			#2		
IIV		Once annually after 2-dose season (starting after 6 months of age)								

[a] If longer than 6 months since the first dose.

[b] Dose may be necessary depending on the vaccine used.

DTaP, diphtheria, tetanus, acellular pertussis; HepA, hepatitis A; HepB, hepatitis B; Hib, *Haemophilus influenzae* type b; HPV, human papillomavirus; IIV, inactivated influenza vaccine; IPV, inactivated poliovirus; MenACWY, meningococcal serotypes ACWY; MenB, meningococcal serotype B; MMR, measles, mumps, and rubella; PCV13, pneumococcal conjugate vaccine; RV, rotavirus; Tdap, tetanus, diphtheria, acellular pertussis; Var, varicell; WWC, well-child check

ANTICIPATORY GUIDANCE

Anticipatory guidance may be considered information about physical and behavioral changes the family can anticipate between the current visit and the next regularly scheduled well exam. Or parents and caregivers might have questions or concerns about those items that can affect growth or development. Common areas of anticipatory guidance and education include dietary recommendations, sleep hygiene (including sudden infant death syndrome [SIDS], which is also referred to as *"sudden unexpected infant death [SUID]"* prevention), anticipated growth patterns and expected changes in development, and what all those changes may mean for families and patients. Safety is a major aspect of pediatric care, so a large focus of education surrounds safety practices such as carseat use, bicycle safety, pedestrian safety, water safety, choking hazards, toxic ingestion prevention, sun safety, and accident prevention. For preteens and teens, distracted driving, mitigating high-risk behaviors, contraception, and drug and alcohol abuse are hot topics.

AGES AND STAGES

With pediatrics having such a wide variation in ages and abilities, it can be helpful to group ages with stages of development and common parental concerns. The following section briefly describes the various ages and stages of pediatrics to help you remember key developmental features and anticipatory guidance for those ages. Additionally, Appendix 4.1 provides a brief chart view of the various WCC ages with age-appropriate recommendations for nutrition, voiding, sleep, development and guidance suggestions.

BIRTH TO 1 MONTH

The first month of life is a roller coaster ride for both the newborn and the family. There are the up-and-down emotions of being giddy with joy to tearful with the baby blues; the adjustment to a new addition; and the physical, physiological, and emotional demands of the postpartum period. Breastfeeding support is a primary focus at the 3- to 5-day check and adequate weight gain and family adjustment typically dominate the 2-week well visit. Well visits in the first month of life should focus on the following:

- Encouraging families to initiate and continue exclusive breastfeeding with a recommendation for feeding 8 to 12 times in a 24-hour period based on hunger cues
- Educating mothers on the changes that occur at the breast with continued breastfeeding, such as less engorgement, milk being made on demand in response to suckling, and milk let-down sensations, which are just as important as caring for sore nipples, perceptions of low milk supply, and proper latch
- Reviewing practices to reduce SIDS, such as putting the baby on his or her back to sleep, keeping baby swaddled until able to roll over, and never sharing a bed
- Counseling families on infant breathing patterns and avoiding swings or bouncers that can allow the infant's unsupported neck to collapse the airway
- Reviewing signs of respiratory distress is imperative at this stage

2 TO 6 MONTHS

Once adjusted, families typically find great contentment during the first 6 months of an infant's life. They are able to establish some routines, sleep begins to improve, and development is overt and tangible. Physically, infants at this stage are growing rapidly. Motor development quickly moves an infant from a supine, helpless position to a sitting, grasping position, and there are increasing signs of connection between the baby and the parents. However, one of the normal developmental stages that parents may not anticipate is crying.

A crying infant can be very distressing for parents, so educating families at this stage about crying as a developmental milestone is essential. The anticipatory guidance at this stage centers on the following:

- Teaching families that the "crying" milestone peaks at 2 months and then begins to lessen; crying at this stage is unexpected and unexplainable; may not stop no matter what is done; can appear as though it is painful; can be long lasting; and occurs more frequently in the afternoons and evenings;[2] the most influential advice may very well be to discuss "never shake a baby," support systems, and walk-away techniques
- Reviewing soothing techniques for the developmental stage of crying
- Screening and discussing maternal crying/postpartum depression symptoms
- Explaining how and when to introduce complementary foods
- Reminding parents to be mindful of increasing infant mobility and keeping a hand on the infant at all times to reduce fall risks

9 TO 12 MONTHS

Nine to 12 months is a time of slowed physical and gross motor development and increased social–emotional and cognitive growth. In addition to changes in social–emotional development, the child will display an increasing autonomy (self-feeding, holding toys, sitting unsupported, pulling to a stand, and maybe even taking those first few steps). Having repeated successes and autonomy often means that infants are even more determined to accomplish a goal; however, they are still quite developmentally dependent and the disconnect between their motor abilities, their communication skills, and their wants can create great frustration for the infants. Although there are early signs of foundational language, such as stringing together sounds like "da-da," it is far from what is needed to express emotion. Consequentially, 9- to 12-month-olds revert to crying for communication. Anticipatory guidance at this stage centers on the following:

- Discussing the expanding diet and reviewing choking hazards, portion sizes, and healthy foods and drinks
- Preparing for erupting teeth by discussing oral health care and safe teething remedies
- Helping parents in their new role of setting limits by reviewing the difference between discipline and punishment (discipline is teaching about wanted behavior; punishment is control over bad behaviors via fear) and providing techniques for discipline, such as redirection and time-outs
- Guiding parents on the do's and dont's, such as do read and introduce books to the infant, do provide safe spaces for exploration, do lower the mattress on the crib, but do not smoke around the child, do not leave the child unattended, and do not use a walker[3]

15 TO 24 MONTHS

This stage may very well be the most explosive developmentally of all the stages. Physically, growth is somewhat stable, but there is great refinement in the gross and fine motor skills. Toddlers build their independence and begin walking and running between activities, exploring previously uninteresting corners and cabinets of the house, and explaining their findings with an expanding vocabulary. Their play moves from playing alone to playing in parallel with other toddlers, but stranger apprehension may have them hiding behind their mothers' legs in unfamiliar situations. In addition to safety, the anticipatory guidance at this stage centers on:

- Reading aloud to a child; this is the single most important factor in early literacy development, which correlates to increased expressive and receptive language skills, reading ability, and academic success
- Exploring the world; Toddlers should be given safe spaces to explore and structured outdoor play; caution parents to watch their fearless toddlers closely, as their exuberance and inexperience can lead to falls/injuries
- Educating on elimination; you should share with parents that toilet training should start only when the toddler is developmentally ready, which is signaled by an interest and desire to learn, staying dry for 2-hour periods, being able to pull pants down and up, knowing the difference between wet and dry, and communicating when he or she knows he or she needs to have a bowel movement; reassurance around the variable speed and acumen of this developmental skill should be given routinely

3 YEARS OLD

Having gained great motor control, the 3-year-old has developed the coordination to ride a tricycle, dress and undress, draw with some precision, and prepare a bowl of cereal. He or she has an extensive vocabulary that is 75% understandable, understands 2-step commands, and has begun to learn how to take turns, making interactive play easier to facilitate. At this stage, children crave attention and will use their new found vocabulary and growing intelligence to say funny things to make adults laugh. They make friends easily, yet they can be fickle about foods, sleep, and being offered help with daily tasks. Melt downs are not uncommon. Much of the anticipatory guidance at this stage centers on the following:

- Helping parents balance the freedom a 3-year-old needs to explore, with the limits that he or she needs to stay safe, organized, and functional
- Reminding parents that children demonstrate more desirable behaviors when given firm limits with the freedom to make choices within those limits, such as which shoes to wear out of two choices

4 YEARS OLD

Four year olds are "big kids" with big imaginations. Physically, their growth continues at a modest pace, but their coordination is improving. They typically attend preschool or day care and are beginning to recognize letters and sounds, print their names with a mature pencil grasp, draw pictures, and play collaboratively with friends. They may ride a bike with training wheels and are the gregarious, "who, what, when, and why" kids with an insatiable curiosity. Their magical thinking brings imaginary friends to life and goofy details to a story. The anticipatory guidance for 4-year-old WCCs may focus on the following:

- Gun safety, including safe storage (out of the house or locked with the safety in place and ammunition in separate storage area)[3]
- Strangers, including giving parents the tools to discuss how to respond to grown-up strangers
- Private areas, including "good touch/bad touch" and private areas are those covered by a bathing suit; no adults should ask kids to help them with their private parts; and so on
- School preparation, including encouraging families to play games with their children that help with identifying letters and sounds, reading together, and providing age-appropriate chores that will help children develop the skills to get ready to attend school

5 to 6 Years Old

This stage marks a dramatic shift in development from primarily outward development to more cognitive development. The visual difference between the first day and the last day of kindergarten may be only a few inches or pounds, but the cognitive changes are tremendous. School-aged children must undertake cognitive and psychosocial tasks to have educational and social achievement and must shift from "taking it all in" to differentiating between important and unimportant information. The kindergartener must work on self-regulation, impulse control, following the rules, and making friends. There is also a shift from isolated developmental tasks to activities that require integration of multiple skills, such as sitting still; following directions; managing time; and sequencing the execution of a task, which requires persistence and sustained attention. When they are not in school, they love to climb trees, hop and skip, ride a bike, and practice printing with improved precision. They play cooperatively with others and may even join their first sports team. They show off their counting skills and letter decoding, as they learn simple arithmetic and reading. The anticipatory guidance for this stage centers on:

- Encouraging parents to create routines around homework to reinforce concepts being taught in school; activities such as reading nightly even if it is not assigned; helping with homework, but not doing it for them; creating a space and a time in the routine to do the homework; and so on will bolster concepts taught in school
- Educating children and parents about healthy habits that include providing five servings of fruits and vegetables a day, limiting screen time to 2 hours a day, engaging in 1 hour of exercise/activity a day, and limiting sugar-sweetened beverages[4]

● Emphatically reminding families to require the use of a helmet when riding a bike, scooter, skateboard, or roller skates

7 TO 10 YEARS OLD

Well established in school routines, 7- to 10-year olds have now made the transition to school life, gained small doses of independence, and improved simple executive functions. They have also transitioned from a learning-to-read stage to a reading-to-learn mindset and school performance has become the developmental gauge. This is also the time that learning disabilities and attention deficit hyperactivity disorder (ADHD) may become apparent. Inquiring about school performance, inability to keep up with grade-level expectations, or teacher concerns can uncover these issues.

Same gender friendships and activities that require increased coordination and physical skill dominate the playground at recess. The elementary school child displays slow and steady growth and by late childhood (8–9 years old in females and 9–10 years old in males) may exhibit some prepubertal changes, such as body odor, increased oil production on the facial skin, axillary hair, and acne (blackheads and pimples). For females, late childhood marks the onset of puberty with thelarche (initial breast development) occurring on average between 8 and 10 years old, depending on genetics and ethnicity. This increases feelings of modesty and may change the dynamic of the WCC (e.g., draping appropriately during the exam, asking siblings to step out of room, giving opportunity to talk with provider alone). The anticipatory guidance for this age centers on:

● Encouraging families to talk daily about school issues, including bullying, concerns about school performance, or praise of school successes.
● Instructing parents on praising their children for responsible behavior, allowing children to make age-appropriate decisions, enjoying activities together, and giving them chores to help them gain competence and see their importance to the family and the community.
● Supervising children online and reviewing Internet safety, a key point to cover with kids and parents, as increasing independence and a world of handheld devices may soften the boundaries previously set by a family; kids should be supervised whenever they are online, should have only game choices that are age-appropriate, screen time should be limited, and Internet filters should be employed; remind kids that "browsing the Internet" can be potentially harmful and is not a good use of time.

11 TO 14 YEARS OLD

The physical and social–emotional changes associated with tweens and early teens are some of the most dramatic since the toddler years. Although girls may begin pubertal changes between 9 and 10 years old, the majority of the hormonal and physical changes occur in the tween and early teen years. Puberty, like other developmental phases, follows a fairly predictable pattern for both males and females. The rapid growth and physical changes create an increased nutritional demand, a shift in sleep cycles, increasing myelination of the brain's frontal lobe, and emotional lability. Adjusting to increased responsibility and independence, burgeoning love interests, and rising school demands, the middle school or junior high patient can appear distracted, introverted, or may be difficult to engage in conversation. A large focus of the anticipatory guidance for this stage is around:

- Asserting independence, as this is a major task of early adolescence; Providing tweens and teens with an opportunity to talk directly with you one-on-one offers the opportunity to provide tweens and teens with age-appropriate, evidence-based health information and encourages them to make their own conclusions about how to handle the information; this approach is far more effective than "lecturing" or "telling them what to do."
- Providing a safe space for tweens/teens to talk about issues and concerns without judging them, which will help them feel supported
- Talking with tweens/teens about how difficult it can be to juggle new responsibilities, emerging independence, school demands, and social interests, which can allow them an opportunity to articulate their priorities and work through the barriers that are keeping them from reaching their goals
- Reminding tweens of the importance of quality sleep and that sleep should not be ignored when juggling multiple priorities; chronic sleep deprivation can lead to poor judgment, poor academic performance, and poor concentration

15 TO 18 YEARS OLD

At 15 to 18 years old, teens are now making their way through the halls of high school trying to navigate the unstable landscape of social status, peer and opposite-sex relationships, and identity formation. Although most of the physical change of puberty is complete by 15, patients' outward appearances and brain development continue to change. These teens experiment with appearance via hairstyles, clothing, jewelry, makeup, tattoos, and piercings, all in an effort to overcome self-consciousness and develop an identity. Depression, anxiety, and suicidality rise in this age group, so screening for (and intervening when necessary) mental health issues is universally recommended for all teens. Toward the later end of this stage, teens are preparing for life after high school, whether that is working, going to college, or attending a trade school. They are developing the ability to make judgments using sound reasoning, but may resort to more emotional decision-making, which continues to lead to risk-taking behaviors, especially as related to sexual exploration, illegal substances, and driving. Anticipatory guidance in this stage really focuses on risk mitigation, including:

- Having candid conversations about prescription and illicit drugs; Prescription drug overdoses have recently become one of the leading killers of

teens (surpassing motor vehicle accidents in some states); This conversation, although difficult at times, can provide teens with reliable, evidence-based information upon which to make decisions
- Providing an opportunity to discuss sexual activity and safe-sex practices, sexually transmitted infections, and family-planning options; With 20% of teens experiencing an unintended pregnancy or sexually transmitted infection, discussing safe sex and the benefits of long-acting reversible contraceptives (LARCs) may feel uncomfortable at first, but teens will be grateful for the opportunity to receive quality information about these topics from you
- Educating patients and parents about the risks of newly licensed teens, driving at night, and texting and driving, as motor vehicle accidents are one of the leading causes of death in this age group
- Using the teen's long-term goals as a springboard for discussing how choices and behaviors can either help or hurt his or her ability to reach those goals, which may allow the teen to open up to more discussions

Key Points

- The history, including diet, elimination, sleep, and family adjustments, combined with objective data, such as the developmental milestones and growth charts, are key areas that should be reviewed in a WCC.
- Physical exam components are variable and change with the age of the patient.
- Screening tests and immunizations are an important component of the well visit.
- Understanding the ages and stages of pediatrics can help to create a gestalt about what to expect, what kids are capable of doing, and how you can guide parents/patients.

REFERENCES

1. Goldenring JM, Cohen E. Getting into adolecent heads. *Contemporary* Pediatrics. http://www.contemporarypediatrics.com/pediatrics/getting-adolescent-heads/page/0/3. Published July 1, 1988.
2. Barr M. What is the period of PURPLE crying? The Period of PURPLE Crying website. http://purplecrying.info/what-is-the-period-of-purple-crying.php
3. Hagan JF, Shaw JS, Duncan PM, eds. *Bright Futures: Guidelines for Health Supervision of Infants, Children, and Adolescents.* 4th ed. Elk Grove, IL: American Academy of Pediatric; 2017.
4. MaineHealth. Let's go!'s response to latest national childhood obesity data. https://mainehealth.org/news/2018/03/lets-gos-response-to-latest-national-childhood-obesity-data. Published March 9, 2018.

Electronic Resources

Bright Futures Periodicity Schedule:
https://www.aap.org/en-us/professional-resources/practice-transformation/ managing-patients/Pages/Periodicity-Schedule.aspx
CDC Immunization Schedule:
https://www.cdc.gov/vaccines/schedules/hcp/child-adolescent.html
HHS/USDA Pediatric Calorie Requirements by Age and Activity level:
https://www.nhlbi.nih.gov/health/educational/wecan/downloads/calreqtips.pdf

Appendix 4.1 Well-Child-Check Charts by Age

2 Months Old

Nutrition	
Breastfeeding	8–12 times per day (on-demand cues)
	10 minutes of active feeding
Bottle-feeding	Feeds less frequently than breastfed infant
	3–4 oz. q3–4hr
Vitamins	Vitamin D (400 IU) daily if breastfeeding
	Prenatal vitamins for mother
Dairy	Breast milk or lactose-based formula

Source: American Heart Association. Dietary recommendations for healthy children. https://www.heart.org/en/healthy-living/healthy-eating/eat-smart/nutrition-basics/dietary-recommendations-for-healthy-children. Last reviewed April 16, 2018.

Elimination	
Urination	6–8 wet diapers per day
Stooling	Breastfed: Yellow, loose, and seedy; may be irregular and infrequent Formula-fed: Tan to brown; 3–4 stools per day

Sleep	
Position	Put on back for sleeping
Quantity	4–5 hours per night; 2–3 naps Total: 12–16 hours
Sleep site/safety	AAP recommends cosleeper or crib with room sharing; no bedsharing
	Snug mattress and narrow crib slats
	No plush toys, blankets, pillows, bumpers in sleeping area
	No bottles to bed

Family	
Family, including siblings	Division of responsibility
	Parental time with each other
	Parental time with other children (W/O infant)

(continued)

(continued)

Family	
Outside support	Ask about support networks
	Childcare if parent returning to work
Adjustment to age or stage	Ask about/screen for maternal depression and sleep
	Colic and crying
Money	Any food insecurity
	WIC supplements, if needed and qualify

Developmental Milestones	
Physical Development	
Gross motor	Lifting head up
	Pushing up from prone position
Fine motor	Grasping objects
	Brings hands to midline/mouth
Communication/Language Development	
Verbal	Coos
Nonverbal	Differentiation of cry
Cognitive/Intellectual Development	
Intelligence	None to note
Problem solving	Indicates boredom with crying/fussiness
Social–Emotional Development	
Connection	Social smile
	Responds to parents' voices
	Follows parents' faces and/or light with eyes
Self-regulation	Hands to midline/mouth

Screenings and Immunizations	
Screenings	EPDS
	ASQ
Immunizations	HepB, IPV, DTaP, Hib, PCV13, Rotavirus

Anticipatory Guidance	
Continue to offer breast milk (or formula) as primary nutrition	Nighttime awakenings can occur at 4 months
Vitamin D, if not using	Continue to put back to sleep in a crib or cosleeper, no bed sharing
Hold complementary foods until 4–6 months	

(continued)

(continued)

Anticipatory Guidance	
Avoid passive smoke exposure	Postpartum depression si/sx
Turn hot water heater to <120°F	Colic and infant crying; techniques to
Sun safety	handle
Car seat (backward-facing infant	Rolling and increased mobility → fall
carrier in the back seat)	risk → need to keep one hand on
Do not allow bottle grazing	baby at all times

AAP, American Academy of Pediatrics; ASQ, Ages and Stages Questionnaire; DTaP, diphtheria, tetanus, acellular pertussis; EDPS, Edinburgh Postpartum Depression Screen; HepB, hepatitis B; Hib, *Haemophilus influenzae* type b; IPV, inactivated poliovirus; PCV13, pneumococcal conjugate vaccine; WIC, Women, Infants, and Children.

4 Months Old

Nutrition	
Breastfeeding	6–10 times per day (more routine feedings)
	Easily distractible, so may need low stimuli during feeds
Bottle-feeding	6–8 feeds per day
	30–32 oz. per day
Natural foods	Hold complementary foods until 6 months if breastfeeding
	Rice cereal OK as first food
Vitamins	Vitamin D (400 IU) daily if breastfeeding
	Prenatal vitamins for breastfeeding mother
Iron sources	May need to screen and supplement LBW and preemies
Dairy	Breastmilk or lactose-based formula

Elimination	
Urination	6–8 wet diapers per day
Stooling	Breastfed: Yellow, loose, and seedy; may be irregular and infrequent Formula-fed: Tan to brown; 3–4 stools per day

Sleep		
Position	Put on back for sleeping	
Quantity	5–6 hours per night; 2–3 naps	Total: 12–16 hours

(continued)

(continued)

Sleep	
Sleep site and safety	AAP recommends cosleeper (a device that attaches to the bed) or in a crib in the parent's room (room sharing); no bedsharing Snug mattress and narrow crib slatsNo bottles, plush toys, blankets, pillows, bumpers in sleeping area Stop swaddling when infant begins rolling

Family	
Family, including siblings	Division of responsibility Parental time with each other Parental time with other children (without infant)
Outside support	Ask about support networks Childcare if parent returning to work
Adjustment to age or stage	Ask about/screen for maternal depression and sleep Returning to work/childcare decisions
Money	Any food insecurity WIC supplements, if needed and qualify

Developmental Milestones	
Physical Development	
Gross motor	Sits with support Pushes up on elbows/rolls from front to back
Fine motor	Reaching for objects/bats at objects Brings hands together in clapping motion
Communication/Language Development	
Verbal	Babbles more expressively and spontaneously Imitates sounds
Nonverbal	Clearer behavior to indicate needs
Cognitive/Intellectual Development	
Intelligence	Responds to changes in environment
Problem solving	Indicates boredom with crying/fussiness
Social–Emotional Development	
Connection	Smiles spontaneously Laugh and squeal develop
Self-regulation	Solidified self-consoling skills

Screenings and Immunizations	
Screenings	EPDS ASQ
Immunizations	HepB, IPV, DTaP, Hib, PCV13, Rotavirus

Anticipatory Guidance	
Continue to offer breast milk (or formula) as primary nutrition source	Stooling may change with addition of complementary foods
Vitamin D, if not using	Postpartum depression si/sx
Offer only one food at a sitting until sure that it is well tolerated	Begin weaning night-time feeds
Avoid passive smoke exposure	Continue to put back to sleep in a crib or cosleeper, no bed sharing
Turn hot water heater to <120°F	Colic and infant crying; techniques to handle
Sun safety	Rolling and increased
Car seat (backward-facing infant carrier in the back seat)	mobility → fall risk → need to keep one hand on baby at all times
No bottle propping	

AAP, American Academy of Pediatrics; ASQ, Ages and Stages Questionnaire; DTaP, diphtheria, tetanus, acellular pertussis; EPDS, Edinburgh Postpartum Depression Screen; HepB, hepatitis B; Hib, *Haemophilus influenzae* type b; IPV, inactivated poliovirus; LBW, low birth weight PCV13, pneumococcal conjugate vaccine; WIC, Women, Infants, and Children.

6 Months Old

Nutrition	
Feeding	Breastmilk or formula feed 4–6 times per day (routine feedings)
	Typically take 24–32 oz. per day with complementary feedings
	Breastfeed before offering complementary food
	May begin complementary foods once tongue thrust disappears
	Rice cereal (usually the first food) or pureed foods can be offered 2–3 times per day
	OK to start on sippy cup with water (no juice) with solid feedings
Vitamins	Vitamin D (400 IU) daily if breastfeeding
	Prenatal vitamins for breastfeeding mother
Iron sources	Baby's iron stores diminishing, so introduce iron-fortified cereals or pureed red meat; 1 oz. of iron-fortified cereal = daily requirement
Teeth	First teeth erupt; begin oral healthcare for baby (brush/wash teeth BID)

Elimination	
Urination	6–8 wet diapers per day
Stooling	Breastfed: May be irregular and infrequent; may become more odiferous and change to brown/pasty with addition of solids
	Formula-fed: Tan to brown; 3–4 stools per day

Sleep	
Position	Put on back for sleeping
Quantity	"Sleeping through night" Total: 12–16 hours
	6–8 hours per night; 2–3 naps
Sleep site and safety	AAP recommends cosleeper or crib with room sharing; no bedsharing
	Snug mattress and narrow crib slats
	No bottles, plush toys, blankets, pillows, bumpers in sleeping area
	Stop swaddling when infant begins rolling

Family	
Family, including siblings	Typically clearer role definitions by this time
	If siblings helping with infant → Discuss sibling safety
Outside support	Early support systems begin to fade, but ↑ demands on time from infant → may need respite time
	Childcare, if parent returning to work
Adjustment to age or stage	Ask about/screen for maternal depression and sleep
	Returning to work/childcare decisions
Money	Any food insecurity
	WIC supplements, if needed and qualify

Developmental Milestones	
Physical Development	
Gross motor	Sits with minimal support
	Rolls back to front
Fine motor	Holds blocks/toys (likes toys that require two hands)
	Object transfer
Communication/Language Development	
Verbal	Single consonant vocalizations (ah, eh, oh)
	Vocal turn taking
Nonverbal	Points with index finger
	Smiles responsively
Cognitive/Intellectual Development	
Intelligence	Recognizes own name and turns toward sounds
Problem solving	Visual and oral exploration helps develop learning
Social–Emotional Development	
Connection	Interacts with people (especially parents)
	Tries to talk to image in mirror
Self-regulation	Grasps a toy for comfort
	Oral exploration/visual exploration for calming

Screenings and Immunizations	
Screenings	EPDS
	ASQ
Immunizations	HepB, IPV, DTaP, Hib, PCV13, Rotavirus, influenza (if seasonally appropriate)

Anticipatory Guidance	
Continue breast milk (or formula) as the primary nutrition source	Do not allow bottle grazing
Offer only one food at a sitting until sure that it is well tolerated	Stooling may change with addition of complementary foods
Avoid honey until 1 year of age (infant botulism risk)	Night-time feeds should be weaned
Avoid passive smoke exposure	Continue to put back to sleep in a crib or cosleeper, no bed sharing
Turn hot water heater to <120°F	Postpartum depression si/sx
Sun safety	Walkers are fall risk and not recommended
Car seat (backward-facing infant carrier in the back seat)	Increased mobility → fall risk → need to keep one hand on baby at all times

AAP, American Academy of Pediatrics; ASQ, Ages and Stages Questionnaire; DTaP, diphtheria, tetanus, acellular pertussis; EPDS, Edinburgh Postpartum Depression Screen; HepB, hepatitis B; Hib, *Haemophilus influenzae* type b; IPV, inactivated poliovirus; PCV13, pneumococcal conjugate vaccine; WIC, Women, Infants, and Children.

9 Months Old

Nutrition	
Feeding	Breastfeeding 4–5 times per day
	Bottle-feeding 3–4 times per day (16–24 oz./d with complementary feedings)
	Solids can be offered as three meals per day; three snacks per day
	Sippy cup with water (no juice)
	Offer new foods as snacks
	Increased self-feeding
	High chair for solids; arms for milk/formula
Iron sources	1 oz. of iron-fortified cereal = daily requirement; serve with fruit with vitamin C for increased iron absorption
Grains	Continue grain cereals; add in whole grain, cooked pasta; Cheerios
Teeth	Usually have two to four teeth; begin looking for dental home

Elimination	
Urination	8–12 times per day
Stooling	Usually less frequent than before due to slower transit time

Sleep	
Position	Continue to put on back for sleep, but decreased SIDS risk
Quantity	Longer night-time stretches; two to three naps Total: 12–16 hours May see increased night-time awakenings
Sleep site and safety	Most have moved to crib Put mattress on lowest level Always put sides up in the crib, as standing up in crib becomes common

Family	
Family, including siblings	Ask about relationship and date nights for parents Sibling safety → never leave infant alone with sibling
Outside support	Who are the caregivers outside of the parents? Are there resources for childcare for "date nights"?
Adjustment to age or stage	Discipline versus punishment Setting limits Behavior management
Money	Financial supports WIC supplements, if needed and qualify

Developmental Milestones	
Physical Development	
Gross motor	Crawling Pulls to a stand
Fine motor	Pincer grasp Likes to shake, bang, throw, and drop objects
Communication/Language Development	
Verbal	Repetitive consonants and vowels (e.g., ma-ma, da-da, be-be) Understands *no*
Nonverbal	Starts to point objects out
Cognitive/Intellectual Development	
Intelligence	Object permanence
Problem-solving	Likes cause-and-effect toys (drop and dump)
Social–Emotional Development	
Connection	Stranger apprehension Plays peek-a-boo and so-big games

(continued)

(continued)

Developmental Milestones	
Self-regulation	Seeks parents for comfort and as a resource
	May use a transitional object

Screenings and Immunizations	
Screenings	EPDS
	ASQ
Immunizations	Typically none, but catch-up vaccines can be done at this time

Anticipatory Guidance	
Continue breast milk (or formula) as primary nutrition source	Continue iron-fortified foods
Encourage healthy complementary foods	Avoid honey until 1 year of age (infant botulism risk)
Transition to cow's milk (usually whole) at 1 year old	Crib safety
	Encourage routines around sleep
Avoid passive smoke exposure	Water safety, stair safety (never leave unattended near water, gates on stairs, no walkers)
Sun safety	
Car seat (backward-facing infant carrier in the back seat)	
Discipline vs. punishment	Choking hazards (plastic bags, small toy parts, foods—grapes, hot dogs, carrots, popcorn, nuts, etc.)
Remind parents that infants cannot remember "rules"	
Discuss early literacy and the importance of reading aloud	
Provide book resources	

ASQ, Ages and Stages Questionnaire; EPDS, Edinburgh Postpartum Depression Screen; SIDS, sudden infant death syndrome, WIC, Women, Infants, and Children.

12 MONTHS OLD

Nutrition	
Feeding	Encourage continued breastfeeding, if mutually desirable
	Begin weaning off bottle and formula
	Eating less than previously (may eat one large meal, two smaller meals, and two to three snacks)
	Wide variety of foods, including fruits, veggies should be offered
	Food struggles are common
	Snacks should be rich in complex CHO, but minimal sweets
	Like finger foods, but are MESSY EATERS!

(continued)

(continued)

Nutrition	
Vitamins	Vitamin D-fortified whole milk
	Other vitamin supplements not necessary, if eating balanced diet
Grains	Single grain (baby) cereals
	Finger foods (pasta, Cheerios, some crackers)
Teeth	Now has four to eight teeth; routine oral healthcare
	Establish dental home and first visit
Dairy	Transition formula feeders to whole milk in cup; if weaning from breastfeeding or only nursing a few times a day or night, transition to whole milk in a cup 2–3 cups (480–720 mL/d)

Elimination	
Output	Unchanged from previous visits

Sleep		
Position	Back to sleep	
Quantity	Longer nighttime stretches; one to two naps	Total: 12–16 hours
Sleep site and safety	Usually still in a crib	
	May be able to crawl out of the crib, even if mattress on lowest setting	

Family	
Family, including siblings	Ask about routines, as they continue to be very important
Outside support	Who are the caregivers outside of the parents?
	Are there resources for childcare for "date nights"?
Adjustment to age or stage	Encourage time-outs (1 minute per year of age) and redirection for unwanted behaviors
Money	Financial supports
	WIC supplements, if needed and qualify

Developmental Milestones	
Physical Development	
Gross motor	Stands alone; cruises and may take few steps alone
Fine motor	Puts items into and takes items out of containers
Communication/Language Development	
Verbal	Jabbers with inflection of normal speech
	One to three words in vocabulary, in addition to ma-ma and da-da

(continued)

(continued)

Developmental Milestones

Nonverbal	Protodeclarative pointing (points to desired object)
Cognitive/Intellectual Development	
Intelligence	Understands one-command directions, but may not follow Identifies a person on request
Problem-solving	Looks for dropped or hidden objects
Social–Emotional Development	
Connection	Plays games (peek-a-boo and pat-a-cake) and waves bye-bye Strong attachment to parent → separation anxiety
Self-regulation	Continued use of transitional objects

Screenings and Immunizations

Screenings	EPDS ASQ Screening for lead Screening for anemia
Immunizations	Hib, MMR, varicella, HepA, influenza (if seasonally appropriate)

Anticipatory Guidance

Encourage continued breastfeeding, as mutually desirable	Continue iron-fortified foods
Encourage healthy complementary foods	Crib safety
Transition to whole milk at 1 year	Encourage routines around sleep
Avoid passive smoke exposure	Discuss use of time-outs
Turn hot water heater to <120°F	(1 min/y of age) and redirection techniques
Sun safety	Remind parents that infants cannot remember "rules"
Car seat (may vary by state; forward-facing five-point harness at 1 year *and* 20 pounds)	Water safety, stair safety, choking hazards (see 9 months)
Discuss early literacy and the importance of reading aloud	
Provide book resources	

ASQ, Ages and Stages Questionnaire; CHO, carbohydrates; EPDS, Edinburgh Postpartum Depression Screen; HepA, hepatitis A; Hib, *Haemophilus influenzae* type b; MMR, measles, mumps, and rubella; WIC, Women, Infants, and Children.

15 TO 18 MONTHS OLD

Nutrition	
Feeding	Encourage continued breastfeeding, if mutually desirable
	Slowed growth now, so decease in appetite expected
	3 meals per day; 2-3 snacks per day (may skip meals; food jags common)
	Wide variety of foods, including fruits, veggies should be offered
	Should be adding in meat, poultry, beans, and fish over time
	Continue to introduce new flavors and textures
	Uses utensils with more dexterity, but prefers finger foods
	Keep regular schedule of meals/snacks
	Limit juice to <4 oz. per day
	Whole milk in a cup (16–24 oz./d)
Vitamins	Continue vitamin D-fortified whole milk
	Other vitamin supplements not necessary, if eating balanced diet
Iron sources	Meats, like chicken and fish, as well as beans
	Limit milk to ≤24 oz./d to prevent iron-deficiency anemia
Grains	Whole-grain pasta, Cheerios, some crackers
Teeth	Usually has eight teeth; routine oral healthcare

Elimination	
Output	Typically still in diapers, but may begin to transition to pull-ups

Sleep		
Position	Squirmy sleepers	
Quantity	12–14 hours per day; 1–2 naps per day	Total: 11–14 hours
	May have dreams and nightmares	
Sleep site and safety	If crawling out of the crib, may need to consider transition to toddler bed or bed with side rails	

Family	
Family, including siblings	Ask about plans for additional children
	Ask about consistent limits/expectations/discipline
	Any sibling rivalry?
Outside support	Toddler play groups
	Parents with children of same age

(continued)

(continued)

Family	
Adjustment to age or stage	Toddler's independence and mobility may lead to power struggles
	Temper tantrums/breath holding
	Biting, hitting
Money	Financial supports
	WIC, day-care assistance, HeadStart

Developmental Milestones

	15 months	18 months
Physical Development		
Gross motor	Walks well (wide gait)	Walks up steps holding a hand
	Stoops and recovers	Kicks a ball
Fine motor	Stacks two blocks	Stacks two to three blocks
	Drinks from a cup with help	Uses spoon and cup without spilling
Communication/Language Development		
Verbal	3-10 meaningful words	15–20 words with two-word phrases
Nonverbal	Brings objects to adults to show/ask for help	
Cognitive/Intellectual Development		
Intelligence	Understands simple commands	Follows simple commands without cues
		Points to one body part
Problem-solving	Points to specific object when asked, "Where is . . . ?"	
Social–Emotional Development		
Connection	Separation anxiety continues	Kisses and feeds dolls/animals Explores, if parent nearby
Self-regulation	Unpredictable behavior	Is selfish; cries when toys taken away

Screenings and Immunizations

Screenings	ASQ at 15 months
	M-CHAT at 18 months
Immunizations	DTaP, HepA, influenza (if seasonally appropriate)

Anticipatory Guidance

Continue iron-rortified cereal until age 2
Review portion sizes; educate on food jags
Avoid mealtime fights (parents decide what variety of healthy foods to offer at a meal and child decides how much to eat)

Review signs of toilet-training readiness (shows interest, stays dry for 2-hour periods, able to pull pants down and up, knows difference between wet and dry, can communicate when needs to have bowel movement)

(continued)

(continued)

Anticipatory Guidance	
Avoid passive smoke exposure	Transition to toddler bed or bed with side rails
Car seat (laws may vary by state; forward-facing five-point harness)	Poisons out of cabinets, locks on cabinets, medicine storage
Water safety, stair safety, choking hazards (see 9 months)	Gun safety (store out of house; store in locked cabinet with safety in place, store ammunition separately)

Discuss early literacy and the importance of reading aloud

Power struggles—offer de-escalating tips

Screen time and physical activity (60 minutes of activity; limit screen time to 1–2 hours)

ASQ, Ages and Stages Questionnaire; DTaP, diphtheria, tetanus, acellular pertussis; HepA, hepatitis A; M-CHAT, Modified Checklist for Autism in Toddlers; WIC, Women, Infants, and Children.

24 MONTHS OLD

Nutrition	
Feeding	Encourage continued breastfeeding, if mutually desirable
	Slowed growth now, so decrease in appetite expected
	Three meals per day; two to three snacks per day (may skip meals; food jags common)
	1 cup of fruits and 1 cup of vegetables per day
	1–2 oz. per day of meat and beans[a]
	Continue to introduce new flavors and textures
	Keep regular schedule of meals/snacks
	Limit juice to <4 oz. per day
Grains	3 oz. per day with 1.5 oz. from whole-grain sources[b]
Teeth	Usually has 16 teeth; routine oral healthcare
Dairy	Transition to 1% or skim milk
	Recommended daily intake is two servings per day of 1% or skim milk or yogurt (8 oz.) or cheese (1 ½ oz. natural cheese)

[a] 1 oz. = 1 oz. of meat, poultry, or fish, ¼ cup cooked dry beans or one egg.

[b] 1 oz. = 1 slice of bread, 1 cup of ready-to-eat cereal, ½ cup of cooked rice, pasta, or cooked cereal.

Elimination	
Output	Typically still in diapers, but may begin to transition to pull-ups

Sleep

Position	Squirmy sleepers	
Quantity	11–14 hours per day; 1 nap per day May have dreams and nightmares	Total: 11–14 hours
Sleep site and safety	Transition to toddler bed or bed with side rails Bedroom safety	

Family

Family, including siblings	Ask about plans for additional children Ask about consistent limits/expectations/discipline Any sibling rivalry?
Outside support	Toddler play groups Parents with children of same age
Adjustment to age or stage	Toddler's independence and mobility may lead to power struggles Temper tantrums/breath holding Biting, hitting
Money	Financial supports WIC, day-care assistance, HeadStart

Developmental Milestones

Physical Development	
Gross motor	Goes up and down stairs one at a time Throws a ball overhand Jumps up
Fine motor	Stacks five to six blocks Copies a straight line Can help to put clothes on
Communication/Language Development	
Verbal	20–50 words Two-word phrases ½ speech is understandable
Cognitive/Intellectual Development	
Intelligence	Follows two-step commands Names one picture in a book (cat, dog, boy)
Problem solving	Points to specific object when asked, "Where is . . . ?"
Social–Emotional Development	
Connection	Pretend play increases Parallel play (playing alongside another toddler, but not with)
Self-regulation	Attachment to objects

Screenings and Immunizations	
Screenings	M-CHAT
	Lead poisoning screening
	Iron-deficiency anemia screening, if necessary
Immunizations	HepA, influenza (if seasonally appropriate)

Anticipatory Guidance	
Review and encourage iron-fortified foods	Review signs of toilet-training readiness (see
Review portion sizes; educate on food jags	15–18 months)
Avoid passive smoke exposure	Transition to toddler bed or bed with side
Turn hot water heater to <120°F	rails Poisons out of cabinets, locks on
Car seat (may vary by state; forward-	cabinets, medicine storage
facing five-point harness)	Gun safety (store out of house; store in
Water safety, stair safety, choking hazards	locked cabinet with safety in place, store
(see 9 months)	ammunition separately)

Discuss early literacy and the importance of reading aloud
Power struggles—offer de-escalating tips
Screen time and physical activity (60 minutes of activity; limit
  screen time to 1–2 hours)

HepA, hepatitis A; M-CHAT, Modified Checklist for Autism in Toddlers; WIC, Women, Infants, and Children.

3 Years Old

Nutrition	
Feeding	Highly active, so continue with three meals a day; two to three snacks a day (keep regular schedule of meals/snacks to avoid grazing and overeating throughout the day)
	May become picky eaters or get stuck on a food for several days
	Snacks should be CHO-rich and nutrient dense
	1 ½ cups of vegetables and fruits per day
	3–4 oz. per day of meat and beans[a]
Grains	4–5 oz. per day with ½ coming from whole-grain sources[b]
Added sugar/salt	Not recommended for preschoolers, but OK to have occasional treats
	Limit sugar-sweetened beverages to no more than 4 oz. per day (dilute)
Teeth	Usually have all primary teeth in (20 teeth)
	BID brushing with pea-sized fluorinated toothpaste, parental flossing
Dairy	Recommended daily intake is two servings per day of 1% or skim milk or yogurt (8 oz.) or cheese (1 ½ oz. natural cheese)

[a] 1 oz. = 1 oz. of meat, poultry, or fish, ¼ cup cooked dry beans or one egg.

[b] 1 oz. = 1 slice of bread, 1 cup of ready-to-eat cereal, ½ cup of cooked rice, pasta, or cooked cereal.

Elimination	
Output	Typically eliminating independently

Sleep		
Quantity	Naps may become less frequent	Total: 10–13 hours
Routine	Consistent bedtime with routine May need a transitional object	
Sleep site safety	Typically in a toddler bed or bed with side rails Bedroom safety	

Family	
Family, including siblings	Ask about plans for additional children Ask about consistent limits/expectations/discipline Play with siblings (sharing/turn-taking)
Outside support	Toddler play groups Parents with children of same age
Adjustment to age or stage	Transition to preschool/ECE Negotiating with parents; power struggles Activity/attention span/energy level of preschooler
Money	Financial supports WIC, day-care assistance, HeadStart

Developmental Milestones	
Physical Development	
Gross motor	Throws a ball overhand Balances on one foot for 1 second Pedals a tricycle
Fine motor	Draws a person with two body parts (head+) Thumb wiggle Towers six to seven blocks
Communication/Language Development	
Verbal	Conversations with pronouns, plurals, and two to three sentences per idea Speech is 75% understandable

(continued)

(continued)

Developmental Milestones	
Cognitive/Intellectual Development	
Intelligence	Names four pictures in a book
	Knows one color
Problem-solving	Prepares cereal
	Names the use of a cup, ball, spoon, and crayon
Social–Emotional Development	
Connection	Interactive play
	Shows affection for friends/family
Self-regulation	Increasingly better at taking turns

Screenings and Immunizations	
Screenings	ASQ
	Vision screening, if child able to cooperate
Immunizations	Typically none, but catch-up vaccines and influenza, if appropriate, can be done at this time

Anticipatory Guidance

Review portion sizes and recommendations for food groups

Educate on picky-eater stage and avoiding mealtime fights

Provide safe and supervised playtime to explore

Car seat safety (forward-facing five-point harness until outgrows height and weight limits)

Occasional accidents when preschooler does not want to stop playing to attend to bowel/bladder function are normal

Routine and limit setting around sleep

May wake due to dreams, nightmares, and night terrors

Poisons out of cabinets, locks on cabinets, medication storage

Gun safety (see 24 months)

Encourage continued reading aloud

Provide community resources (i.e., library) book acquisition

Discuss preparation for/readiness for preschool or ECE

Screen time and physical activity (60 minutes of activity; limit screen time to 1–2 hours)

ASQ, Ages and Stages Questionnaire; BID, bis in die (twice a day); CHO, carbohydrates; ECE, early-childhood education; WIC, Women, Infants, and Children.

4 YEARS OLD

Nutrition	
Feeding	Highly active, so continue with three meals a day; 2–3 snacks a day (keep regular schedule of meals/snacks to avoid grazing and overeating throughout the day)
	More adult-like utensil use and can begin learning to use a knife with supervision
	Snacks should be CHO-rich and nutrient dense
	2 cups of vegetables and fruits per day
	5 oz. per day of meat and beans[a]
Grains	4–5 oz. per day with ½ coming from whole-grain sources[b]
Added sugar/salt	Not recommended for preschoolers, but OK to have occasional treats
	Limit sugar-sweetened beverages to no more than 4 oz. per day (dilute)
Teeth	Usually have all primary teeth (20 teeth)
	BID brushing with pea-sized fluorinated toothpaste, parental flossing
Dairy	Recommended daily intake is two servings per day of 1% or skim milk or yogurt (8 oz.) or cheese (1 ½ oz. natural cheese)

[a] 1 oz. = 1 oz. of meat, poultry, or fish, ¼ cup cooked dry beans or one egg.

[b] 1 oz. = 1 slice of bread, 1 cup of ready-to-eat cereal, ½ cup of cooked rice, pasta, or cooked cereal.

Elimination	
Output	Typically eliminating independently; occasional daytime and night-time enuresis

Sleep		
Quantity	Naps may become less frequent	Total: 10–13 hours
Routine	Consistent bedtime with routine	
	May need a transitional object	
Sleep site and safety	Typically in a toddler bed or bed with side rails	
	Bedroom safety	

Family	
Family, including siblings	Ask about consistent limits/expectations/discipline
	Play with siblings (sharing/turn-taking)
Outside support	Preschool teachers/day-care providers
	Parents with children of same age

(continued)

(continued)

Family	
Adjustment to age or stage	Transition to preschool/ECE
	Negotiating with parents; power struggles
	Activity/attention span/energy level of preschooler
Money	Financial supports
	WIC, day-care assistance, HeadStart

Developmental Milestones	
Physical Development	
Gross motor	Hops
	Pedals a bike with training wheels
Fine motor	Mature pencil grasp
	Copies a cross or circle; draws a person with two to four body parts
	Dresses and undresses without assistance
Communication/Language Development	
Verbal	Tells a story
	Talkative with animated conversations
	Speech is 100% understandable
Cognitive/Intellectual Development	
Intelligence	Defines five words and counts up to 5
	Knows four colors
Problem-solving	Plays card and board games
	Knows what to do if cold, hungry, tired
Social–Emotional Development	
Connection	Enjoys make-believe play (magical thinking)
	Insatiable curiosity (asks why, when, where, how questions)
	Collaborative play and developing friendships
Self-regulation	Identifies emotions in themselves

Screenings and Immunizations	
Screenings	ASQ
	Vision screening
	Hearing screening
Immunizations	IPV, DTaP, MMR, varicella, influenza (if seasonally appropriate)

Anticipatory Guidance	
Review portion sizes and recommendations for food groups	Occasional accidents are normal
Educate on picky-eater stage and avoiding mealtime fights	Routine and limit setting around sleep
	May wake due to dreams, nightmares, and night terrors
Safe and supervised playtime to explore	Poisons out of cabinets, locks on cabinets, medication storage
Car seat safety (Forward-facing five-point harness)	Gun safety (see 24 months)

(continued)

(continued)

Anticipatory Guidance
Encourage continued reading aloud
Discuss preparation for/readiness for preschool or ECE
Screen time and physical activity (60 minutes of activity; limit screen time to 1–2 hours)

ASQ, Ages and Stages Questionnaire; BID, bis in die (twice a day); CHO, carbohydrates; ECE, early-childhood education; IPV, inactivated poliovirus; MMR, measles, mumps, and rubella; WIC, Women, Infants, and Children.

5 TO 6 YEARS OLDS

Nutrition	
Feeding	Three meals a day; one to two snacks a day
	Snacks should be CHO-rich and nutrient dense
	1–1 ½ cups[a] of vegetables and fruits per day
	3–4 oz. per day of meat and beans[b]
Grains	4–5 oz. per day with ½ coming from whole-grain sources[c]
Added sugar/salt	Limit sugar-sweetened beverages to no more than 4 oz. per day (dilute)
Teeth	Usually begin to lose baby teeth at 5–6 years old
	BID brushing with fluorinated toothpaste, flossing once daily
Dairy	Recommended daily intake is two servings per day of 1% or skim milk or yogurt (8 oz.) or cheese (1 ½ oz. natural cheese)

[a] ½ cup = 1 serving.
[b] 1 oz. = 1 oz. of meat, poultry, or fish, ¼ cup cooked dry beans or one egg.
[c] 1 oz. = 1 slice of bread, 1 cup of ready-to-eat cereal, ½ cup of cooked rice, pasta, or cooked cereal.

Elimination	
Output	Nocturnal enuresis may still be an issue, but most kids are dry throughout the day

Sleep	
Quantity	10–12 hours per night
	Naps typically eliminated from daily routine
Routine	Typical bedtime is 7–8 p.m.
	Wake up around 6–8 a.m.
	Routines are still important, but have likely changed slightly
Sleep site	Typically have moved to a regular bed

Family	
Family, including siblings	Ask about consistent limits/expectations/discipline
	Ask about chores
Outside support	Starting kindergarten, so working with school as a support
	After-school care
Adjustment to age or stage	Transition to kindergarten; adhering to a schedule/routines
	Testing previously established rules
	Increased interest in spending time with friends rather than family
Money	WIC assistance ends at 5
	Parents may be considering returning to work

Developmental Milestones		
	5 years	**6 years**
Physical Development		
Gross motor	Hops on one foot	Skips
	Rides bike	Climbs trees; tests physical ability
Fine motor	Draws person with six body parts	Draws person with more than six body parts
	Prints some letters and numbers	
	Copies a square	Prints most letters with precision
		Copies a triangle
Communication/Language Development		
Verbal	Good articulation	Accelerated expressive language
Cognitive/Intellectual Development		
Intelligence	Can count to 10+	Understands number concepts
	Magical thinking and imagination	Begins more concrete thinking
Problemsolving	Begins to sequence and organize	Basic adding and subtracting
Social–Emotional Development		
Connection	Listens and attends to others	Increased attention to things outside of the home
	Explores gender identity	
	Cooperative play (sharing)	
Self-regulation	Better self-discipline and impulse control	Expresses positive and negative feelings about family members
	Obeys rules	Understands the need for rules

Screenings and Immunizations	
Screenings	ASQ until 5 years old
	Hearing screening
	Vision screening
Immunizations	Typically none, but catch-up vaccines and influenza, if appropriate, can be done at this time

Anticipatory Guidance	
Review portion sizes and recommendations for food groups	Night time enuresis may still be normal for some 5-year-olds
Encourage five servings of fruits and vegetables per day	Routine bedtime and awakening times help with school routine
Discourage sugar-sweetened beverages	Good touch/bad touch (on bathing suit areas, no adult should make kids keep a
Bike safety and helmets	secret, no adults should need help with
Booster seat (may switch to booster seat with lap belt)	private parts)
Discuss school readiness and encourage good school habits	
Screen time and physical activity (60 minutes of activity; limit screen time to 1–2 hours)	

ASQ, Ages and Stages Questionnaire; BID, bis in die (twice a day); CHO, carbohydrates; WIC, Women, Infants, and Children.

7 TO 10 YEARS OLD

Nutrition	
Feeding	Three meals a day; one to two snacks a day
	1 ½–2 ½ cups[a] of vegetables per day
	1 ½ cups[a] of fruits
	4–5 oz. per day of meat and beans[b]
	Limit sugar-sweetened beverages
Grains	4–6 oz. per day with ½ coming from whole-grain sources[c]
Teeth	By 8 years old, the bottom and top four primary incisors replaced by permanent teeth, with break in tooth eruption between 8 and 10 years old, BID brushing with fluorinated toothpaste, flossing daily
Dairy	Recommended daily intake is two to three servings per day of 1% or skim milk, yogurt, or cheese

[a] ½ cup = 1 serving.
[b] 1 oz. = 1 oz. of meat, poultry, or fish, ¼ cup cooked dry beans or one egg.
[c] 1 oz. = 1 slice of bread, 1 cup of ready-to-eat cereal, ½ cup of cooked rice, pasta, or cooked cereal.

Sleep		
Quantity	9–11 hours per night	
Routine	Typical bedtime is 8–9 p.m.	
	Wake up around 6–8 a.m.	
	Routines, especially around waking time, important for school	
Sleep site and sleep hygiene	Regular bed	No electronics at bedtime
	No TV in bedroom	Minimize white light

Growth	
Growth	Boys' growth is slow and steady; gain 10 pounds between ages of 7–10 Girls' height growth spurt begins near 9–10 years

Family	
Family, including siblings	More involved chores that require more time, concentration, and attention to detail Family time with special activities May be more physically aggressive with siblings
Outside support	Parents of child's friends After-school care Teacher/school support
Adjustment to age or stage	Adhering to a schedule/routines Increasing school demands Increased time with friends rather than with family
Money	Increasing importance to children, as desired items are more costly Money sometimes equated to social status/peer acceptance

Developmental Milestones		
	7-8 years old	9-10 years old
Physical Development		
Motor	Improved coordination	Improved strength, flexibility, and physical skill
Communication/Language Development		
Verbal and written	Increased vocabulary Can tell a coherent narrative with beginning, middle, end	Understands metaphors, similes, and figures of speech Word play and jokes
Cognitive/Intellectual Development		
Intelligence	Thinking becomes reversible Improved memory	Improved executive processing Categorizes memories, recalls
Problem solving	Ability to consider two or more aspects of a problem	Tries new approaches to problem-solving more readily
Social–Emotional Development		
Connection	Fantasy play is internalized Wider net of same-gender friends	Ritualized play with friends Hero/role model is real person
Self-regulation	Increased coping skills; some control over feelings	More adept at appraising a situation and using coping skills

Screenings and Immunizations	
Screenings	Hearing and vision screening Dyslipidemia screening at 10 years old
Immunizations	Typically none, but influenza, if appropriate, can be done at this time

Anticipatory Guidance

Review portion sizes and recommendations for food groups	Bike helmets and traffic safety
Encourage five servings of fruits and veggies per day	Internet safety (supervised online, limit game choices to age-appropriate, avoid "browsing the Internet," computer in family space, Internet filters, etc.)
Discourage sugar-sweetened beverages	
Bullying (decreased self-esteem leads to poorer school performance; coping strategies)	Self-esteem promotion (participate in activities together, praising, modeling responsibility, age-appropriate decision-making, etc.)
Discuss the signs of ADHD and learning disabilities (may be identified during this time in school)	
	Sexual education (pubertal changes, hygiene, delaying sexual behavior, answer questions with concrete answers, encourage questions and open forum)
Chores (increasing independence and responsibility increases sense of competence)	

ADHD, attention-deficit hyperactivity disorder; BID, bis in die (twice a day).

11 TO 14 YEARS OLD

Nutrition

Feeding	Three meals a day; one to two snacks a day 2–2 ½ cups[a] of vegetables per day 1 ½ cups[a] of fruits 5 oz. per day of meat and beans[b] Limit sugar-sweetened beverages
Grains	5–6 oz. per day with ½ coming from whole-grain sources[c]
Teeth	Permanent tooth eruption (28) usually occurring until ~13 years Highest rate of caries during tween years
Dairy	Recommended daily intake is three servings per day of 1% or skim milk, yogurt, or cheese

[a] ½ cup = 1 serving.

[b] 1 oz. = 1 oz. of meat, poultry, or fish, ¼ cup cooked dry beans or one egg.

[c] 1 oz. = 1 slice of bread, 1 cup of ready-to-eat cereal, ½ cup of cooked rice, pasta, or cooked cereal.

Sleep

Quantity	Recommendation is for 8–10 hours per night, but only 15% get this much Naps are rare, so teens who take 2–3 hour afternoon naps may have underlying problems with sleep hygiene, depression, or school issues
Routine	Have a shift in sleep–wake cycle (staying up later and sleeping in) Routine bedtime and waking time should extend into weekends with only about 60 minutes of extra sleep allowed
Sleep site and sleep hygiene	Make bedrooms "tech free" No electronics near bedtime

Growth	
Growth	Girls: Growth spurt (height) occurs at ~11.5 years (usually 1 year after onset of puberty) and peak weight gain usually 6–9 months later Boys: Growth spurt (both height and weight) occurs ~13.5 years (usually 2 years after onset of puberty)

Family	
Family and friends	Privacy for the adolescent? Tween's family responsibilities—appropriate or overwhelming? Recent changes in family or peer group structure/dynamic?
Outside support	Do you know the parents of tween/teen's friends? Family counseling, if needed, for battling parents/teens? Coaches, teachers, counselors, friends for tween/teen?
Adjustment to age or stage	Move toward independence Puberty (physical and emotional changes) School/activity schedule/homework
Money	Increasing importance to tweens, as desired items are more costly Money sometimes equated to social status/peer acceptance

Developmental Milestones	
Physical Development	
Puberty	May feel gangly and awkward May develop body image concerns with changes in adipose tissue Increased interest in sexual anatomy, breast/penis size, menstruation, nocturnal emissions, and masturbation
Communication/Language Development	
Verbal and written	Increased ability to express self through writing, speech, drawings Adopts peer language and slang Picks up on nonverbal cues more easily
Cognitive/Intellectual Development	
Intelligence	Abstract thinking and creativity
Problem solving	Beginning to use deductive reasoning (if this, then that)
Social–Emotional Development	
Connection	Creates new support group of same-gender peers with strong emotional feelings toward peers (love–hate relationships) May be more introspective, feel disconnected from adults
Self-regulation	Lack of impulse control can lead to risk-taking Emotional lability (wide mood and behavior swings)

Screenings and Immunizations	
Screenings	Depression screening Alcohol and drug use assessment
Immunizations	HPV, MCV, Tdap, and influenza (if seasonally appropriate)

Anticipatory Guidance	
Discuss healthy food choices with the tween	School success (decreased risky behaviors; emphasize importance of school; praise positive efforts)
Ensure adequate Ca++ and vitamin D intake with growth spurt	
Limit soda and sugar intakeMinimum of 8 hours a night with good sleep hygiene	Sexuality (onset of fertility + curiosity + risk-taking → discuss abstinence, sexual pressure, pregnancy prevention, STI prevention)
High-risk activities (open forum to discuss concerns/worries; skills for navigating peer pressure situations)	
	Body image issues (disordered eating; obesity; muscle development; gynecomastia; asymmetric breast development)
Phone/texting/social media (create a plan for phone/Internet use; signs of addiction; increased risk of depression)	Mood regulation (how to deal with stress, signs of depression/anxiety, angry outbursts, disagreements with parents
Phone/texting/social media (create a plan for phone/Internet use; signs of addiction; increased risk of depression)	

HPV, human papillomavirus; MCV, meningococcal vaccine; STI, sexually transmitted infection; Tdap, tetanus, diphtheria, acellular pertussis.

15 TO 18 YEARS OLD

Nutrition	
Feeding	3 meals a day 2 ½ cups of vegetables per day[a] 2 cups of fruits[a] 5 ½ oz. per day of meat and beans[b] Limit sugar-sweetened beverages
Vitamins	Adolescents tend to fall short of their daily quotas of calcium, iron, zinc, and vitamin D; supplement if not able to get from diet
Grains	6 oz. per day with ½ coming from whole-grain sources[c]
Teeth	Third molars (wisdom teeth) begin to erupt at 17–18 years BID brushing with fluorinated toothpaste, flossing QD
Dairy	Recommended daily intake is three servings per day of 1% or skim milk, yogurt, or cheese

[a] ½ cup = 1 serving.

[b] 1 oz. = 1 oz. of meat, poultry, or fish, ¼ cup cooked dry beans or one egg.

[c] 1 oz. = 1 slice of bread, 1 cup of ready-to-eat cereal, ½ cup of cooked rice, pasta,or cooked cereal.

Sleep	
Quantity	Should get a minimum of 8 hours per night Short (20–30 minute) naps may help keep normal sleep cycle at night
Routine	Routine bedtime and waking time should extend into weekends

(continued)

(continued)

Sleep	
Sleep site/sleep hygiene	Make bedrooms "tech free," especially at bedtime Avoid caffeine, smoking, alcohol, and drugs at night Bed should be used only for sleeping—not a study pod, a reading nook, or a gaming chair

Growth	
Growth	Growth slows after the peak height velocity (males) and peak weight velocity (for females) When close to adult stature, growth decelerates to ~1 cm/y

Family	
Family and friends	Where is teen living? What are the rules/expectations/boundaries for teen around household help, homework, extracurricular activities, curfew, dress, dating, etc.
Outside support	Do you know the parents of teen's friends? Family counseling, if needed, for battling parents/teens? Other support such as coaches, teachers, counselors, friends?
Adjustment to age or stage	Increased independence with decreased family involvement Learning to drive Sexual feelings and relationships
Money	May start working after school or on weekends to earn own money

Developmental Milestones	
Physical Development	
Postpuberty	Body image concerns continue, so experiments with appearance May appear older than developmental age
Communication/Language Development	
Verbal and written	May be opinionated about political and philosophical viewpoints May have a "you do not understand" attitude toward parents
Cognitive/Intellectual Development	
Intelligence	Abstract thinking Introspection
Problem solving	Improving executive function Developing ability to make judgments using sound reasoning, but may resort to more emotional decision-making
Social–Emotional Development	
Connection	Has a somewhat labile relationship with parents Expanding peer groups to include opposite-gender peers, with increasing interest in romantic relationships
Self-regulation	Still impulsive and does not always use logic to regulate decisions Begins to demonstrate resiliency when faced with life stressors Major developmental task is becoming comfortable with one's sexuality, learning to express and control sexual drives

Screenings and Immunizations

Screenings	Depression screening
	Alcohol and drug use assessment
	HIV screening
	STI screening, if sexually active
Immunizations	MCV and influenza (if seasonally appropriate)

Anticipatory Guidance

Encourage healthy food choices and review dangers of skipping meals	Discuss that sexuality is a normal developmental stage; offer skills to navigate and how to say "no"; review contraception, STI prevention
Provide evidence-based information on weight loss, if necessary	Signs and symptoms of depression
Review importance of 8 hours per night of sleep and sleep hygiene	Older teens should begin discussing posthigh school plans and how current academics and activities are helping to meet this goal
Driving: Review distracted driving; encourage seatbelt use; discourage driving under the influence	Recommend 60 minutes of physical exercise daily
Illicit substances: Discuss alcohol abuse/binge drinking; prescription drug misuse; illicit substance/marijuana use	

BID, bis in die (twice a day); MCV, meningococcal vaccine; QD, quaque die (every day); STI, sexually transmitted infection.

5

Urgent Management in Pediatrics

ACUTE ASTHMA EXACERBATION, BRONCHIOLITIS, EPIGLOTTITIS, AND TRACHEITIS

Overview and Presentation

- The approach to the management of a pediatric patient with an asthma exacerbation in the ED/urgent care is described here. There are many established scores or protocols developed to determine what medications should be administered, whether the patient should be admitted or discharged, and what medications may be prescribed for the patient to take at home after discharge. Asthma symptoms severity scores, such as the Pediatric Respiratory Assessment Measure (PRAM), the Pediatric Asthma Severity Score (PASS), and the Respiratory rate–Accessory muscle use–Decreased breath sounds (RAD) score, help to guide treatment and assist with decision-making regarding hospital admittance of a patient.[1] When patients present to an urgent care or ED with asthma exacerbation, an initial brief assessment is necessary to guide intervention. Patients and their families may use the Childhood Asthma Control Test (C-ACT) and bring the results of this self-administered survey with them to help explain their symptoms and the severity of their symptoms over the previous 4 weeks.

- A common asthma masquerader in infants and toddlers is bronchiolitis. Bronchiolitis is a lower respiratory tract viral infection that usually involves children younger than 2 years old and causes inflammation of the bronchioles, which results in small airway obstruction, air trapping, and atelectasis. The most common cause of bronchiolitis is the respiratory syncytial virus (RSV).[2] Patients will present within 3 to 5 days of symptom onset with worsening lower respiratory symptoms after a few days of upper respiratory prodromal symptoms such as nasal congestion, rhinorrhea, and cough.

- Epiglottitis is a now rare, acute-onset upper respiratory infection that causes inflammation of the supraglottis, epiglottis, and/or aryepiglottic folds. Patients can present with a mild sore throat and fever to severe upper airway obstruction. In the past, *Haemophilus influenzae* type b was the most common etiology of epiglottitis. With the widespread use of the *H. influenzae* type b vaccine, most epiglottitis is now caused by parainfluenza viruses, *Streptococcus pyogenes, Streptococcus pneumoniae*, and *Streptococcus aureus*.

- Bacterial tracheitis is a rare but potentially life-threatening disease that can occur in isolation or as a secondary infection of viral croup. Bacterial tracheitis occurs primarily during the viral infectious seasons of autumn and winter and may be seen in a wider range of ages than typical croup.

Diagnostic Evaluation

- A brief history and physical examination, including respiratory rate, heart rate, use of accessory muscles, pulmonary function testing or spirometry, pulse oximetry, and auscultation, should be completed when the patient first arrives. Many pediatric patients with asthma exacerbation will be unable to attempt pulmonary function testing so you may have to go by respiratory rate, accessory muscle use, and auscultation findings alone. Breath sounds can range from wheezing; rhonchi; stridor; and barking, "seal-like" coughs. These sounds can often narrow your differential diagnosis.

- Assessment of the patient during this evaluation will determine into which category of asthma severity he or she belongs and will guide your treatment. Most patients will fall into a mild, moderate, or severe category with some severe enough to be categorized as impending or actual respiratory arrest and should be directly admitted to the pediatric intensive care unit (PICU).

- Bronchiolitis is a clinical diagnosis. Based on the season of the year and the presence of the virus in the community, RSV can be suspected with varying degrees of certainty. When bronchiolitis is not accompanied by infiltrates on chest x-ray, there is little likelihood of a bacterial component.

- For younger patients presenting with acute onset of dyspnea, pharyngitis, drooling, wheezing, and/or stridor (both of the last two symptoms are often audible without a stethoscope), fever and increased work of breathing, a comprehensive history, and physical exam can usually quickly narrow your differential diagnosis. X-rays are not usually necessary to help with the diagnosis of epiglottitis and should not take the place of airway management. Look for "the tripod sign" (upright patient leaning forward with hands on knees and neck hyperextended), drooling, and restlessness in children with epiglottitis. These patients usually require airway management with intubation to protect their airway during severe inflammation. If airway x-rays are done, look for the typical "thumb sign" that shows a swollen epiglottis.

- The presentation for bacterial tracheitis differs from epiglottitis by an absence of preferred posture, dysphagia, or drooling, but patients tend to be similarly toxic in appearance. Leukocytosis often is prominent in patients with bacterial tracheitis. Blood cultures are usually negative, but tracheal cultures reliably reveal the bacterial pathogen. Plain radiographic imaging of the upper airway may show a "steeple" sign of the upper trachea or subglottis on an anterior view.

Management

- Patients in the mild–moderate asthma categories should be given oxygen to achieve SaO_2 $\geq$90% and an inhaled short-acting beta2-agonist (SABA) by nebulizer or metered dose inhaler (MDI) three times in the first hour. They can then be given oral or injectable systemic corticosteroids if there is no immediate response. These patients should have regular, repeated assessments throughout treatment. Patients with severe exacerbation will receive similar treatment with high-dose SABA plus ipratropium by nebulizer or MDI every 20 minutes or continuously for 1 hour along with oral systemic corticosteroids. If, after 1 hour, a moderate–severe patient is not improving, the patient should continue to receive SABA and additional adjunct therapies, and providers should consider admitting the patient to the appropriate hospital floor or the ICU.[3] Most patients are discharged to home from the ED or urgent care setting and should have the following information:
  - Continue treatment with inhaled SABA and oral corticosteroid.
  - Continue inhaled corticosteroid (ICS). For those not on long-term control treatment, consider initiation of an ICS.
  - Include patient and parent education about a review of medications, inhaler technique, environmental control measures, review of an action plan, plus recommendation for close medical follow-up.
  - Schedule follow-up appointment with primary care provider or asthma specialist in 1 to 4 weeks.[3]
- Management of bronchiolitis usually centers around humidified oxygen, fluids, and symptomatic treatments. There are mixed opinions among experts regarding use of beta$_2$-agonist, especially for longer durations.
- Establishing an airway by endotracheal or nasotracheal intubation or, less often, by tracheostomy is indicated in patients with epiglottitis, regardless of the degree of apparent respiratory distress, because as many as 6% of children with epiglottitis without an artificial airway die, compared with fewer than 1% of those with an artificial airway.[4] Racemic epinephrine and corticosteroids are considered ineffective but patients should be given antibiotics parenterally pending culture reports, because 10% to 40% of *H. influenzae* type b cases are resistant to ampicillin. Epiglottitis improves after a few days of antibiotics, and the patient may be extubated while intravenous (IV) antibiotics should be changed to oral antibiotics and continued for at least 10 days.

- Stabilization of the patient with bacterial tracheitis should be similar to the management of epiglottitis. Suction removal of copious secretions is both therapeutic and diagnostic when sent for culture and Gram stain. Intubation may be necessary, especially with the risk of further mucosal injury and edema from suctioning of the airway. Toxic patients are typically treated with vancomycin, with or without clindamycin. Extubation can be safely performed when the child's temperature has returned to normal, a leak is present around the endotracheal tube. and the secretions have markedly decreased.[4]

ASPIRATED FOREIGN BODY

Overview and Presentation

- Choking is a leading cause of morbidity and mortality among children, especially those younger than 4 years old. The most common objects that children choke on are food, coins, balloons, and toys. The foods most frequently associated with pediatric fatal choking are hot dogs, seeds, nuts, candy, and certain types of fruits and vegetables.[5]

Diagnostic Evaluation

- A positive history must never be ignored, whereas a negative history may be misleading. Choking or coughing episodes accompanied by new-onset wheezing are highly suggestive of an airway foreign body. Because nuts are the most common bronchial foreign body, you should always specifically question the parents about nuts. If there is any history of eating nuts, bronchoscopy should be carried out promptly. Posteroanterior and lateral chest x-rays, along with abdomen, are first-line imaging, whereas a CT can help define radiolucent foreign bodies such as fish bones. If there is a high index of suspicion, bronchoscopy should be performed despite negative imaging studies. History is the most important factor in determining the need for bronchoscopy.[5]

Management

- Complete obstruction asphyxiates the child unless it is promptly relieved with the Heimlich maneuver. The treatment of choice for airway foreign bodies is prompt endoscopic removal with rigid instruments.

BACTEREMIA AND SEPSIS

Overview and Presentation

- Bacteremia is the presence of bacteria in the blood. If left untreated, it can progress to sepsis. Bacteremia can present with subtle signs and symptoms and often with only a fever. Pediatric patients with increased risk for bacteremia and sepsis are those who are underimmunized, of low birth weight, preterm, attend day care, and those with immune deficiencies.

- Sepsis is a clinical syndrome characterized by the systemic inflammatory response syndrome (SIRS), immune dysregulation, and end-organ dysfunction. Its broad scope goes beyond what we are able to cover in this chapter. We discuss the clinical presentation of neonatal early-onset sepsis ($\leq$3 days of birth), late-onset sepsis (after 3 days of life), as well as sepsis in older children and adolescents. Definitions for sepsis are continually being updated. A widespread inflammatory response that may or may not be associated with infection, SIRS has specific diagnostic criteria, including:
  - ○ General Signs and Symptoms: Core temperature changes of less than 36°C or more than 38.5°C, tachycardia, tachypnea, altered mental status, significant peripheral edema, and/or hyperglycemia in the absence of diabetes[6]
  - ○ Evidence of Inflammation: Leukocytosis or leukopenia, normal white blood cell (WBC) count with more than 10% immature cells, c-reactive protein (CRP) more than 2 standard deviations above normal, procalcitonin more than 2 standard deviations above normal
  - ○ Hemodynamics/Organ Dysfunction: Arterial hypotension, arterial hypoxemia, acute oliguria, creatinine increase, coagulation abnormalities, thrombocytopenia, hyperbilirubinemia, and decreased tissue perfusion identified through hyperlactatemia or decreased capillary refill/mottling
  - ○ Additional signs to consider for the diagnosis of sepsis in neonates and infants: poor color, poor responsiveness, poor feeding, and increased irritability or sleepiness[7]
- Early-onset neonatal sepsis has a 3% to 40% mortality rate[8] depending on birth weight and race, with African American, preterm, low-birth-weight babies having the highest risk; late-onset type sepsis is more likely to be complicated with meningitis.
- For early-onset sepsis, prolonged rupture of membranes (>18 hours) and a diagnosis of chorioamnionitis in the mother increases the risk for sepsis in the newborn. Delivering mothers are assessed for Group B *Streptococcus* (GBS) status and if there is confirmation of GBS carrier state or infection during pregnancy, maternal fever/chorioamnionitis during labor, baby born before culture can be done, or there is history of no prenatal care, a sepsis workup is advised.
- Early-onset sepsis occurs in a neonate in the first 3 days of life and is usually the result of transmission from the mother during labor. Late-onset sepsis occurs in a newborn after the first 3 days of life until 2 to 3 months of life. This usually occurs via horizontal transmission. There are various sepsis risk calculators, and for this population, you can use the Kaiser Neonate Sepsis Risk calculator (neonatalsepsiscalculator.kaiserpermanente.org).

- Sepsis can be caused by bacterial, viral, fungal, parasitic, and rickettsial infections. Bacteria and viruses are the most frequently identified pathogens,[6] with GBS the most common organism in neonates and *Escherichia coli* the most common organism in preterm babies.
- Routine immunization of infants against *H. influenzae* type b and *S. pneumoniae* has resulted in a dramatic decrease in the incidence of sepsis in young children due to these organisms.

Diagnostic Evaluation

- Workup for early-or late-onset neonatal sepsis should include blood cultures, complete blood count (CBC) with differential and CRP. If the neonate presents with tachypnea or labored breathing, a chest x-ray will be added. If the neonate is found to have a positive blood culture and/or has central nervous system (CNS) activity, such as seizures or lethargy, and can tolerate the procedure, a lumbar puncture (LP) should be performed. It is best to perform an LP before starting antibiotics.

Management

- Mothers who have positive GBS cultures should have prophylaxis penicillin before or during labor. There are alternative antibiotics for those who are penicillin-allergic. Mothers who have chorioamnionitis are treated with antibiotics during labor to prevent sepsis in the newborn. The newborn should then be observed for 48 hours after birth for any signs of sepsis.
- The American Academy of Pediatrics recommends that high-risk newborns be treated with IV antibiotics for 48 hours until cultures are negative. Newborns who do have lab-confirmed sepsis and meningitis should receive IV antibiotics for 10 days and 14 days, respectively.
- Older children presenting with signs and symptoms suspicious for sepsis should have immediate treatment with IV antibiotics. Antibiotics should be selected based on the most likely cause of the infection. Although it is most desirable to obtain blood cultures before starting antibiotics in order to guide type and duration of treatment, it is imperative for patients with sepsis to receive early and aggressive control of any source of infection. This may include surgical drainage of abscesses or removal of infected foreign bodies.

Concussion or Mild Traumatic Brain Injury

Overview and Presentation

- Concussion, also referred to as "mild traumatic brain injury (mTBI)," generates more than 2 million emergency and outpatient visits annually,[9] with effects that impair the child's ability to function physically, cognitively, and psychologically.

- Typically, a child or adolescent with a concussion or mTBI will present with a history of a relatively low-impact trauma involving the head, neck, or upper body. A whiplash-like history is common, as is direct impact.
- Given the heightened awareness about concussion and TBIs, many times these patients will present to the urgent care or ED for initial evaluation, but will have subsequent follow-up with a primary care provider.

Diagnostic Evaluation

- On initial presentation, healthcare providers must determine whether the patient is at higher risk for intracranial injury from a concussion or mTBI. Use of clinical decision tools is very helpful in determining whether the child is at lower risk for intracranial injury. This child can then be assessed with a validated symptom score rating scale, such as the Graded Symptom Checklist or the Postconcussion Symptom Scale.[10]
- The patients at higher risk for intracranial injury (and the need for more invasive diagnostic testing) are children:
  - Younger than 2 years old
  - With vomiting
  - With loss of consciousness
  - Who experienced a severe mechanism of injury
  - With severe or worsening headache
  - With amnesia
  - With a Glasgow Coma Scale (GCS) score of less than 15
  - With clinical suspicion for skull fracture[11]
- Used appropriately, after informed discussions with the family about the risks versus benefits of a head CT, a head CT may identify serious intracranial pathology such as epidural hematoma, subdural hematoma, intracranial hemorrhage, subarachnoid hemorrhage, intraventricular hemorrhage, cerebral edema, and depressed skull fractures.
- Skull x-rays, MRI, and single-photon emission CT (SPECT) scans should not be used routinely for diagnosis of mTBI.[9]

Management

- Pediatric mTBI recovery is highly variable, but the majority of children resolve within 1 to 3 months postinjury. Some of the factors that may play into the recovery trajectory of patients include the following:
  - History of previous concussion
  - Premorbid lower cognitive ability
  - Preexisting neurologic disorders, psychiatric diagnoses, and/or learning difficulties
  - History of preinjury symptoms, such as migraine headaches, depression, or sleep disorders
  - Family or social stress[9]
- Educating families and patients on the unique course of recovery seen by all patients, symptoms of postconcussion syndrome, and possible

educational and athletic modifications are important for patient outcomes. Although there is no consensus on the timing or duration of modification, patients should be encouraged to restrict their physical and cognitive activity the first several days after a TBI, with graduated increases in cognitive activity. Family members, providers, athletic trainers, and educators can all monitor for exacerbation of symptoms. After patients are fully reintegrated into their cognitive activities, a progressive return-to-play protocol can be instituted for athletes.[12] Clearance for return to full physical activity can be given when the patient is able to maintain pre-TBI activities without exacerbation of symptoms.[10]

- Validated symptom scores are useful for assessing recovery from a TBI and can inform a provider's return-to-learn and return-to-play decisions.[13]
- The most common symptoms following a TBI include headaches, dizziness, sleep disturbances, mood lability and cognitive impairment.
  - ○ Recommendations for managing headaches include nonnarcotic analgesia (i.e., ibuprofen or acetaminophen) for children with painful headache following acute mTBI. Counseling for the family regarding the risks of analgesic overuse, including rebound headache, should be discussed. Chronic headaches following mTBI should be referred for multidisciplinary evaluation and treatment.[9]
  - ○ Dizziness is a sign of vestibular and oculomotor dysfunction that may be correlated with longer duration mTBI symptoms. Even though there are pharmacologic agents for dizziness, these are not recommended in post-TBI patients. Referral to vestibular therapy is the preferred management.[9]
  - ○ Sleep disturbances are common in TBI patients and may manifest as poor sleep quality, shorter sleep durations, and more frequent awakenings during sleep. Emphasizing appropriate sleep hygiene is a crucial management component for TBI patients, but if despite these measures a patient continues to have problematic sleep, the patient should be referred to a sleep specialist.
  - ○ Cognitive impairments may be a direct result of the TBI or may be a manifestation of other sequalae. Understanding whether the cognitive impairments are secondary to another problem, such as headache, poor sleep, easy distractibility, and so on, will determine the best course of management. Formal neuropsychological evaluations can assist in determining etiology of cognitive impairment if an etiology is not readily apparent.
- Patients whose symptoms do not resolve in an expected course of 4 to 6 weeks should be referred to specialist for further evaluation and management.

DIABETIC KETOACIDOSIS

Overview and Presentation

- Diabetic ketoacidosis (DKA) is a severe acute metabolic complication of type 1 diabetes, but may also occur in type 2 diabetes, though not as commonly. The most common precipitating factor is a failure to use insulin, although other stressors, such as infections, illness, trauma, and certain drugs (SGLT2 inhibitors, antipsychotics), might also lead to DKA. Many of these factors are associated with the release of epinephrine, which blocks any residual insulin action and stimulates the secretion of glucagon. The insulin deficiency—coupled with glucagon excess—decreases uptake of glucose by cells. This, along with the gluconeogenesis caused by the increased glucagon, causes severe hyperglycemia (plasma gluocose levels higher than 200 mg/dL). The hyperglycemia causes an osmotic diuresis and dehydration characteristic of the ketoacidotic state.[14]

Diagnostic Evaluation

- DKA is defined by the presence of *all* of the following factors in a patient with diabetes, as outlined in a consensus statement from the International Society for Pediatric and Adolescent Diabetes in 2018:
  - ○ Hyperglycemia: Blood glucose >200 mg/dL (11 mmol/L)
  - ○ Metabolic acidosis: Venous pH <7.3 or serum bicarbonate <15 mEq/L (15 mmol/L)
  - ○ Ketosis: Presence of ketones in the blood (>3 mmol/L) or urine ("moderate or large" urine ketones); the severity of DKA can be categorized according to the degree of acidosis
- Neurologic assessment: All patients should have a rapid assessment of level of consciousness at presentation using the GCS. This should be followed by a more detailed assessment for the more subtle signs of cerebral edema, which include headache (especially sudden onset), altered or sluggish pupillary responses, age-inappropriate incontinence, as well as vomiting, restlessness, irritability, or drowsiness. Decreased heart rate, increased blood pressure, and opisthotonic posturing are late signs in the evolution of cerebral edema. The neurological assessment should be repeated hourly throughout treatment or until the patient is clinically recovered from ketoacidosis and his or her mental status examination is normal.[15]
- The anion gap can be used as an index of the severity of the metabolic acidosis and is calculated from the following equation:
  Anion gap = Sodium – (chloride + bicarbonate); a normal anion gap is 12 ± 2.

Management

- As DKA is a state of hyperosmolar dehydration, the volume depletion is caused by urinary losses from osmotic diuresis (due to osmotic action of glucose and ketones in the urine), as well as gastrointestinal losses from vomiting and/or diarrhea, if present. The overall volume deficit in children with DKA is typically between 5% and 10%. Fluid administration is required, but administration should proceed cautiously to minimize the risk for cerebral edema. The goals of initial volume expansion are to restore the effective circulating volume by acutely replacing some of the sodium and water loss, and to restore glomerular filtration rate to enhance clearance of ketones and glucose from the blood. The main principles of management are to administer insulin and to correct the fluid and electrolyte abnormalities of hypovolemia and whole-body sodium and potassium depletion.[15]

Envenomations, Animal and Arthropod Bites, and Sting Reactions

Overview and Presentation

- Pediatric patients may present with complaints of a recent bite or sting. There are different insects and animals that can inflict painful wounds that can become infected or cause anaphylaxis. In an urgent care or ED setting, you frequently will see patients who have stings or bites caused by bees, wasps, yellow jackets, ticks, spiders, and other arthropods. Patients also often present with scratch and bite injuries caused by cats, dogs, and rabbits.

Diagnostic Evaluation

- For arthropod stings and bites, a good history and physical exam are key to guiding your clinical decision-making process. Assess the patient for anaphylaxis and monitor for any changes in status. The presentation of a spider bite may range from a 1-mm, slightly erythematous lesion to a 10-cm, asymmetrically shaped maculopapular lesion with the "red, white, and blue" sign of a brown recluse spider. Some arthropod bites may require lab serology to assess for infection and to guide further treatment. If you are ordering lab work for tick-borne illness, make sure the timing of the blood draw is appropriate and labs will adequately diagnose your patient. For example, to diagnose a patient with Lyme disease, the blood draw timing is key to observe the rise of antibody levels to *Borrelia burgdorferi*.
- For cat and dog wounds, in addition to taking a good history and physical, you may need to consider diagnostic imaging such as plain film x-rays or MRI. If the patient presents with a dog bite wound to an extremity, consider whether the patient has had crush injuries and/or deep puncture wounds that could cause periosteal injury, ultimately leading to osteomyelitis. There should be a high suspicion of infection in these types of injuries, especially in wounds caused by cats.

Management

- If the patient has any history of allergy to arthropod bites or stings, consider giving an injection from an EpiPen and monitor for any signs of anaphylaxis. Whether or not the patient has signs, symptoms, or history of allergy to the offending insect, you should consider prescribing and/or administering a glucocorticoid such as dexamethasone or prednisolone.
- Discuss the physical exam findings with the patient and his or her family and give anticipatory guidance regarding what symptoms to watch for after discharge.
- For dog and cat bites or deep scratches, use copious amounts of saline to irrigate the wound and debride the wound edges. You should approximate wound edges slightly, but do not close lacerations unless they are large and could be disfiguring. You may consider performing a swab of the wound before the patient begins antibiotics, but most mild to moderate infections will respond to amoxicillin–clavulanate. For patients with penicillin allergy, you may consider trimethoprim–sulfamethoxazole and/or clindamycin.[16]

EYE COMPLAINTS: ORBITAL INJURIES AND PERIORBITAL CELLULITIS

Overview and Presentation

- Approximately 30% of blindness in childhood is the result of injuries, and boys are the most vulnerable.[17] The clinical findings for eye injuries and infections range from vision-threatening to common conditions. Rapid recognition and treatment of ocular chemical burns, orbital compartment syndrome, or open-globe injuries are essential to the preservation of vision. The most common complaints seen in the pediatric ED include corneal abrasions, corneal or conjunctival foreign body, and periorbital cellulitis.
- Patients presenting with corneal abrasions report severe eye pain and reluctance to open the eye due to photophobia and/or foreign-body sensation. Corneal abrasions without other serious eye injuries typically have normal visual acuity, normal pupillary response, and a staining defect on fluorescein examination.
- Periorbital cellulitis produces erythema and swelling of the tissues surrounding the globe, whereas orbital cellulitis involves the intraorbital structures. Patients presenting with periorbital cellulitis complain of eyelid edema, erythema, warmth, and tenderness with possible visual impairment. Conjunctival chemosis (a nonspecific sign of eye irritation with conjunctiva edema), decreased visual acuity, impaired extraocular movements, injection, proptosis, and restricted ocular motility with pain

on attempted eye movement are usually present. Signs of optic neuropathy may be present in severe cases of orbital cellulitis.[18] The most common cause of periorbital cellulitis and orbital cellulitis in children is paranasal sinusitis.[19]

Diagnostic Evaluation

- Begin assessment of orbital injuries by obtaining a full history before proceeding with visual acuity testing and a focused physical exam. Abrasions are detected by instilling fluorescein dye directly into the eye and inspecting with a slit lamp, ophthalmoscope with blue filtered light, or a handheld Woods lamp. If there is any history of high-velocity projectile injuries, you should consider the presence of a retained foreign body. During the history and physical exam, consider a referral to an ophthalmologist if you discover:
  - ○ Hyphema (presence of blood in the anterior chamber of the eye)
  - ○ Inferior or superior lid margin laceration
  - ○ Laceration involving the canaliculus
  - ○ Deep superficial lid laceration
  - ○ Distorted pupil
  - ○ Significant periorbital ecchymosis
  - ○ Abnormal eye movements
- Clinical examination for periorbital cellulitis will show lack of proptosis, normal ocular movement, and normal pupil function. A CT will demonstrate edema of the eyelids and subcutaneous tissues anterior to the orbital septum. Orbital cellulitis must be recognized promptly and treated aggressively. All patients require CT imaging of the orbit, including the surrounding CNS, preferably with intravenous contrast.

Management

- Most superficial eyelid lacerations may be repaired by the primary clinician and should not require referral.
- Corneal abrasions are treated with a topical antibiotic ointment until the epithelium is completely healed. The use of an eye patch does not improve healing time or reduce pain.
- Treatment for periorbital cellulitis involves antibiotic therapy and careful monitoring for signs of sepsis and local progression. Hospitalization and systemic antibiotic therapy are usually indicated for those with orbital cellulitis. Parenteral antibiotics must be started immediately, and if there is no evidence of improvement or if there are signs of progression, sinus drainage may be required.

FRACTURES AND DISLOCATIONS

Overview and Presentation

- The most common fractures in the pediatric population are buckle fracture and greenstick fracture. The most common location is within the upper extremity, including fingers, hand, wrist, forearm, humerus, and clavicle. Most injuries occur from a fall onto outstretched hand (FOOSH) and you will frequently see it abbreviated this way on patient reports. Clavicle fractures are usually the result of a fall on the affected shoulder or direct trauma to the clavicle. The most common site for fracture is the junction of the middle and lateral clavicle.

- Common dislocations in the pediatric population are the knee joint (patellofemoral), elbow (nursemaid's elbow), and finger (proximal interphalangeal and distal interphalangeal joints).

Diagnostic Evaluation

- Clinicians will often have a good idea of the patient's diagnosis with only a good history and physical exam, but it is usually necessary to order anterior–posterior (AP) and lateral x-rays of the injured site to know type of fracture, displacement, angulation, rotation, and injury to the growth plate. Assessing for these findings can place the injury into one of the five Salter–Harris classifications shown in Figure 5.1. Many EDs are using ultrasound (US) to assess for musculoskeletal injuries, including fractures, soft tissue injuries, vascular injuries, and compartment syndrome.

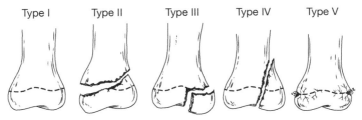

| Type I | Type II | Type III | Type IV | Type V |

FIGURE 5.1   Salter–Harris physeal injury classification system.
Type I: Fracture extends through the growth plate causing separation through the physis; prevalent in younger children. Type II: Fracture begins in the physis and extends through the metaphysis; most common type of fracture and prevalent in older children. Type III: Fracture begins below the physis and moves through the epiphysis and into the joint; prevalent in older children. Type IV: Fracture passes through the metaphysis, physis, and epiphysis. Type V: Crush injury at the physis caused by compressive forces or a stress injury.

Management

- Most type I and II fractures can be managed with casting and splinting techniques and do not require surgical consult. Referral to an orthopedic surgeon is recommended if the patient has a type III-V Salter–Harris fracture. Applying a brace, splint, or cast will be necessary to keep the joint supported, secure, and reduce the patient's use of the extremity. Check with your preceptor for his or her preferred method of treatment, including reduction with sedation, splinting/casting, pain management, and follow-up appointments. Clavicle fractures are usually treated with a figure-of-eight splint or a simple sling. If a fracture is tenting the skin, the skin is open, or the fracture is resulting in neurovascular compromise, surgery is indicated. Most fractures will heal within 3 to 6 weeks.
- Reduction of dislocations can usually be performed in the urgent care or ED without sedation.

HEADACHE AND MENINGITIS

Overview and Presentation

- Meningitis is inflammation of the meninges secondary to viral, fungal, or bacterial infection. Infants presenting with meningitis typically have nonspecific histories, including fever and a bulging fontanelle, whereas older children may present with fever, photophobia, headache, altered level of consciousness, and stiff neck. The most common organisms in infants younger than 30 days are GBS and *E. coli*, whereas *S. pneumoniae* is most common across all age groups. The most common viral organisms are enteroviruses.[20]
- Headache is one of the most common complaints in all age groups, including children, and usually increases in incidence with increasing age. Rarely does a child present to an urgent care or ED with complaints of a nontraumatic headache, but when they do viral illness, sinusitis, or migraine are the most common causes.[21,22] Life-threatening causes of headache are those that may result in brain injury or death from various mechanisms, including inflammation, increased intracranial pressure, and/or hypoxia. These may include infections, tumors, hemorrhage, and carbon monoxide poisoning. Children with intracranial tumors complaining of headache have many other symptoms and neurologic signs.[23]

Diagnostic Evaluation

- A comprehensive history is essential for determining the etiology of the headache. Physical exam findings that are highly suggestive of meningitis include nuchal rigidity, Kernig's sign, and Brudzinski's sign. Cerebrospinal fluid culture is the gold standard for diagnosis of bacterial meningitis. In most patients with meningitis who do not have focal neurologic findings, an LP may be safely performed without a prior CT scan. The presence of focal neurological signs, papilledema, seizures, and depressed mental status are associated with increased complications from an LP, and a CT scan should replace the LP for these patients. Two or three blood cultures should be obtained for all patients who are being evaluated for a CNS infection, even when antimicrobial therapy has already been administered. The blood cultures can improve the identification of the causative organisms.

- For the typically healthy child or adolescent who presents with headache without trauma, a comprehensive history and physical will guide further workup and management. The majority of children with headache and normal neurologic examinations who present emergently do not require neuroimaging studies. Experts suggest that neuroimaging in the ED is warranted for children with the following clinical features:
  - ○ Worst headache/thunderclap headache
  - ○ Abnormal neurologic examination (e.g., altered mental status, ataxia, or focal neurologic examination)
  - ○ Skin lesions suggestive of neurocutaneous syndromes
  - ○ Age younger than 3 years with unexplained severe headache[24]
- For these children, a CT scan of the brain should be performed, which does not require sedation in most children, and generally identifies any condition that requires immediate attention.
- Other lab studies or imaging may be ordered based on findings within the history and physical. If the patient has a history of headache and is presenting with changes in symptoms or signs, additional labs, or imaging studies may be ordered as directed by the new clinical features.
- The emergency evaluation of a child with headache should include an LP in the following situations: suspected meningitis, encephalitis, subarachnoid hemorrhage not diagnosed on neuroimaging, and for suspected idiopathic intracranial hypertension.

Management

- Adequate and prompt treatment of bacterial meningitis is critical to outcome. Early initiation of parenteral antimicrobial therapy should not be delayed pending an LP. Dexamethasone has been implemented as adjunctive treatment for *H. influenzae* type b and pneumococcal meningitis. All patients should be admitted to the hospital, with strong consideration of admitting the patient to the PICU. Referral should also be made to an infectious disease specialist. If the patient has experienced seizures or there is altered mental status, a referral should also be made to a pediatric neurologist.
- Management of headache usually depends on the underlying etiology. Treatment of the common causes of headache in the emergency setting usually include antibiotics, anti-inflammatories, migraine-specific

analgesics, and patient education. Many patients presenting with migraine or tension-related headaches should be educated about diet, fluid intake, sleep hygiene, food triggers, and the appropriate use of prescription and over-the-counter medications. Patients may need additional instruction about keeping a headache diary and referral to a pediatrician or a specialist to manage their chronic or recurrent symptoms.

OSTEOMYELITIS AND SEPTIC JOINT INFECTIONS

Overview and Presentation

- Osteomyelitis is a relatively common diagnosis in childhood. Rapid recognition of this bone infection in younger patients is important, especially if the physis is damaged. Bacteria are the most common agents in acute infections. *Staphylococcus aureus* is the most common organism in osteomyelitis in all age groups. Community-acquired methicillin-resistant *S. aureus* (MRSA) makes up more than half of all *S. aureus* isolates obtained from children, whereas GBS and *E. coli* are also important pathogens. Older infants and children usually present with fever, pain over affected site, refusal to use, and localizing signs such as edema, erythema, and warmth. When the affected bone is in the lower extremities, limp or refusing to bear weight are often seen. The most common bones to become infected are the long bones, such as femur, tibia, and humerus.[25]
- Septic joint infections, or septic arthritis, should be quickly recognized as it too has the potential to cause permanent destruction. Before the development of the conjugate vaccine, *H. influenzae* type b accounted for more than half of all septic arthritis in infants and children.[26] Septic joint infections are more common in young children as half of all cases occur by 24 months of age and three fourths of all cases occur by 5 years of age. Sexually active adolescents and neonates are at risk for gonococcal septic arthritis. Clinical presentation depends on the age of the patient and early signs and symptoms can be subtle. Erythema, edema, and warmth of the skin are often seen earlier than it might be with osteomyelitis, as the joint infection is more superficial than the deep bone infections. The exception to this is an infection of the hip because of the deep location of the joint. Older infants and children may present with fever, localized joint pain, and refusal to use the extremity. Joints of the lower extremity make up 75% of all cases of septic arthritis.

Diagnostic Evaluation

- The workup for osteomyelitis depends on blood cultures and imaging studies. Blood cultures are vital for diagnosis and antibiotic treatment can be delayed until cultures are obtained. There are no laboratory tests specific for osteomyelitis although a CBC, erythrocyte sedimentation rate (ESR), and a CRP can be helpful in initial diagnosis and monitoring treatment. X-rays play an essential role in the evaluation as they help to establish a site of infection and can also rule out other causes of symptoms, such as trauma and foreign bodies[26] The gold standard for diagnostic imaging within osteomyelitis is MRI although CT and radionuclide imaging are valuable in specific instances.

- Blood cultures should be obtained in all suspected cases of septic arthritis. The technique that remains the gold standard for diagnosing joint infections is aspiration of the joint fluid for Gram stain and culture. Most large joint spaces are relatively easy to aspirate but US can be used to help insure needle placement as well as be beneficial for diagnostic imaging. X-rays, US, CT, MRI, and radionuclide studies can assist with determining the diagnosis.

Management

- Initial empirical antibiotic treatment for osteomyelitis and septic arthritis is based on knowledge of the likely pathogen for the patient's age as well as locale. In neonates, an antistaphylococcal penicillin and a broad-spectrum cephalosporin provide coverage for MRSA, GBS, and Gram-negative bacilli. In older infants and children, the primary pathogens are *S. aureus* and *Streptococcus*. Special situations will dictate deviation from the usual course of antibiotics. For example, immunocompromised patients, those with sickle cell disease, and those with penicillin allergies may receive various antibiotic substitutes such as clindamycin, vancomycin, azithromycin, or rifampin. The duration of antimicrobial therapy for osteomyelitis will be individualized depending on the isolated pathogen and the clinical course, but the minimal duration is 21 to 28 days even though 4 to 6 weeks of treatment may be required.
- Duration of antibiotic therapy for septic arthritis is typically 10 to 14 days. Initial IV antibiotics can be changed once the culture report is provided, the patient is afebrile for 48 to 72 hours, and the patient is clearly improving.
- Infection of the hip is considered a surgical emergency due to the precarious nature of the blood supply to the femoral head.
- All children treated for osteomyelitis and septic arthritis should have long-term follow-up as sequelae of skeletal infections may not become noticeable for months or years.

OVARIAN AND TESTICULAR TORSION

Overview and Presentation

- Torsion of the testis and ovaries can be true surgical emergencies. If surgical or manual detorsion is not attempted, the patient could lose function due to arterial infarction. Female and male patients usually present with localized pain, nausea with or without vomiting, and radiation of pain to the abdomen.

- The primary risk factor for ovarian torsion is an ovarian mass, particularly a mass that is 5 cm in diameter or larger. Because many of these masses are associated with the reproductive cycle or reproductive hormones (e.g., corpus luteum), the risk of torsion is increased in adolescents of reproductive age.

- Testicular torsion is the most significant condition causing acute scrotal pain and is a true surgical emergency. Torsion of the testis is a diagnosis that can usually be made clinically without imaging or laboratory studies. The best chance of testicular recovery is surgical detorsion within 6 hours following the onset of pain.[27]

Diagnostic Evaluation

- A female pediatric patient who presents with sudden onset of pelvic pain, nausea with/without vomiting, and an adnexal mass should prompt a high index of suspicion for ovarian mass with torsion. Color doppler flow US is used frequently to assess for ovarian cystic masses, ovarian hypertrophy, and decreased blood flow to ovary[28] One series studying the effectiveness of US in diagnosing ovarian torsion yielded a positive predictive value of 87.5% and specificity of 93.3%, corroborating the potential for expeditiously making this diagnosis.[29] Promising findings, incorporating both grayscale and color Doppler sonography, are a twisted vascular pedicle and the "whirlpool sign".[30] US may also help to rule out appendicitis and a tubo-ovarian abscess. Additional studies should include urine pregnancy test, CBC, basic metabolic panel (BMP), and MRI if the US is equivocal.

- Male patients who present with acute onset of scrotal pain, nausea/vomiting, and have positive findings on exam should be examined by an emergency medicine attending physician or you should consult a urologist. US should be considered if it does not delay transfer to higher level care. Manual detorsion should not be attempted without specific direction from urology. A normal Doppler US does not rule out testicular torsion. A patient has a low probability of torsion if both testes are palpable, there is no nausea/vomiting, only mild pain but with a positive cremasteric reflex and positive Prehn's sign. You should consider an alternative diagnosis for these patients and treat their pain appropriately. If, after further testing, you are still concerned about torsion, consult urology. Alternative diagnosis may include torsion of appendix testis, epididymitis or orchitis, vasculitis, testicular mass, and inguinal hernia. If there are additional signs or symptoms that warrant further testing, consider urinalysis, urine culture, and urine polymerase chain reaction (PCR) for *Neisseria gonorrhoeae* and *Chlamydia trachomatis* for sexually active patients.

Management

- Surgical evaluation is the mainstay of treatment if ovarian/fallopian torsion is present on diagnostic imaging. Direct visualization is necessary to confirm the presence of torsion and evaluate the viability of the ovary and fallopian tube. Several studies have found that detorsion and ovarian conservation lead to continued ovarian function for most patients, and they do not lead to ovarian necrosis or an increased risk for ovarian vein embolus.[31]
- The best chance of testicular recovery is surgical detorsion within 6 hours following the onset of pain.

OVERDOSE AND ACUTE TOXIC INGESTION

Overview and Presentation

- Toxic exposures occur frequently in children and adolescents and in many instances the toxic agent is readily identified. However, in an important minority of exposures, a history of poisoning is not provided. Common patterns of pediatric poisoning consist of measuring and dispensing errors and exploratory ingestions in children younger than 6 years of age, and intentional ingestions and recreational drug use in older children and adolescents.[32]

Diagnostic Evaluation

- The approach to the poisoned child begins with initial evaluation and stabilization followed by a thorough evaluation to attempt to identify the agent(s) involved and assess the severity of exposure. In any patient with altered mental status, a glucose level should be obtained early and naloxone administration should be considered. Clinicians caring for a patient who may have ingested one or more toxic substances should consider consulting with the local poison control center.
- Pertinent laboratory tests include complete metabolic panel (CMP) to assess electrolytes as well as renal and liver function and a urine pregnancy test for all female adolescent patients. A quantitative concentration of intoxicants (a drug panel) may be ordered if the patient's history is specific enough to point to a likely ingestion or coingestion. These panels can help to narrow the differential or confirm intoxication with a drug, whereas serum N-acetyl-para-aminophenol level should be checked in most pediatric cases as acetaminophen is readily available in many over-the-counter analgesics and cough-and-cold preparations.[33] An EKG should help to assess cardiopulmonary status and may help to focus the differential diagnosis. A chest x-ray or abdominal x-rays can help provide further clues for inhaled or ingested agents.

Management

- Management of the poisoned patient should include full assessment, supportive care, antidotes (if available), decontamination, and enhanced elimination.

References

1. Arnold DH, Gebretsadik T, Abramo TJ, et al. The RAD score: a simple acute asthmaseverity score compares favorably to more complex scores. *Ann Allergy Asthma Immunol.* 2011;107(1):22-28. doi:10.1016/j.anai.2011.03.011

2. Coates BM, Camarda LE, Goodman DM, Bordini BJ. Wheezing, bronchiolitis, and bronchitis. In: Kliegman RM, ed. *Nelson Textbook of Pediatrics.* 20th ed. Philadelphia, PA: Elsevier; 2016:2044–2050.

3. Third Expert Panel on the Diagnosis and Management of Asthma. Expert panel report 3: guidelines for the diagnosis and management of asthma. Washington, DC: United States Department of Health and Human Services http://www.nhlbi.nih.gov/guidelines/asthma/asthgdln.pdf. Published August 28, 2007.

4. Roosevelt GE. Acute inflammatory upper airway obstruction (croup, epiglottitis, laryngitis, and bacterial tracheitis). In: Kliegman RM, ed. *Nelson Textbook of Pediatrics.* 20th ed. Philadelphia, PA: Elsevier; 2016:2032–2034.

5. Chapin M, Rochette L, Annest J, et al. Nonfatal choking on food among children 14 years or younger in the United States, 2001–2009. *Pediatrics.* 2013;132(2):275–281. doi:10.1542/peds.2013-0260

6. Kawasaki T. Update on pediatric sepsis: a review. *J Intensive Care.* 2017;5:47. doi:10.1186/s40560-017-0240-1

7. Goldstein B, Giroir B, Randolph A. International pediatric sepsis consensus conference: definitions for sepsis and organ dysfunction in pediatrics. *Pediatr Crit Care Med.* 2005;6(1):2–8.doi:10.1097/01.PCC.0000149131.72248.E6

8. Tesini BL. Neonatal sepsis. *Merck Manual Professional Version* [online]. https://www.merckmanuals.com/professional/pediatrics/infections-in-neonates/neonatal-sepsis. Updated July 2018.

9. Lumba-Brown A, Yeates KO, Sarmiento K, et al. Centers for Disease Control and Prevention guideline on the diagnosis and management of mild traumatic brain injury among children. *JAMA Pediatr.* 2018;172:e182853. doi:10.1001/jamapediatrics.2018.2853

10. Halstead ME, Walter KD. Sport-related concussion in children and adolescents. *Pediatrics.* 2010;126(3):597–615. doi:10.1542/peds.2010-2005

11. Kuppermann N, Holmes JF, Dayan PS, et al. Identification of children at very low risk of clinically-important brain injuries after head trauma: a prospective cohort study. *Lancet.* 2009;374(9696):1160–1170. doi:10.1016/S0140-6736(09)61558-0

12. McCrory P, Meeuwisse W, Johnston K, et al. Consensus statement on concussion in sport: the 3rd International Conference on Concussion in Sport held in Zurich, November 2008. *Br J Sports Med.* 2009;43:i76–i84. doi:10.1136/bjsm.2009.058248

13. Centers for Disease Control and Prevention. HEADS UP to health care providers. https://www.cdc.gov/headsup/providers/index.html

14. Ellenson LH, Pirog EC. The female genital tract. In: Kumar V, Abbas A, Aster J, eds. *Robbins and Cotran Pathologic Basis of Disease.* 9th ed. Philadelphia, PA: Elsevier Saunders; 2015:1113–1114.

15. Dunger DB, Sperling MA, Acerini CL, et al. ESPE/LWPES consensus statement on diabetic ketoacidosis in children and adolescents. *Arch Dis Child.* 2004;89(2):188–194. doi:10.1136/adc.2003.044875

16. Ki V, Rotstein C. Bacterial skin and soft tissue infections in adults: a review of their epidemiology, pathogenesis, diagnosis, treatment and site of care. *Can J Infect Dis Med Microbiol.* 2008;19(2):173–184. doi:10.1155/2008/846453

17. Olitsky SE, Hug D, Plummer LS, et al. Injuries to the eye. In: Kliegman RM, ed. *Nelson Textbook of Pediatrics.* 20th ed. Philadelphia, PA: Elsevier; 2016:3064–3068.

18. Gerstenblith AT, Rabinowitz MP, eds. *The Wills Eye Manual: Office and Emergency Room Diagnosis and Treatment of Eye Disease.* 6th ed. Philadelphia, PA: Lippincott Williams & Wilkins; 2012:159–164.

19. Olitsky SE, Hug D, Plummer LS, et al. Orbital infections. In: Kliegman RM, ed. *Nelson Textbook of Pediatrics.* 20th ed. Philadelphia, PA: Elsevier; 2016:3062–3064.

20. Somand DM, Meurer WJ. Central nervous system infections. In: Walls R, Hockberger R, Gausche-Hill M, eds. *Rosen's Emergency Medicine: Concepts and Clinical Practice.* 9th ed. Philadelphia, PA: Elsevier; 2018:1328–1340.

21. Burton LJ, Quinn B, Pratt-Cheney JL, Pourani M. Headache etiology in a pediatric emergency department. *Pediatr Emerg Care.* 1997;13(1):1–4. doi:10.1097/00006565-199702000-00001

22. Lewis DW, Qureshi F. Acute headache in children and adolescents presenting to the emergency department. *Headache.* 2000;40(3):200–203. doi:10.1046/j.1526-4610.2000.00029.x

23. The Childhood Brain Tumor Consortium, Gilles FH. The epidemiology of headache among children with brain tumor: headache in children with brain tumors. The childhood brain tumor consortium. *J Neuro-Oncol.* 1991;10(1):31–46. doi:10.1007/BF00151245

24. American College of Radiology. ACR appropriateness criteria®: headache—child. https://acsearch.acr.org/docs/69439/Narrative/Updated 2017.

25. Kaplan SL. Osteomyelitis. In: Kliegman RM, ed. *Nelson Textbook of Pediatrics.* 20th ed. Philadelphia, PA: Elsevier; 2016:3322–3327.

26. Kaplan SL. Septic arthritis. In: Kliegman RM, ed. *Nelson Textbook of Pediatrics.* 20th ed. Philadelphia, PA: Elsevier; 2016:3327–3330.

27. Children's Hospital Colorado. Acute painful scrotum: algorithm—suspicion for testicular torsion. https://www.childrenscolorado.org/globalassets/healthcare-professionals/clinical-pathways/acute-scrotum.pdf. Published September 27, 2016.

28. Stark JE, Siegel MJ. Ovarian torsion in prepubertal and pubertal girls: sonographic findings. *Am J Roentgenol.* 1994;163(6):1479–1482. doi:10.2214/ajr.163.6.7992751

29. Graif M, Itzchak Y. Sonographic evaluation of ovarian torsion in childhood and adolescence. *Am J Roentgenol.* 1988;150(3):647–649. doi:10.2214/ajr.150.3.647

30. Vijayaraghavan SB. Sonographic whirlpool sign in ovarian torsion. *J Ultrasound Med.* 2004;23(12):1643–1649. doi:10.7863/jum.2004.23.12.1643

31. Oelsner G, Cohen SB, Soriano D, et al. Minimal surgery for the twisted ischaemic adnexa can preserve ovarian function. *Hum Reprod.* 2003;18(12):2599–2602. doi:10.1093/humrep/deg498

32. Gummin DD, Mowry JB, Spyker DA, et al. 2016 annual report of the American Association of Poison Control Centers' National Poison Data System (NPDS): 34th annual report. *Clin Toxicol.* 2017;55(10):1072-1254. doi:10.1080/15563650.2017.1388087

33. Erickson TB, Thompson TM, Lu JJ. The approach to the patient with an unknown overdose. *Emerg Med Clin North Am.* 2007;25(2):249–281. doi:10.1016/j.emc.2007.02.004

Electronic Resources

CDC HEADS UP Provider Resources:
https://www.cdc.gov/headsup/providers/index.html
Childhood Asthma Control Test:
https://www.asthma.com/additional-resources/childhood-asthma-control-test.html
RAD score: a simple acute asthma severity score compares favorably to more complex scores (Compares RAD to PRAM and PASS scores):
https://www.ncbi.nlm.nih.gov/pmc/articles/PMC3760486

6

Common Procedures in Pediatrics

Although numerous procedures are performed in daily practice in the ambulatory pediatric and inpatient pediatric setting, these are not necessarily specific to pediatrics, such as immunization administration, phlebotomy, finger or heel sticks for point-of-care (POC) tests, throat swabs, nasal swabs, lumbar punctures, wound debridement, and laceration repair. In the interest of providing pediatric-specific procedures, the following are considered the most common ambulatory pediatric procedures that you may be asked to observe or perform during your pediatrics rotation.

BLADDER CATHETERIZATION

Bladder catheterization is a relatively common procedure in pediatrics, but can be more difficult to perform on the female infant and the very young child due to anatomical size and cooperation. When done properly, bladder catheterization causes minimal pain and emotional trauma.

Indication
The procedure is quite useful for obtaining a sterile urine sample, especially in children not yet toilet trained, as a catheterized urine specimen is superior to a bag urine specimen because it reduces the risk of contamination. In addition, an indwelling catheter is useful for monitoring urine output in hospitalized children and emptying a distended or painful bladder that does not empty on its own. The common complications of a bladder catheterization include pain during or after the procedure, voiding dysfunction after the procedure, urinary tract infection (UTI), and urethral trauma.

Equipment

- Absorbent pad/chuck
- Fenestrated drape
- For short-term catheterization, such as to obtain a urine specimen, use a straight catheter (sometimes referred to as a "French [Fr] catheter") to size; #8 Fr feeding tube may also be used for all ages with #5 Fr feeding tube used for newborns and/or premature infants
  - #4 to 6 Fr (for newborns)
  - #6 to 8 Fr (for infants)
  - #10 to 12 Fr (for prepubertal children)
  - #10 to 14 Fr (for adolescents)
- Indwelling Foley catheters to size
  - #5 to 8 Foley (for 0–5 years old)
  - #8 to 10 Foley (for 5–10 years old)
  - #10 Foley (for 10–14 years old)
  - #10 to 14 Foley (for >14 years old)
  - #5 Fr straight catheter kit may be needed for premature infants
- Sterile 2% lidocaine jelly
- Sterile lubricant
- Sterile gloves
- Sterile swabs
- Cleaning solution (chlorhexidine gluconate solution or povidone–iodine swabs)

Procedure

1. Prepare the family and the child for the procedure. This includes instruction on pelvic muscle relaxation whenever possible.

   > **CLINICAL PEARL:** Ask preschoolers and young children to blow bubbles and to press hips against bed to relax the pelvic and periurethral muscles.

2. Position the child at the end of the table and ask the parent/caregiver to stand near the child's head.
   a. Girls should be placed in a frog-leg position for optimal positioning.
   b. Boys should be lying comfortably with knees bent and hanging over the edge of the table, so that you can lean against the legs and try to control lower body movement.
3. Before cleansing girls, you can apply 2% lidocaine jelly by gently separating the labia and appling the jelly to the perimeatal area.
4. Wait about 3 minutes for the anesthetic to begin numbing the area.
5. While waiting, you can don your sterile gloves and drape a sterile field, lubricate the catheter with sterile jelly, and position it on your sterile tray at the ready for insertion.

6. Using sterile technique, clean the urethral meatus in a downward motion.
    a. Because identifying the urethral meatus in infant girls can be difficult, this can also help you identify the meatus, as the meatus "opens" briefly with each downward motion. Located midline just superior to the vaginal introitus, the urethral meatus in infant girls can sometimes be hidden by the superior portion of the hymen.
    b. Use a fresh cotton ball soaked in cleaning solution or povidone–iodine swab each time, repeating until the meatus is clearly visualized.
7. Once cleaned, you will gently retract the labia or foreskin (only retract far enough to visualize the urethral meatus, so as to avoid causing a paraphimosis) with your thumb and forefinger of your nondominant hand.
8. Using your dominant hand, place the catheter tip in the urethral meatus, and then gently advance the catheter until you feel resistance at the external urethral sphincter. Pause and allow the sphincter to relax before trying to advance into the bladder.
9. Remove the straight catheter slowly and smoothly, pinching the lumen until you have a collection device available to hold the sterile sample.
10. Once the urine flow stops, gently remove the catheter from the urethra and clean the external genitalia of iodine, if used.

Foreign-Body Removal from Ears and Nose

Children are notorious for placing small objects in small orifices, in particular the ear canal and the nose. This activity occurs primarily with children under the age of 8 years old. Foreign bodies, such as beads, buttons, pebbles, popcorn kernels, small toys, and button batteries, are often found incidentally or because a child has complained of mildly irritating symptoms.[1] Having a full sensation or decreased hearing are typical of ear foreign bodies, whereas nasal foreign bodies typically present with foul-smelling, purulent nasal discharge.

Indication

Any foreign body that can be well visualized and has a high chance of successful removal is an indication for a removal attempt in the primary care office. The shape of the object will often determine the type of removal method attempted and the propensity for successful removal in the ambulatory pediatric setting.[1] If the object cannot be removed within one to two attempts, the likelihood of successful removal declines rapidly with each additional attempt, and the child should be referred to an otolaryngologist for further evaluation and if sedation or anesthesia is necessary.[1]

> **CLINICAL PEARL:** Multiple foreign bodies are not uncommon, so be sure to check opposite ear, nares, and oropharynx for other foreign bodies.

Equipment

The equipment required depends on the foreign body location and removal method, but typical equipment for foreign body removals may include the following:

- Otoscope with removable lens
- Nasal speculum
- Headlamp
- Alligator forceps
- Curette
- Hooked probe
- Topical vasoconstrictor (nose)
- Viscous lidocaine (2%)
- Bag valve mask (Ambu bag)
- Syringe
- Balloon angiocatheter—20 gauge
- Emesis basin
- Soft-tipped suction catheter and suction equipment
- Magnet for metallic foreign bodies

Procedure

Whether mechanical removal, irrigation, or suction is used for the foreign-body removal depends upon the type of object to be removed. See Table 6.1 for a list of possible objects and their associated removal techniques.

1. Prior to removal of a foreign body in the nose, spray phenylephrine in the nostril to reduce edema. You may also use viscous lidocaine dropped or syringed into the nose or ear canal for anesthesia.
   a. Avoid placing too much lidocaine or phenylephrine spray, as it can obstruct visualization and can make the object slippery.
2. You will need to wait approximately 3 minutes for the area to become anesthetized.
3. Mechanical removal is ideal for easily visualized, nonspherical, and non-friable foreign bodies.
   a. Forceps
      i. Ear: If it is easily visible and can be grasped with forceps, position the patient so that you can maneuver freely. Insert the otoscope into the ear canal and note the location and depth of the foreign object. Move the otoscope lens to one side and carefully introduce forceps through the otoscope speculum. Advance the forceps incrementally through the external auditory canal until the foreign body can be

TABLE 6.1 Common Foreign Bodies Found in Pediatrics and Removal Techniques

Foreign Body	How to Remove	Notes
BB pellet	Magnet	
Bead	Suction or irrigation	If there is enough room to slip a thin balloon-tip catheter (i.e., a 5 Fr) past the foreign body, you can then inflate the balloon and gently pull the inflated catheter out, pulling the object with it; however, this is more difficult to perform in the ear than the nose
Button	Alligator forceps or toothed thumb forceps	
Button battery	Strong magnet, but if not available immediate removal by ENT specialist	Do not irrigate an area suspected to have a button battery, as the electrical current may cause liquefaction necrosis
Chewing gum	Acetone	Use only in the ear canal
Food particles	Suction or irrigation	Irrigation is contraindicated for organic matter that might swell and enlarge in the auditory canal
Insects	Suction or mechanical removal (if it can be removed whole)	Mineral oil, microscope oil, or alcohol can be used to immobilize or kill the insect prior to removal
Styrofoam	Acetone	Acetone to the ear canal will dissolve Styrofoam; however, due to the strong vapors, it should not be used for nasal foreign bodies

ENT, ear, nose, and throat.

Source: Kwong AO. Ear foreign body removal procedures. In: Meyers AD, ed. *Medscape*. https://emedicine.medscape.com/article/80507-overview. Updated May 8, 2018; Fischer JI. Nasal foreign bodies. In: Dronen SC, ed. *Medscape*. https://emedicine.medscape.com/article/763767-overview. Updated June 6, 2019.

    grasped. Gently withdraw the forceps, with attached foreign body, from the auditory canal.

  ii. Nose: With a sufficient light source, slowly advance forceps into the nose and grasp the object.

  iii. If the object is magnetic, use a small, strong magnet grasped by alligator forceps, advance it toward the object until attraction occurs, and then slowly and gently remove the object.

    b. Hooked probes (i.e., right-angle hook) can be used for objects that are easily visualized but difficult to grasp. Place the hook behind the foreign body and swivel the hook so that the hook angle is behind the object, then pull the object forward.

4. Balloon dilation is used primarily in the nose and is best for small, round objects. Lubricate the catheter with 2% lidocaine jelly and insert it past the foreign body. Inflate the balloon with 2 mL to 3 mL of air depending on the size of the child and then slowly withdraw the catheter, pulling the object with it.

5. Suction
    a. Ear: If the object is better removed with suction, advance the suction catheter tip through the otoscope toward the object and, once touching the object, apply the suction and slowly remove the catheter, bringing the object along with it.
    b. Nose: The process used is similar to the ear, but performed without the otoscope.

6. Irrigation is reserved primarily for auditory canal foreign bodies, but occasionally saline irrigations may be done in the nose.
    a. To irrigate, first attach a 20-gauge angiocatheter to a 60-mL syringe and drape the patient to keep him or her dry.
    b. An assistant or a cooperative patient can hold an emesis basin under the affected ear to collect irrigation runoff.
    c. Place the catheter tip gently into the external auditory canal, paying attention not to advance it too far.
    d. Hold the catheter tip in position and slowly inject warmed irrigation fluid, watching for the foreign body to wash out with the irrigation runoff.

7. If the object is large, obstructive, and in the nostril and the patient is old enough to cooperate, positive pressure ventilation can be used to remove the object.
    a. The patient can "blow" the nose while you or the parent obstruct the opposite nostril.
    b. The parent can block the unobstructed nostril, place his or her mouth on the child's mouth, and blow a rapid puff of air.
    c. Positive pressure ventilation can also be done by occluding the unobstructed nostril and using a bag valve mask to give the rapid puff of air.

CLINICAL PEARL: Topical benzocaine, procaine, or lidocaine preparations are an alternative pain reliever for children 2 years and older but should not be used in children with tympanic membrane perforation.

NEBULIZER TREATMENT

A nebulizer is a delivery vehicle for medications that need to be aerosolized. The nebulization of the medication allows the medications to be inhaled into the small airways of the lungs. Although most bebulizer treatments are commonly associated with asthma medications, they can be used for some antibiotics and mucolytics commonly available only as a liquid formulation.

Indication
The indications for use of a nebulizer are children who are too ill or too young to use a metered-dose inhaler with spacer, when medications need to be administered via aerosol, or when larger doses of medications are necessary.[2] The most common indications in ambulatory pediatrics are acute asthma exacerbation, cough, wheezing, and shortness of breath. Nebulized isotonic saline, however, can be used for nasal congestion, and epinephrine can be administered in the ED setting for croup.

Equipment
- Prefilled vial of albuterol or budesonide
- Nebulizer (cup device that hooks to the tubing)
- Tubing
- Compressor
- Mouthpiece or face mask (for children under the age of 5)

Procedure
1. After auscultating the lungs for adventitious sounds, you may decide that a nebulizer treatment is warranted for a patient, especially if there are wheezes on auscultation.
2. Place the compressor where it is out of the reach of the child, but where you can reach the power switch.
3. Wash your hands.
4. Measure the correct dose of medication (or open a prefilled tube by twisting the top off the tube) and add the medications to a clean (typically prepacked) nebulizer cup.
5. Close the top of the nebulizer cup.
6. Connect the air tubing from the compressor to the nebulizer base.
7. Attach a mouthpiece or face mask to the nebulizer.
8. Turn on the compressor and verify that a fine mist flows from the mouthpiece/mask.

9. Instruct the patient to sit in an upright position or have the parent hold the child upright, as the nebulizer chamber should be kept upright to ensure that the air passes through the medication chamber.
10. Instruct the patient to breathe normally. Deep breathing is not necessary. Warn parents that some children do not like the feel of the mask on their face/head and may cry and try to remove it. Assure parents that infants and small children who cry are still getting adequate medication delivery, as long as the mask is held in place over the nose and mouth.
11. Once misting stops, the treatment is complete.
12. If the child is old enough and is able to cooperate, instruct the patient to gargle with warm water after the treatment.
13. Allow the patient to sit comfortably for 3 to 5 minutes after the treatment and then auscultate the lungs again.
14. If symptoms are improved, but not completely resolved, you can repeat the nebulizer treatment. Typically, symptoms that are not significantly improved after two nebulizer treatments should be evaluated in a more acute care setting.

Pneumatic Otoscopy

An important tool in pediatrics, pneumatic otoscopy is a physical exam technique that can be done to determine tympanic membrane (TM) mobility, even when the TM appears normal.[3] Abnormal TM mobility can lead to conductive hearing loss and potentially affect speech development.

Indication
Pneumatic otoscopy is indicated if you suspect acute otitis media (AOM) or otitis media with effusion; in the presence of otorrhea; in a child with upper respiratory tract infection symptoms, ear pain, irritability or sleep difficulties; or with concerns for hearing loss.[4] Pneumatic otoscopy can also differentiate a retracted TM from a perforated TM and can assess eustachian tube function.

Equipment
- Otoscope with pneumatic bulb
- Ear speculums in various sizes (speculum tips with rubber rings can be helpful for creating a seal)

Procedure
1. Choose an ear speculum that will fit tightly into the ear canal without creating trauma.
2. Attach the speculum to the otoscope and gently insert it into the ear canal. Typically, a snug speculum will straighten the external canal bringing the TM into full view.

3. Gently squeeze the bulb of the pneumatic apparatus to apply positive pressure to the eardrum and release the bulb to exert negative pressure. Watch the movement of the eardrum with both positive and negative pressure.

   a. A normal eardrum should move briskly with positive and negative pressure.

   b. An eardrum with positive pressure in the middle ear (i.e., AOM) may move sluggishly or not at all when positive pressure is applied to the TM.

   c. When the TM is retracted secondary to negative middle ear pressure (i.e., eustachian tube dysfunction), TM movement is greater when the bulb is released than when the bulb is compressed.

Reduction of Subluxed Radial Head (Nursemaid's Elbow)

This condition is typically seen with toddlers. A nursemaid's elbow is the displacement of the annular ligament into the radiohumeral joint caused by a sudden pull of an extended arm/elbow. The child typically cries at the onset of the displacement, but ongoing pain is not usually noted.

Indication

Radial head subluxation should be considered in any toddler with a mechanism consistent with possible displacement of the annular ligament, who holds his or her arm in flexion and pronation against his or her body and refuses to use the arm *without* deformity or signs of trauma.[5] An attempt at reduction of the subluxated radial head can be done after you have performed a thorough exam of the extremity and have confirmed that there is no point tenderness, swelling, ecchymosis, or suspicion of fracture.

Equipment

- None

Procedure

There are two different methods to reduce a subluxed radial head, both of which are discussed in the following. The hyperpronation technique has been found to be more effective and less painful, but if one method fails, knowing how to do the other method may result in successful reduction.[6]

Hyperpronation Method

1. Place the child in parent's lap with his or her back to the parent's chest.
2. Flex the elbow to 90 degrees.
3. Grasp the patient's wrist with one hand and stabilize the elbow with your other hand, placing your thumb over the radial head.

4. Once stabilized, firmly hyperpronate the wrist.
5. You may feel a click on the radial side of the elbow and the child may scream.
6. Allow the child to sit with parent for 10 to 30 minutes and then reexamine the elbow to ensure that range of motion has returned.

SUPINATION–FLEXION METHOD

1. Place the child in parent's lap with his or her back to the parent's chest.
2. Grasp the affected hand as though you are going to shake the child's hand.
3. Put your other hand under the affected elbow and place your thumb over the radial head.
4. Slowly pronate the wrist and extend the elbow.
5. Fully flex the elbow, keeping the forearm in pronation.
6. As with the hyperpronation technique, a palpable or audible click is associated with a high probability of successful reduction.
7. Reexamine the elbow in 10 to 30 minutes to ensure that range of motion has returned.

ELECTRONIC RESOURCES

Bladder catheterization in a female pediatric patient:
https://www.youtube.com/watch?v=6DjBz_7dCEo
Ear foreign body removal (various techniques):
https://emedicine.medscape.com/article/80507-overview#a7
Nasal foreign body removal (various techniques):
https://emedicine.medscape.com/article/763767-overview#a8
Pneumatic otoscopy:
https://www.nejm.org/doi/full/10.1056/NEJMvcm0904397
Preparing a nebulizer treatment:
https://www.youtube.com/watch?time_continue=128&v=idjeYf9C5IU

Radial Head Subluxation Reduction

Supination–Flexion technique:
  https://www.merckmanuals.com/enca/professional/multimedia/video/v2337072(
Hyperpronation technique:
  https://emedicine.medscape.com/article/104158-technique#c3

REFERENCES

1. Heim SW, Maughan KL. Foreign bodies in the ears, nose, and throat. *Am Fam Physician.* 2007;76(8):1185–1189. https://www.aafp.org/afp/2007/1015/p1185.html
2. National Jewish Health. Using a nebulizer. https://www.nationaljewish.org/treat ment-programs/medications/asthma-medications/devices/nebulizers/instructions. Published February 2015.
3. Pichichero ME, Poole MD. Assessing diagnostic accuracy and tympanocentesis skills in the management of otitis media. *Arch Pediatr Adolesc Med.* 2001;155(10):1137–1142. doi:10.1001/archpedi.155.10.1137

4. Shakh N, Hoberman A, Kaleida PH, et al. Diagnosing otitis media—otoscopy and cerumen removal. *N Engl J Med.* 2010;362:e62. doi:10.1056/NEJMvcm0904397
5. Buttaravoli P, Leffler SM, eds. *Minor Emergencies.* 3rd ed. Philadelphia, PA: Elsevier Saunders; 2012.
6. Lent GS, Lamb RP. Reduction of radial head subluxation technique. In: Schraga ED, ed. *Medscape.* https://emedicine.medscape.com/article/104158-technique#c1. Updated March 26, 2018.

7

Common Abbreviations in Pediatrics

The following are common abbreviations seen in pediatrics.

AAP: American Academy of Pediatrics
abx: Antibiotic
ADD: Attention deficit disorder
ADHD: Attention deficit hyperactivity disorder
AFOSF: Anterior fontanelle open, soft, and flat
AGA: Average for gestational age
Alk Phos: Alkaline Phosphatase
ALT: Alanine aminotransferase
AOM: Acute otitis media
AP: Anterior–posterior (usually in reference to imaging positioning)
AS: Atrial stenosis
ASD: Autism spectrum disorder or atrial septal defect
AST: Aspartate aminotransferase
ASQ: Ages and stages questionnaire
BMI: Body mass index
BMP: Basic metabolic panel
BP: Blood pressure
BV: Bacterial vaginosis
BUN: Blood urea nitrogen
CBC: Complete blood count
CBC w/diff: Complete blood count with differential
CC: Chief complaint
C/C/E: Clubbing, cyanosis, or edema
CDC: Centers for Disease Control and Prevention
CHD: Congenital heart disease/defect

CMP: Comprehensive metabolic panel

CNS: Central nervous system

CRAFFT: A mneumonic for the words about which this high-risk behavior screening tool asks, including C: Have you ever ridden in a CAR driven by someone (including yourself) who was "high" or had been using alcohol or drugs? R: Do you ever use alcohol or drugs to RELAX, feel better about yourself or fit it? A: Do you ever use alcohol/drugs while you are by yourself, ALONE? F: Do you ever FORGET things you did while using alcohol or drugs? F: Do your family or FRIENDS ever tell you that you should cut down on your drinking or drug use? T: Have you gotten into TROUBLE while you were using alcohol or drugs?

CT: Computed tomography

CTAB: Clear to auscultation bilaterally

CV: Cardiovascular

CVD: Cardiovascular disease

CVP: Cardiovascular and pulmonary

CXR: Chest x-ray

DD: Developmental delay

DKA: Diabetic ketoacidosis

DOI: Day of illness

DOL: Day of life

Dx: Diagnosis

Dz: Diseas

ED: Emergency department

EKG: Electrocardiogram

ESR: Erythrocyte sedimentation rate (an acute-phase reactant laboratory test)

FB: Foreign body

FOC: Father of child

FP: Femoral pulse

FSH: Follicle stimulating hormone

FT: Full term

FT4: Free T4

FTT: Failure to thrive

G&D: Growth and development

GBS: Group B *Streptococcus*

GC/CT: Gonorrhea and chlamydia

GDD: Global developmental delay

GERD: Gastroesophageal reflux diseas

HC: Head circumference

Hct: Hematocrit

HEENT: Head, eyes, ears, nose, throat

HFMD: Hand–foot–mouth disease

Hgb: Hemoglobin

H/H: Hemoglobin and hematocrit

HI: Homicidal ideation

H&P: History and physical
HPI: History of present illness
HR: Heart rate
HSM: Hepatosplenomegaly
HSP: Henoch–Schonlein purpura
HSV: Herpes simplex viru
IBD: Inflammatory bowel disease
I&D: Incision and drainage
IEP: Individualized education plan
IGF-1: Insulin-like growth factor 1
I&O: Intake and output; usually in reference to intake and elimination
IUGR: Intrauterine growth restriction
IV: Intravenous
IZ: Immunization
JIA: Juvenile idiopathic arthritis
LARC: Long-acting reversible contraception
LGA: Large for gestational age
LH: Lutenizing hormone
LLL: Left lower lobe
LOC: Loss of consciousness
LP: Lumbar puncture
LUL: Left upper lobe
MAI: Minor acute illness
MCH: Mean corpuscular hemoglobin
M-CHAT: Modified checklist for autism in toddlers
MCHC: Mean corpuscular hemoglobin concentration
MCV: Mean corpuscular volume
MGM: Maternal grandmother
MMM: Moist mucous membranes
MOC: Mother of child
MRI: Magnetic resonance imaging
MSK: Musculoskeletal
NAAT: Nucleic acid amplification test
NAD: No acute distress
NAT: Nonaccidental trauma (child abuse)
NC: Nasal cannula
NC/AT: Normocephalic, atraumatic
NKDA: No known drug allergies
NTND: Nontender and nondistended
O/B: Ortolani/Barlow maneuver
OFC: Occipital–frontal circumference; synonymous with HC
O/P: Oropharynx
ORT: Oral rehydration therapy
OT: Occupational therapist

OTC: Over the counter (reference to medications that can be purchased without a prescription)

PERRL: Pupils are equal, round, and reactive to light

PFT: Pulmonary function test

pH: Acidity or alkalinity of a solution

PHQ: Patient health questionnaire

PID: Pelvic inflammatory disease

PMHx: Past medical history

PO: Per os (by mouth)

POC: Parents of child or point of care

POCUS: Point-of-care ultrasound

PPE: Preparticipation exam

PROM: Premature rupture of membranes

PRN: Pro re nata (as needed)

PS: Pulmonary valve stenosis

Pt: Patient

PT: Physical therapist

PTA: Prior to admission

q: Every

RAD: Reactive airway disease

R/B/A: Risks, benefits, and adverse outcomes

RBC: Red blood cell

RDW: Red blood cell distribution width

RLL: Right lower lobe

ROM: Range of motion

ROS: Review of systems

RR: Respiratory rate

RRR: Regular rate and rhythm

RSV: Respiratory syncytial virus

RTC: Return to clinic

RUL: Right upper lobe

Rx: Prescription

Rxn: Reaction

SBI: Serious bacterial infection

SCM: Sternocleidomastoid (muscle in the neck)

SES: Socioeconomic status

SGA: Small for gestational age

SI: Suicidal ideation

SIDS: Sudden infant death syndrome

SLP: Speech–language pathologist

SOAP: Subjective, objective, assessment, and plan (refers to a type of note used in practice)

SOB: Shortness of breath

SpO$_2$: Oxygen saturation (expressed as a percentage of oxygenated hemoglobin compared to the total amount of hemoglobin in the blood)

s/p: Status post
SROM: spontaneous rupture of membranes
s/s: Signs and symptoms
SSO: Spanish-speaking only
STAT: Immediately or instantly (derived from the latin word *statim* and usually refers to care or lab results)
STI: Sexually transmitted infection
Sz: Seizure
T&A: Tonsillectomy and adenoidectomy
TAPVR: Total anomalous pulmonary venous return
TGA: Transposition of great arteries
TM: Tympanic membrane
T_{max}**:** Highest temperature recorded
ToF: Tetralogy of Fallot
TPN: Total parental nutrition
TSH: Thyroid stimulating hormone
TTG IgA: Tissue transglutimase antibody
UA: Urinalysis
UOP: Urine output
US: Ultrasound
UTD: Up to date; usually in reference to immunizations
UTI: Urinary tract infection
VCUG: Voiding cystourethrogram
V/D/D: Vomiting, diarrhea, and dehydration
VSD: Ventral septal defect
WBC: White blood cell
WCC: Well-child check
WD/WN: Well developed and well nourished
WHO: World Health Organization
WIC: Women, infants, and children; governmental nutritional assistance program
WOB: work of breathing
yo: Year old

Index